Sepsis

Guest Editor

R. PHILLIP DELLINGER, MD

CRITICAL CARE CLINICS

www.criticalcare.theclinics.com

Consulting Editor
RICHARD W. CARLSON, MD, PhD

October 2009 • Volume 25 • Number 4

SAUNDERS an imprint of ELSEVIER, Inc.

W.B. SAUNDERS COMPANY
A Division of Elsevier Inc.

Elsevier Inc. • 1600 John F. Kennedy Blvd., • Suite 1800 • Philadelphia, Pennsylvania 19103-2899

http://www.theclinics.com

CRITICAL CARE CLINICS Volume 25, Number 4
October 2009 ISSN 0749-0704, ISBN-13: 978-1-4377-1204-9, ISBN-10: 1-4377-1204-5

Editor: Patrick Manley
Developmental Editor: Donald Mumford

Critical Care Clinics (ISSN: 0749-0704) is published quarterly by Elsevier Inc., 360 Park Avenue South, New York, NY 10010-1710. Months of issue are January, April, July, and October. Business and Editorial Offices: 1600 John F. Kennedy Blvd., Suite 1800, Philadelphia, PA 19103-2899. Customer Service Office: 6277 Sea Harbor Drive, Orlando, FL 32887-4800. Periodicals postage paid at New York, NY and additional mailing offices. Subscription prices are $222.00 per year for US individuals, $366.00 per year for US institution, $111.00 per year for US students and residents, $274.00 per year for Canadian individuals, $454.00 per year for Canadian institutions, $320.00 per year for international individuals, $454.00 per year for international institutions and $161.00 per year for Canadian and foreign students/residents. To receive student/resident rate, orders must be accompanied by name of affiliated institution, date of term, and the *signature* of program/residency coordinator on institution letterhead. Orders will be billed at individual rate until proof of status is received. Foreign air speed delivery is included in all *Clinics* subscription prices. All prices are subject to change without notice. POSTMASTER: Send address changes to *Critical Care Clinics*, Elsevier Periodicals Customer Service, 11830 Westline Industrial Drive, St. Louis, MO 63146. **Customer Service: 1-800-654-2452 (US). From outside of the US, call 1-314-453-7041. Fax: 1-314-453-5170. E-mail: journalscustomerservice-usa@elsevier.com (for print support) or journalsonlinesupport-usa@elsevier.com (for online support).**

Reprints. For copies of 100 or more of articles in this publication, please contact the Commercial Reprints Department, Elsevier Inc., 360 Park Avenue South, New York, NY 10010-1710. Tel.: 212-633-3812; Fax: 212-462-1935; E-mail: reprints@elsevier.com.

Critical Care Clinics is also published in Spanish by Editorial Inter-Medica, Junin 917, 1[er] A, 1113, Buenos Aires, Argentina.

Critical Care Clinics is covered in *MEDLINE/PubMed (Index Medicus), EMBASE/Excerpta Medica, Current Concepts/Clinical Medicine, ISI/BIOMED, and Chemical Abstracts.*

Printed and bound by CPI Group (UK) Ltd, Croydon, CR0 4YY

Transferred to Digital Print 2011

Contributors

GUEST EDITOR

R. PHILLIP DELLINGER, MD, MSc
Department of Medicine, University of Medicine and Dentistry of New Jersey; Critical Care Division, Department of Medicine, Cooper University Hospital, Camden, New Jersey; Society of Critical Care Medicine, Des Plaines, Illinois

AUTHORS

ABDULLAH AL NAQBI, MD
Department of Critical Care Medicine, Li Ka Shing Knowledge Institute, St. Michael's Hospital, University of Toronto, Toronto, Ontario, Canada

BRIAN CASSERLY, MD
Division of Pulmonary and Critical Care Medicine, The Memorial Hospital of Rhode Island, Pawtucket, Rhode Island

R. PHILLIP DELLINGER, MD, MSc
Professor of Medicine, Robert Wood Johnson Medical School, University of Medicine and Dentistry of New Jersey, New Jersey; Head, Division of Critical Care Medicine, Cooper University Hospital, Camden, New Jersey

ROY D. GOLDFARB, PhD, FAPS
Professor of Medicine and Physiology, Division of Cardiology, Cooper University Hospital, University of Medicine and Dentistry of New Jersey—Robert Wood Johnson Medical School, One Cooper Plaza, Camden, New Jersey

SERGE GOODMAN, MD, PhD
Senior Anesthesiologist, Department of Anesthesiology and Critical Care Medicine, Hadassah Hebrew University Medical Center, Jerusalem, Israel

STEVEN M. HOLLENBERG, MD
Director, Divisions of Cardiovascular Disease and Critical Care Medicine, Coronary Care Unit, Cooper University Hospital, Camden, New Jersey

ALAN E. JONES, MD
Assistant Director of Research, Department of Emergency Medicine, Carolinas Medical Center, Charlotte, North Carolina

ANAND KUMAR, MD
Section of Critical Care Medicine, Section of Infectious Diseases, Associate Professor, Department of Medicine, Medical Microbiology and Pharmacology/Therapeutics, University of Manitoba, Manitoba, Canada; Section of Critical Care Medicine, Section of Infectious Diseases, Associate Professor, University of Medicine and Dentistry, New Jersey

Steroid Therapy of Septic Shock 825

Charles L. Sprung, Serge Goodman, and Yoram G. Weiss

Despite their potential benefits, corticosteroids have adverse affects and the benefits and risks must be balanced in determining whether they should be used or not. Some of the serious adverse affects noted in patients with critically illness have included superinfections and critical illness polyneuromyopathy. This article reviews the subject of steroid treatment of patients with septic shock and weighs the advantages and disadvantages of steroid treatment. It reviews and contrasts several low- and high-dose steroid studies, and makes recommendations for future practice.

Genetic Polymorphisms in Sepsis 835

Allen Namath and Andrew J. Patterson

This article is meant to serve as a summary of scientific advances from the past 5 years with regard to genetic polymorphisms in sepsis. It is also meant to highlight some of the discoveries that may improve our ability to identify vulnerable patients at earlier time points in sepsis, when interventions are more likely to have a positive effect. The article begins with an overview of polymorphism studies and a discussion of candidate gene versus genome-wide association studies. Next, an overview of polymorphisms associated with sepsis is presented. The overview includes detailed descriptions of E-selectin, apolipoprotein E, and C-reactive protein polymorphisms and a table in which numerous other sepsis-related polymorphisms are introduced. An examination of consortia-based projects that have the potential to catalyze sepsis research is included as is a preview of technological advancements that are likely to strongly influence sepsis studies in the near future. The article concludes with a brief consideration of ethical and social issues relevant to human genomic studies.

Performance Improvement in the Management of Sepsis 857

Christa Schorr

Performance improvement in medicine based on evidence-based guidelines is a persistent challenge for clinicians. Challenges include deficiencies in collaboration, resistance to change, complex algorithms, inadequate resources, and inability to collect data and provide feedback. In severe sepsis this is further compounded by the perceived importance of early intervention and considerable conflicting literature. The bundle concept first adopted for mechanically ventilated patients and then for central line insertion, has now been applied to care for the patient with severe sepsis. The bundle concept in severe sepsis facilitates the provision of best practice consistent care to eligible patients with a structure to measure compliance. Time sensitive bundle indicators allow for uniform data collection and reporting. Successful modification of clinical practice may require months or years. The success of the program relies upon the cross-departmental collaboration and support generated before implementation and the ability to deliver timely feedback to facilitate change in performance.

Multicenter Clinical Trials in Sepsis: Understanding the Big Picture and Building a Successful Operation at Your Hospital **869**

R. Phillip Dellinger, Christa Schorr, and Stephen Trzeciak

The environment for clinical trials in sepsis has long been identified as challenging and full of road blocks and land mines. Unlike many other diagnoses (ie, cancer, acute myocardial infarction) relevance of animal studies and predictive capability of phase II trials for dose generation is less clear. The members of the investigative team must realize the essentials for success in a multicenter clinical trial. It is also useful and important to understand the big picture of clinical trial development as well as properly functioning interfaces among sponsor, contract research organizations, and investigative sites. Because early enrollment into sepsis clinical trials is usually required, collaboration between emergency medicine and critical care is needed.

Index **881**

Preface

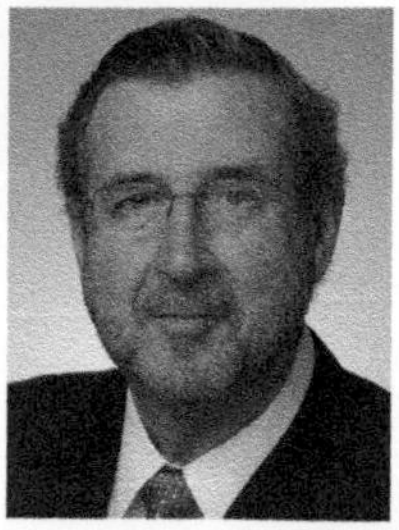

R. Phillip Dellinger, MD, MSc
Guest Editor

Severe sepsis remains a difficult condition to characterize and is often a difficult disease to treat. Morbidity and mortality remains unacceptably high. Although the history of sepsis goes back to the origins of modern medicine, only in the last 40 years is the septic state beginning to be unraveled.

In this issue of *Critical Care Clinics of North America*, the history, characterization, pathophysiology, and treatment of sepsis and severe sepsis are reviewed and updated based on the most recent medical literature. The issue also addresses performance improvement methods and multicenter clinical trial issues (both as to design and for the benefit of participating investigative centers).

This issue is focused on adult patients and is intended for the multiple specialties (critical care, emergency medicine, infectious diseases, surgery, internal medicine, and others) and disciplines (physicians, nurses, clinical pharmacologists, and others). But most importantly it is for the benefit of the septic patient, whose health care providers may learn from this issue and through that learning make a difference in outcome for that patient.

R. Phillip Dellinger, MD, MSc
Department of Medicine
University of Medicine and Dentistry
NJ, USA

Critical Care Division
Department of Medicine
Cooper University Hospital
Camden, NJ, USA

Society of Critical Care Medicine
700 Lee Street
Suite 200
Des Plaines, IL 60016, USA

E-mail address:
dellinger-phil@cooperhealth.edu (R.P. Dellinger)

Crit Care Clin 25 (2009) xiii
doi:10.1016/j.ccc.2009.08.008 criticalcare.theclinics.com

The Evolution of the Understanding of Sepsis, Infection, and the Host Response: A Brief History

Steven M. Opal, MD[a,*]

KEYWORDS

• Sepsis • History of medicine • Infection
• Microbiology • Immunology

Homo sapiens (literally meaning "wise man") and immediate prehominid ancestors have been at risk of death from infection since first descending from the trees (about 3 million years ago) and first adapting a predatory lifestyle on the African plains. Despite intellect, communication skills, and tool-making ability, thin skins and relative absence of body hair inevitably put early humans at risk for cuts and scratches. Death from bleeding and wound infections undoubtedly plagued early humans.[1] An appreciation for the problem of sepsis starts at the very beginning of recorded time. Early writings from the Middle East, China, and Greece indicate that waves of epidemics and sudden death in previously healthy people were noted as having special significance long before the germ theory of disease was first postulated. The history of sepsis has been recently reviewed in *Critical Care Clinics* in an excellent paper by Funk and coworkers.[2] Rather than recapitulating this material over again, the current article focuses on the evolution of understanding about the fundamental nature of infection and the host response that leads to sepsis.[3]

SEPSIS

The primary determinants of lethality for the small, scattered bands of hunter-gatherer populations of humans that existed over the first 150,000 years of the species' existence were likely starvation, injury, predation, and hypothermia. Contagious diseases had a minor role in the evolution of the host response to pathogens in these early

[a] The Warren Alpert School of Medicine of Brown University, BioMed Center, Brown and Meeting Street, Providence, RI 02912, USA
* Infectious Diseases Division, Department of Medicine, Memorial Hospital of RI, 111 Brewster Street, Pawtucket, RI 02860.
E-mail address: steven_opal@brown.edu

Crit Care Clin 25 (2009) 637–663
doi:10.1016/j.ccc.2009.08.007 criticalcare.theclinics.com
0749-0704/09/$ – see front matter

years. Human collective fate was irrevocably altered about 8 to 10,000 years ago when quite suddenly a highly developed immune system became a major selective advantage. Inhabitants of the Fertile Crescent in what is now the modern day Middle East first successfully domesticated plants and animals forever changing human history. Domestication of plant and animal species produced five major outcomes: (1) reduced risk of starvation,(2) establishment of fixed dwellings for maintaining fields of crops,(3) improved nutrition with accelerating fecundity rates in women,(4) use of beasts of burden for labor and transportation, and (5) greater proximity to animals and to other humans with the attendant risk of transmission and spread of zoonotic infections to humans.[4]

The domestication of plants and animals created agrarian societies with ample food supplies, which greatly improved fertility rates and survival, particularly in childhood. A massive population explosion of humans resulted that continues unabated even today. The division of labor that followed permitted a blossoming of civilization innovation, the arts, written language, science, trade, and governments.

Increased population density also created opportunities for massive and repeated epidemic diseases. Human habitations with poor sanitation, absent sewage disposal, proximity to domesticated animals, and lack of understanding about public health created ideal conditions for epidemics. In the absence of any effective treatment, strong selection pressures created by repeated epidemics favored a highly active innate and acquired immune response system in humans. This highly evolved immune response helped localize and combat infection, but it also created a propensity to excessive systemic inflammation when generalized infection occurred.[1] The same system of rapid activation of coagulation and inflammation that was a selective advantage to human ancestors, now becomes a liability to severely injured, critically ill patients at risk for sepsis in the critical care setting.

Crossing species barriers (zoonoses) is a precarious undertaking for pathogens, but once accomplished, the pathogen finds unfettered access to a highly susceptible new host species. Extensive epidemics originating in farm animals and spreading to humans typified the early age of domestication with devastating and predictable results. Endemic camel pox became epidemic human smallpox; bovine rinderpest became human measles; bovine tuberculosis became human tuberculosis; animal forms of brucellosis and salmonellosis became human brucellosis, typhoid fever, and so forth, infections that likely resulted in human disease epidemics. This ongoing process is still relevant today as evidenced by recent examples animal pathogens entering human populations (eg, HIV from simian immunodeficiency virus from nonhuman primates[5] or severe acute respiratory disease from civet cats).[6]

Peridomestic rodent populations, adapted to feeding on the copious amounts of garbage accumulating around towns and cities, became efficient reservoirs for the vector-borne diseases, such as epidemic typhus and plague. Large fixed populations of humans also created conditions for efficient airborne transmission of respiratory pathogens and sexually transmitted diseases.[7] Strong selection forces favored a vigorous innate and adaptive immune response and provided a survival advantage that shaped the human genome. A potent immune response and coagulation system was the best and only viable protection against infection until only a few generations ago.

THE CONCEPT OF CONTAGION: THE EARLY YEARS

The Ancient Greeks, Romans, and Chinese suffered devastating plague epidemics dating back thousands of years. The term "sepsis" (meaning "I rot")[8] was first coined by Greek writers, and Hippocrates used the term to connote a state of odiferous decay and autointoxication that was often lethal. He believed, as did the Egyptians, that this autointoxication state primarily emanated from the colon (ie, the first "gut-motor" hypothesis of sepsis). Cleansing of the colon by enema (also known as "physic") was thought to have a medicinal value. Such enemas were often provided by the patients' caregiver, thereby giving rise to the term "physician" (one who administers enemas). The toll of severe infection and sepsis on human history is incalculable. It is likely that the first European pandemic of plague in 541 hastened the end of the Roman Empire plunging Europe into the Dark Ages. Ironically, the second plague epidemic (the "Black Death") in 1346 likely contributed to the end of the Middle Ages. This epidemic depopulated up to two thirds of the population of Eastern Europe. It also destroyed the confidence in the social contract and religious fabric that dominated much of medieval Europe. This societal upheaval gave rise to the Renaissance and the dawn of the Age of Enlightenment.

A general appreciation for disease resistance on re-exposure to the same disease process was also well appreciated even in ancient times. The Greek historian Thucydides recorded that smallpox survivors did not get reinfected during subsequent epidemics of smallpox. Some form of acquired immunity developed, the nature of which remained obscure for two more millennia. The Chinese made similar observations and exploited this finding to begin the early form of immunization known as "variolation." They used dried smallpox lesions to purposely introduce a milder form of the disease through inserting powdered scabs under the skin or in the nose of susceptible hosts. This process began as early as the tenth century in China and was shown to be remarkably successful in reducing the mortality of smallpox from approximately 30% to less than 3%.[7]

This innovative protective measure to prevent death and disfigurement from smallpox was then introduced into parts of Africa and the Middle East. In 1721, Cotton Mather first introduced this practice to the American colonies after witnessing variolation from his African slave, Onesimus. The major breakthrough in smallpox vaccination using cross-protective immunity from vaccinia cowpox was introduced into clinical use by Edward Jenner's work on vaccination in 1796. This technique rapidly replaced variolation and was instrumental in the eradication of smallpox worldwide by 1980.[7,9]

The intercontinental exchange of people and pathogens during the age of exploration to Africa and the new world in the sixteenth and seventeenth centuries made it clear that some form of "natural resistance" to disease was intrinsic to native populations and lacking in newly exposed populations.[4] Africa was known as a death trap to Europeans and it remained the "dark continent" for centuries as early explorers suffered devastating losses from malaria, trypanosomiasis, and other infections to which indigenous populations had developed relative resistance. African slaves were noted to be much more resistant to tropical diseases, such as yellow fever and malaria, found in the southern colonies of North America when compared with their European counterparts. This became evident when first arriving to the colonies (a process known as "seasoning" by landowner's in search of cheap labor). Africans survived, unlike poor European sharecroppers. Similarly, captured Native Americans transported from the New England colonies and elsewhere to work in the fields in the Caribbean and in the southern colonies were highly susceptible to tropical diseases and rapidly succumbed.[10] The slave trade from Africa became an economic expediency for landowners in need of a healthy labor force.

Conversely, indigenous Amerindian peoples were highly susceptible to smallpox, first introduced into the new world from Europe by the Spanish conquistadors in the early 1500s. Cortez unwittingly unleashed smallpox to the Aztec Empire, and Pizarro brought smallpox with him in his assault against the Inca Empire in Peru, both with the same disastrous outcome for the indigenous peoples.[4] Amherst, a commander of the British troops in 1763 during the French and Indian war, used smallpox as a weapon against the hostile Native American forces in western Pennsylvania. Blankets were deliberately contaminated with the scabs from smallpox victims and left for the Indians in the wintertime. The resulting epidemic decimated the Indians who fought with the French forces. Smallpox contributed to the defeat of the French and maintained the American colonies under British control until 1776.[7]

Back in Europe, a curious, dramatic epidemic of another kind started in 1493.[3] Shortly after Columbus' return voyage from the new world, an epidemic of the "great pox" occurred throughout much of Europe. Great pox was the name ascribed to the skin lesions from secondary syphilis. This term was used to distinguish this entity from the more familiar smallpox. It is likely that some of Columbus' crew contributed to the spread of syphilis throughout Europe in the late 1400s, but they were likely the transmission vector, rather than the original origin of this infectious disease in Europe. Skeletal remains found in both Britain and Greece carry the unmistakable stigma of osseous forms of tertiary syphilis dating back well before Columbus made his famous voyage. Syphilis was likely transported to Europe from the Mediterranean from trade routes established centuries earlier. Syphilis likely existed in Europe but was relatively rare and localized during the medieval period. Transportation over land was difficult and dangerous in this period and the spread of sexually transmitted diseases was severely limited.[7]

Following the Battle of Granada in 1492, Christendom ruled the Iberian Peninsula and throughout Europe. A Papal order then closed all leprosaria in Europe releasing numerous, misdiagnosed, syphilitic patients from leprosaria. These ill people linked up with itinerate armies traveling through Europe. Around this time (1495), the siege of Naples engaged the French forces against the Italian defenders for several years. Mercenary soldiers arrived from many countries and the fortunes of war resulted in the spread of syphilis through prostitutes who serviced both opposing armies during the long siege. Returning troops, likely including some of Columbus' original crew, spread the disease on returning to their respective homelands. This newly recognized and highly virulent form of syphilis caught the attention of a learned few in Europe giving rise to renewed interest in the origin of contagion (**Fig. 1**).[7]

It is worth noting that even in the depths of the Dark Ages in Europe, islands of light and intellect continued to flourish. Even in Europe, isolated pockets of science and intellectual pursuits existed throughout the Middle Ages. The fundamental principles of the scientific method were originally described by Roger Bacon, a Franciscan monk in 1269 (**Fig. 2**). Work in natural sciences continued, but the lack of tools to study things in their fundamental component parts (ie, cells) hampered the understanding of infection and the immune response for centuries.

Using his powers of observation and knowledge of epidemiology, the Italian physician Girolimo Fracastoro (or Hieronymous Fracastorius) wrote a treatise on the germ theory of disease entitled "de Contagione" in 1546 (**Fig. 3**). Fracastorius correctly surmised that tiny, free-living organisms existed ("spores" as he called them). Despite being invisible to human eyes, these disease-causing organisms could be transmitted from person to person or from person to fomite (clothing, towels, utensils, and so forth) to other people, thereby spreading contagious diseases.[3,7] He correctly surmised that syphilis was caused by such a microscopic organism. In his poem entitled "Syphilis sive morbus gallicus" (translated "Syphilis or the French Disease") he described in remarkably accurate detail all the clinical consequences of syphilis in poetic form. The Italians blamed syphilis on the French, hence the name "the French disease."

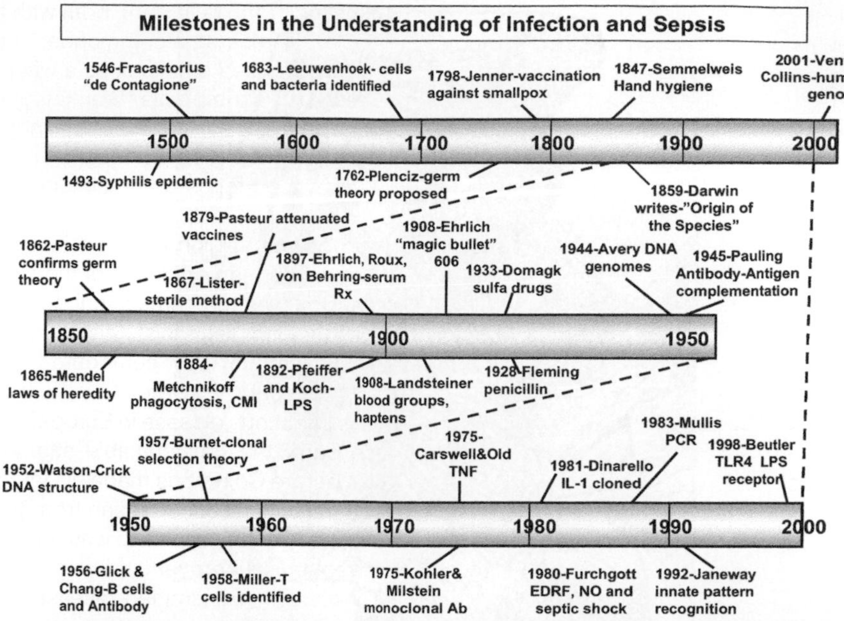

Fig. 1. Milestones in the understanding of infection and sepsis. Ab, antibody; EDRF, endothelial-derived relaxing factor; IL-1, interleukin-1; LPS, lipopolysaccharide; NO, nitric oxide; PCR, polymerase chain reaction; Rx, therapy; TLR, Toll like receptor; TNF, tumor necrosis factor.

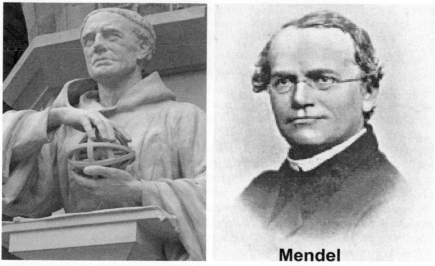

Fig. 2. Roger Bacon (1214–1294). This Franciscan monk laid down the basic tenets of the scientific method (observation, hypothesis, experimentation, and verification) in his 1269 treatise Opus Tertium. Six hundred years later another monk, Gregor Mendel, used this same scientific method to accurately describe the fundamental principles of genetics by studying heritable characteristics of garden peas on the church grounds (1865).

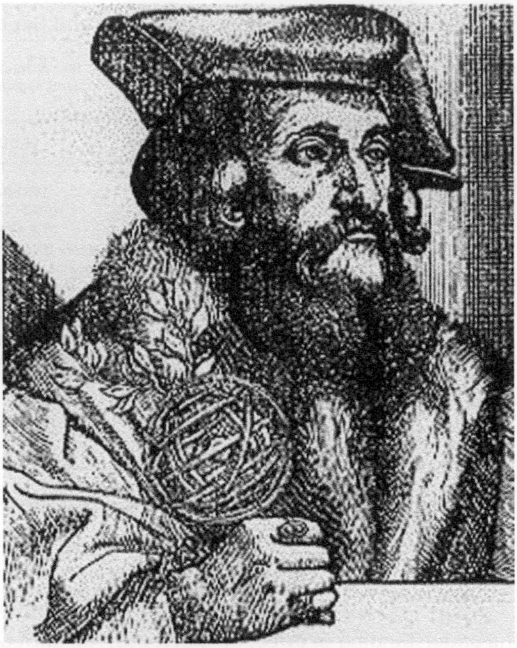

Fig. 3. Girolamo Fracastoro (Hieronymous Fracastorius) (1478–1553). Italian renaissance scholar, scientist, and physician to the Council of Trent. In 1546, he wrote a remarkably prescient treatise, "De contagione," in which he concludes that epidemics are caused by tiny living particles ("spores") that can be transmitted from person to person or by fomites. Regrettably, confirming his hypothesis with a microscope or culture methods took several centuries. He also wrote a famous poem in 1530, "Syphilis sive morbus gallicus" ("Syphilis or The French Disease"), where the multitude of clinical manifestations of syphilis are described. Syphilis is a mythical Greek shepherd who offended Apollo and thereby unleashed epidemic disease among earthly humans as punishment. This poem was so accurate that the disease has been called syphilis ever since.

In return the French blamed syphilis on the Italians referring to it as "the Italian disease." As the disease spread throughout the western world and the Middle East, the disease was routinely blamed on their immediate competitors and adversaries (the Spaniards referred to it as "the Italian disease," the Persians called it "the Christian disease," and so forth).[7]

Regrettably, theories of contagion lacked the tools of scientific proof and the warnings of disease pathogenesis by microorganisms were largely ignored, with tragic consequences. Edmund Hooke first identified microbial pathogens (fungi) in 1680. Antony van Leeuwenhoek was credited with first identifying bacteria using his newly developed microscope in 1683.[11] The critical significance of these tiny forms to human health was not fully appreciated until almost 200 years later when Pasteur and Koch first successfully cultured bacterial organisms from diseased tissue. Despite these technical shortcomings, a number of scientists and physicians correctly hypothesized the existence of microscopic organisms and their contribution to human disease. Plenciz presented a lucid explanation for the clinical observations made up to that time, proposing the germ theory of disease as early as 1762. Henle argued strongly in favor of the idea of germ theory for disease in 1840.[12] The lethal consequences of ignoring scientific ideas and theories about germs before the technology existed for scientific validation is poignantly illustrated by the travails of Semmelweis and Snow.

EPIDEMIOLOGIC CLUES AND MOUNTING EVIDENCE FOR THE GERM THEORY OF DISEASE

In the early 1840s a young Hungarian obstetrician began a series of observations and interventions that would revolutionize the concept of disease causation.[13] Ignaz Semmelweis (**Fig. 4**) was a faculty member of the Lying-In Hospital in Vienna, Austria. The hospital had two obstetric services alternating admissions on an every other day basis. The first clinic was run by physicians and medical students; and the second clinic was run by midwives. The mortality rate from puerperal fever (childbed fever) was such that 1 out of 10 pregnant women could be expected to die shortly after birth from this dreaded complication. Semmelweis observed that the mortality rate was almost fivefold higher in the physician clinic when compared with the midwife clinic. He also noted that the putrid odor associated with women dying of childbed fever was similar to the noxious odor emanating from corpses during autopsies by the faculty and medical students. He noted that the same malodorous smell was found

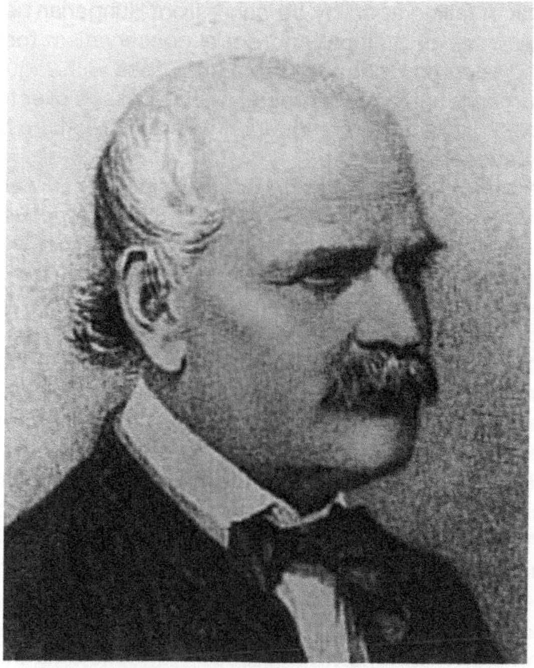

Fig. 4. Ignaz Semmelweis (1818–1865). Hungarian obstetrician who, in 1847, used epidemiologic methods and brilliant insights to demonstrate that hand washing with chlorinated lime solution prevented the spread of "childbed fever." He described his findings before the germ theory of disease was recognized in medicine. He correctly speculated that microorganisms were being transmitted from the hands of doctors to pregnant women, causing puerperal fever, but he was unable to definitively prove his hypothesis. His ideas were rejected by his peers. He developed a deep melancholy and died at age 47 in an insane asylum from sepsis, induced by cuts he received attempting to escape. To this day the "Semmelweis reflex" is used to connote the immediate rejection of a logical but novel idea that runs contrary to prevailing conventional wisdom.

mapped the incidence of cholera in the residents of downtown London and noted their proximity to public water-drawing sites. He observed that the highest incidence of cholera centered on the corner of Broad Street and Cambridge Streets. A pumping station for drinking water was located at this site. The water intake for this pump was drawn from a location just downstream from a large sewer effluent from London into the Thames River. He had the handle removed from the Broad Street pump forcing local residents to seek water from other pumping stations. The epidemic was brought to an abrupt halt. Snow looked at the contaminated water supplies under microscopy and reported some "small, white flocculent particles" that he speculated was likely the cause of cholera. It would take another 30 years before Koch and his colleagues' finally isolated *Vibrio cholerae*, the etiologic agent of this dread epidemic disease.[7]

THE GERM THEORY IS CONFIRMED: THE WORK OF LOUIS PASTEUR

Pasteur essentially proved the germ theory of disease and launched the field of modern microbiology (**Fig. 6**) when he convincingly disproved the theory of "spontaneous generation" in 1857.[16] Many other contemporaries of Pasteur had written earlier about the germ theory. Jakob Henle, Koch's mentor, had proposed the germ theory of disease, but offered no definitive proof. Edmund Klebs argued in favor of

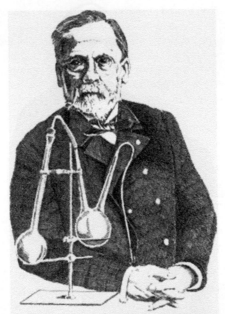

Line drawing- by David Wood

Fig. 6. Louis Pasteur (1822–1895). Pasteur debunked the theory of "spontaneous generation," widely accepted at the time, and firmly established the germ theory of disease by 1862. He developed techniques of sterilization and pasteurization of milk products. He discovered the principles of laboratory attenuation of pathogens as a method to maintain immunogenicity but reduce or eliminate the pathogenicity of microbes for vaccine development. He established the Pasteur Institute as the premier research center for microbiology and immunology. He used this attenuation method to develop the first successful anthrax vaccine (1882) and rabies vaccine (1885).

the germ theory through his studies of wound sepsis. Klebs generated a series of declarative statements, which were later picked up by Koch to generate his famous postulates.[17]

Pasteur showed that heat sterilization, chemical sterilization, or filtration of air and water could maintain organic materials in sterile conditions indefinitely without any microbial growth.[16] Techniques of sterilization of food and instruments and "pasteurization" of milk products were introduced and undoubtedly saved the lives of millions in the generations that followed Pasteur's work. Pasteur inspired Joseph Lister (**Fig. 7**) to use sterile methods to protect the wounds of trauma patients at the orthopedic infirmary in Glasgow, Scotland. Realizing that universal air filtration or heating the patient to maintain sterility were not viable options, Lister investigated the possibility of chemical disinfectants as a way of preventing wound infection. He first demonstrated the value of dilute solutions of carbolic acid in maintaining sterility of bandages, surgical instruments, and the hands of surgeons when caring for injured patients. He tried dilute carbolic acid because local farmers in the area had discovered that this chemical decreased the fetid odor of "night soil" (human excreta), which they used as fertilizer in their fields. Aware of Pasteur's work, Lister correctly speculated that this chemical, and other similar disinfectants, could protect open wounds from microbial contamination. Lister's work was now widely accepted and the use of sterile technique in the care of surgical patients rapidly became an international standard. Lister has succeeded where Semmelweis had failed because the germ theory of disease had gained widespread acceptance by this time through Pasteur's work.[15]

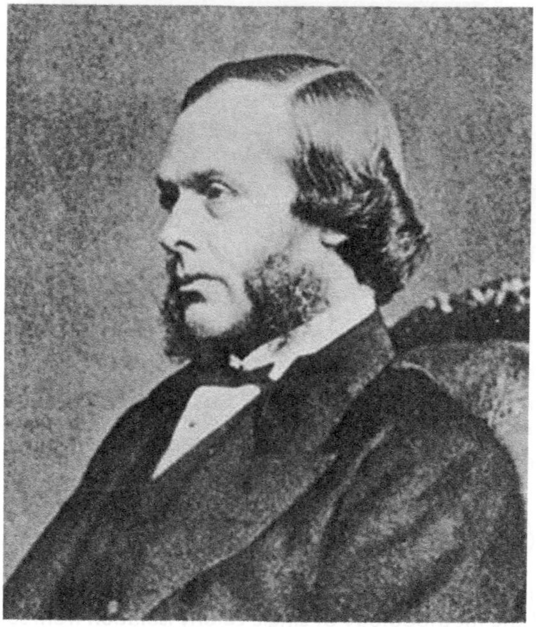

Fig. 7. Joseph Lister (1827–1912). Lister is credited with bringing the idea of chemical sterilization of surgical equipment, dressings, and surgical wounds to prevent infection in the orthopedic ward in Glasgow, Scotland. Using principles set forth by Pasteur's work, he used carbolic acid solutions to chemically sterilize and prevent surgical wound infections (1867). He championed the notion of sterile technique in surgical practice still in use today.

test is still in use today. He found some initial evidence that tuberculin could be a curative agent capable of inducing remission from tuberculosis. When Koch first presented these data at the end of a speech as a preliminary finding, the world immediately seized on the information as the long awaited cure for tuberculosis by the great Robert Koch. Within the next year, hospitals, hotels, and even the streets of Berlin were flooded with tuberculosis patients seeking treatment with tuberculin as a cure for their disease. A national commission was established to confirm the value of tuberculin. Within a year it was clear that tuberculin was not effective in the management of tuberculosis. Koch never formally retracted his claim, but irreparable damage to his career and reputation had already been done. This was a major blow to the meticulous and careful scientist who had overstepped the bounds of his research, making unsubstantiated claims that subsequently were proved to be incorrect.[17]

Despite setbacks, the Koch Institute and its offshoots flourished. Berlin and Frankfurt attracted a superb group of investigators and collaborators to the field of microbiology and immunotherapy. Some of these notable investigators included Paul Ehrlich (**Fig. 9**) (codiscoverer of humoral immunity, antigens, and chemotherapy for infectious diseases); Richard Pfeiffer (**Fig. 10**) (discoverer of bacteriolysis and bacterial endotoxin)[19,20]; Emil von Behring (discoverer of serum therapy for diphtheria and tetanus); and Kitasato and Hata (Japanese scientists who contributed to serum therapy and the discovery of salvarsan [compound 606] for the treatment of syphilis, respectively).

Koch's methodology for bacteriology remains today the clinical standard in microbiology laboratories.[21] Nonculture methods based on nucleic acid testing may displace Koch's culture methods of microbiology in the future,[22] and his famous

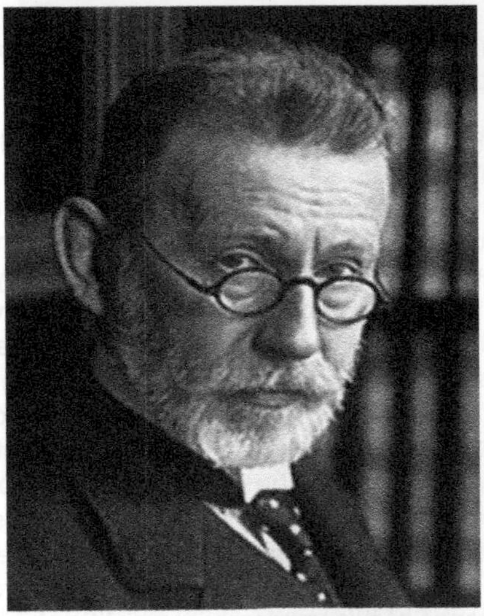

Fig. 9. Paul Ehrlich (1854–1915). German chemist and physician who, along with Emil von Behring, first described the principles of passive and active humoral immunity in 1897. He developed the techniques to titer antibodies efficiently for clinical use in the treatment of diphtheria and other toxigenic diseases. He generated the "side chain theory" for development of antibody diversity. He also developed the "magic bullet" hypothesis in which chemical poisons could be found that could specifically bind to invading microorganisms while leaving human tissues unharmed. He developed the first chemotherapeutic agent for the treatment of syphilis, compound 606 (salvarsan), with a Japanese colleague, Dr Hata.

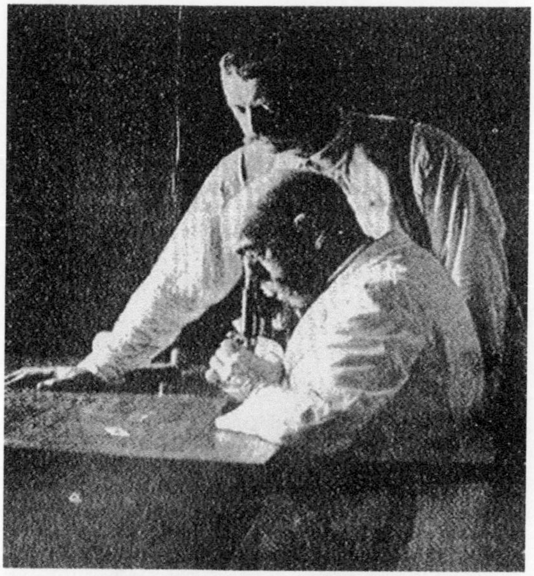

Fig. 10. Richard F.J. Pfeiffer (1858–1945) seen here standing alongside his famous mentor, Robert Koch, as they study a microscope slide. Pfeiffer is credited with first defining the endotoxic principle of the cell wall of gram-negative bacteria and its role as a lethal toxin in bacterial sepsis in 1892. Pfeiffer also described immune serum-induced bacteriolysis (the Pfeiffer phenomenon) and worked on the early development of the typhoid vaccine.

postulates have been revised and revisited on numerous occasions,[23] but Robert Koch and Louis Pasteur remain the two most influential figures in microbiology in history.[16–18]

MODERN ADVANCES IN MICROBIOLOGY, INFECTIOUS DISEASES, AND THE ETIOLOGY OF SEPSIS

Following on the notion of Ehlich's "magic bullet hypothesis" (the idea that a chemical poison could be developed that specifically binds to and kills the invading pathogen without injuring the host),[7] Gerhard Domagk (**Fig. 11**) first introduced sulfa drugs into clinical medicine in 1933.[21] This was a major advance in antimicrobial chemotherapy because it was now possible to cure patients with acute, severe infectious diseases, such as pneumonia, meningitis, and bacteremia, with relative ease through the use of chemotherapeutic agents. The antimicrobial era was launched and aided by Alexander Fleming's famous discovery of the antibacterial properties of *Penicillium notatum* in 1928 (**Fig. 12**). This observation culminated in the successful development of penicillin as a treatment strategy for infection in 1941, with the essential contributions of Florey and Chain.[24]

While progress was being made in the prevention and management of clinical infectious diseases, basic research in microbiology was revealing the fundamental genetic code required for life. Since Darwin's description of natural selection and variation and Mendel's work in defining the laws of genetics, the search was on to determine the biochemical basis for genes that determine the destiny of all life forms.

Avery, McCarty, and MacLeod turned the search for the nature of genes on its head in 1944 when they produced convincing evidence that the genetic material was DNA, and not protein.[25] The complexity and variability of proteins made it seem logical that

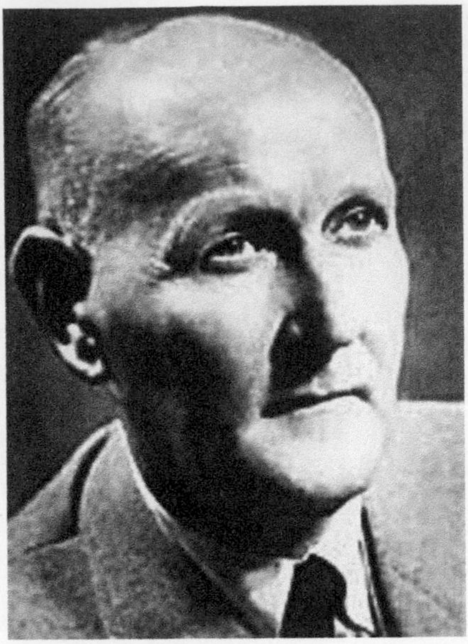

Fig. 11. Gerhard Domagk (1895–1964). This German physician and scientist dedicated himself to finding an effective treatment for gas gangrene after witnessing the horrors of war first hand in the trenches of World War I. He followed up on Ehrlich's earlier work, and in 1928 he first discovers the potential therapeutic value of sulfa drugs as an antibacterial agent. He brings the first antimicrobial "wonder drug" (Prontosil) to the market in 1933. This Nobel Prize laureate (1939) went on to contribute to the successful development of antituberculous drugs. (*Courtesy of* the National Library of Medicine.)

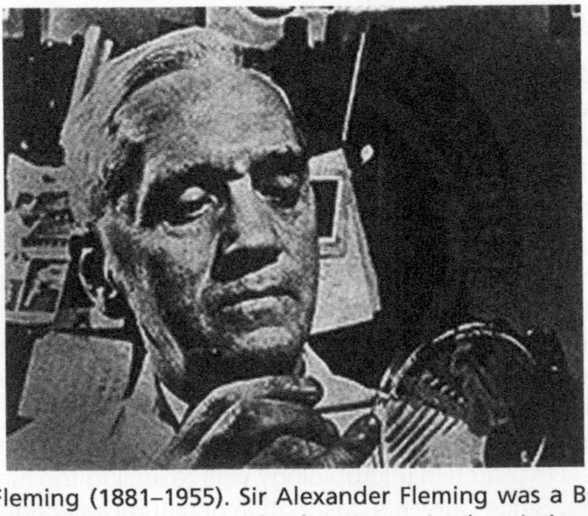

Fig. 12. Alexander Fleming (1881–1955). Sir Alexander Fleming was a British physician and bacteriologist who discovered lysozyme, the first recognized antimicrobial peptide of the innate immune system, in 1922. His most famous discovery was in 1928 when he demonstrated the antibacterial potential of the mold *Penicillium notatum* from a contaminated culture plate of *Staphylococcus aureus*. He shared the Nobel prize in 1945 along with Florey and Chain for their development of penicillin as a treatment for infectious diseases. (*Courtesy of* the National Library of Medicine.)

the genetic code would be protein-based rather than the monotonous series of four nitrogenous bases that make up the structure of DNA. Capitalizing on the finding that *Streptococcus pneumoniae* is naturally competent (able to take up naked DNA), Avery's group used highly purified DNA from a killed, virulent, and encapsulated strain of pneumococci and transformed a rough, unencapsulated, and avirulent serotype of pneumococci into a virulent strain through the transfer of DNA alone. The inheritance of the capsule for virulence was genetically stable and confirmed that DNA encoded the essential genetic traits of bacteria.

This observation enabled Watson, Crick, Franklin (**Fig. 13**), and Wilkins to determine the three-dimensional, molecular structure of the antiparallel, right-handed, double-helical form of DNA. Franklin's famous x-ray crystallography photograph (Photo 51) verified that DNA was held in a double-helical configuration. This allowed Watson and Crick to correctly assemble the chemical structure of DNA using appropriate hydrophilic interactions and correct hydrogen bonding. The structure of DNA, first reported in 1953,[26] was rapidly followed by a biochemical explanation for DNA replication, the central dogma of Watson and Crick (DNA directs RNA, RNA directs protein synthesis, and proteins structures and enzymes directs life), and deciphering of the three codon: anti-codon interacting genetic code that translates nucleic acid sequences to amino acid sequences in protein. This work launched the modern field of molecular biology. The first complete genomic sequencing of a bacteriophage was accomplished by Sanger and coworkers in 1977.[27] The complete genome of a free living organism (*Haemophilus influenzae* Rd) was first accomplished in 1995 by Fleischmann and colleagues,[28] and the first draft of the human genome was completed in 2001 by Collins, Venter, and colleagues.[29,30]

Recent advances in microbiology include the development of recombinant DNA technology, polymerase chain reaction, and development of monoclonal antibodies

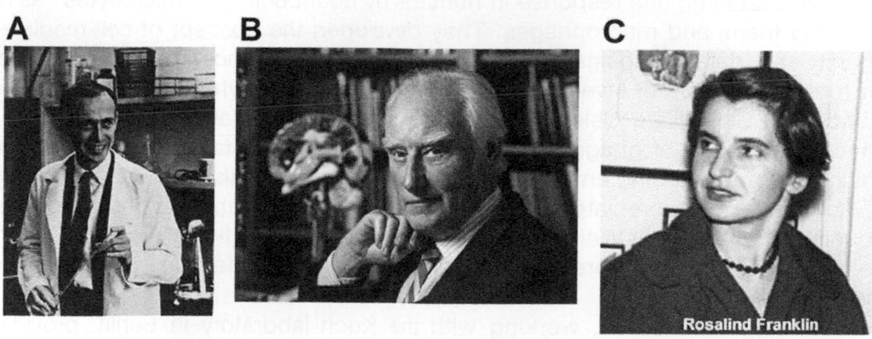

Fig. 13. (*A*) James Watson (1928-). (*Courtesy of* National Library of Medicine.) (*B*) Francis Crick (1916–2004). (*From* Siegel RM, Callaway EM. Francis Crick's legacy for neuroscience: between the α and the Ω. PLoS Biol 2/12/2004: e419; with permission.) (*C*) Rosalind Franklin (1920–1958). (*Courtesy of* Academy of Medical Sciences.) In 1953, Watson and Crick correctly determined the three-dimensional structure of the antiparallel, double-helical nature of DNA. They shared the Nobel Prize along with Maurice Wilkins in 1962. Rosalind Franklin was also instrumental with Wilkins in this discovery by performing the x-ray crystallography that determined that double-helical structure of DNA. She died at age 37 of ovarian cancer before fully receiving the credit due to her for her contributions. Watson and Crick went on to develop the central dogma of Watson-Crick: DNA RNA protein life and the basic elements of the genetic code. Their work launches the "reductionist" view of biology and ushers in the modern era of molecular biology.

that have revolutionized clinical microbiology. These milestones in microbiology are depicted in **Fig. 1**. These technologies now allow the use of nonculture methods to rapidly diagnose difficult-to-culture or noncultivatable organisms after exposure to antimicrobial agents. This methodology is now in clinical use in identifying the causative microorganism responsible for sepsis.[31]

HISTORY OF IMMUNOLOGY

Although it was well known for centuries that humans developed natural resistance to re-exposure to the same pathogen (eg, repeated smallpox outbreaks), the explanation for this resistance remained obscure until the late 1800s. The basic elements of the human immune response were rapidly uncovered with the recognition of the germ theory of disease. The innate immune system coevolved with the coagulation system of multicellular organisms to defend the internal milieu from invasion and from loss of viability from excess bleeding. Adaptive or acquired immunity evolved relatively late in vertebrate evolution through the acquisition of large retro-transposons within the genome. This provided the genetic substrate localized recombination for the diversity to provide specific T- and B-cell responses to a myriad of potential pathogens. Mammals and avian species have adaptive immune responses with immunologic memory with targeted immune responses to previously exposed pathogens.

Innate immunity from myeloid cells was first described in detail by Metchnikoff in the late nineteenth century (**Fig. 14**).[32] He first witnessed phagocytosis of bacteria when studying starfish mesenchymal cells. Metchnikoff was a comparative zoologist who was aware of Darwin's theory of evolution. He speculated that this highly advantageous host defense would likely be selected for by natural selection from invertebrate species to vertebrates.[33] He changed his career and became a human pathologist and microbiologist in search of evidence of phagocytosis in humans. He and his colleagues at the Institute Pasteur confirmed that phagocytosis was an essential part of an innate immune response in humans by neutrophils (or "microcytes" as he referred to them) and macrophages. They developed the concept of cell-mediated immunity as a defense against specific sets of microbial pathogens (ie, *Mycobacterium tuberculosis*). Other investigators had observed phagocytosis before Metchnikoff, including Sir William Osler (**Fig. 15**).[33] This renowned Canadian physician had witnessed evidence of phagocytosis of mineral crystals as far back as 1876. The significance of this finding and the importance of phagocytosis to host defense was not, however, fully appreciated until Metchnikoff developed this concept of cellular immunity in 1884.[32] Osler is also credited for being among the first clinicians to recognize that septic patients were dying from the response to infection, rather than the infection itself.

Von Behring and Ehrlich, working with the Koch laboratory in Berlin, provided evidence that serum factors alone could prevent lethality from bacterial toxins including tetanus and diphtheria.[34] These antitoxins were subsequently shown to be antibodies, and that protection could be passively transferred from one animal to another using serum alone. This formed the basis of the first immune therapy for infectious diseases: passive immunotherapy (or serum therapy) as primary treatment for toxin-mediated infectious diseases. This strategy was widely used by Koch's group and by Roux at the Institute Pasteur. Large animals, such as horses, were used to generate antitoxins through the development of detoxified exotoxins from diphtheria and tetanus.

Von Behring received the Nobel Prize for his seminal work on serum therapy for infectious diseases. Ehrlich and Metchnikoff shared a Nobel Prize in 1908 for their

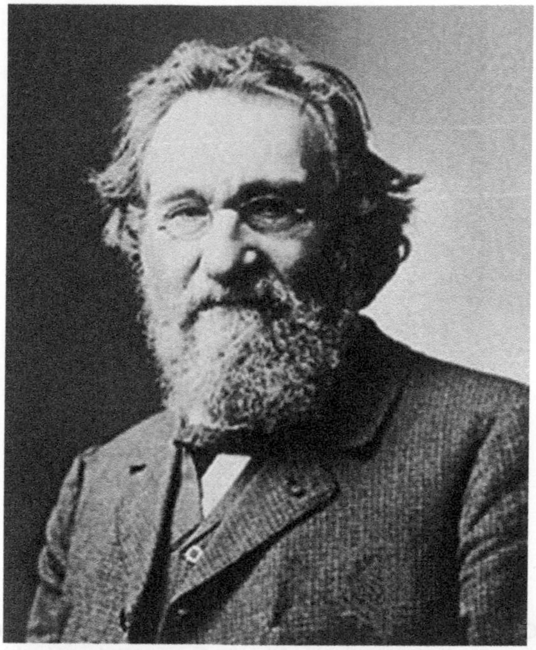

Fig. 14. Elie Metchnikoff (1845–1916). This famous Russian microbiologist and immunologist first observed and appreciated the importance of phagocytosis as a cellular defense mechanism against microbial invasion. He first reported his findings in 1884. He did much of his work at the Pasteur Institute. He recognized the importance of innate and acquired cellular immunity in host response in the prevention and control of infectious diseases. He shared a Nobel Prize with Paul Ehrlich for their respective work on cellular and humoral immunity in 1908.

initial discoveries in describing humoral and cellular immunity.[34–36] Bordet in 1896 first showed the presence of a heat-labile serum factor that contributed to protection induced by heat-stable factors (antibodies) in therapy. Ehrlich similarly recognized this property and referred to it as "complement," a heat-labile serum component that complemented the activity of antibodies. This is the first description of the classical complement system.[37] The alternative complement system was described in 1954 by Pillemer[38] and the third arm of the complement system, the mannose-binding lectin pathway, was recently discovered in 1989 by Super and colleagues.[39]

One of the fundamental problems facing early immunologists was providing an explanation how hundreds of thousands of different antibodies (and T-cell receptors) could be generated to maintain adaptive immunity against a myriad of potential human pathogens and their numerous antigens. Three basic theories to explain antibody diversity (and later T-cell receptor diversity) were postulated: (1) the instruction theory; (2) the natural selection theory; and (3) the germline theory.[40]

The instruction theory was initially attractive because it readily explained the remarkably diverse array of antibodies that can be possibly generated by the human immune system. The hypothesis stated that any antigenic determinants serve as a template for the molding and modeling of a newly created antibody on the cell surface of immune effector cells. This theory predicted that any potential immune cell has the capacity to respond to any antigen by being instructed on the specific

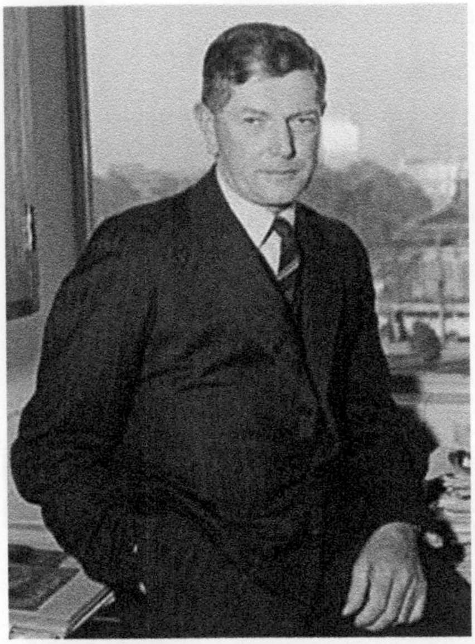

Fig. 17. Sir Frank Macfarlane Burnet (1899–1985). This Australian immunologist is best known for his hypothesis to explain antibody diversity and T cell diversity. The clonal selection theory of Burnet, although controversial when first proposed in the 1950s, has subsequently been shown to be correct and forms the basis of the current understanding of antibody and T cell diversity today. His work was honored with a Nobel Prize in 1960.

practices for resuscitating injured patients with major hemorrhage. This discovery and its application to transfusion therapy undoubtedly saved countless lives since his initial description of blood group antigens in 1908. Landsteiner was also instrumental in describing the nature of antigens and what components were required in a molecule to induce antibody formation. His work on haptens, carrier molecules, and the requisite size and structure of antigens was fundamental to an understanding of humoral immunity.[43]

THE ORIGIN OF B CELLS AND SEGREGATION BETWEEN B CELLS AND T CELLS IN ADOPTIVE IMMUNITY

In the early 1950s, Bruce Glick was studying the effects of bursectomy in chickens at Ohio State University. He observed that the bursa of Fabricius grew rapidly in the first few weeks of life suggesting that it had some important role in chicken development.[44] The function of the bursa remained unknown until a graduate student, Timothy Chang, needed some chickens to raise antibodies to salmonella antigens for another experiment. The only chickens available happened to be bursectomized animals from Glick's laboratory. Surprisingly, they observed no antibody reaction in these animals following immunization. Nonbursectomized animals responded perfectly well to this salmonella antigen.

The significance of this finding was immediately recognized by Glick and Chang, but not to editors of major science journals. They resorted to publishing their seminal discovery on B-cell origin in *Poultry Science* in 1955 and 1956.[44–46] Other investigators confirmed their results and noted that cell-mediated immune responses remained intact in these animals. Francis Miller subsequently demonstrated that cell-mediated immune responses required thymic conditioning.[47] Thymectomy depleted the lymphoid organs of lymphocytes and resulted in absent cell-mediated immune responses.[48] Human immunodeficiency disease equivalents to these B-cell deficiencies and T-cell deficiencies and experimental animal models were rapidly identified.[49,50] The significance of unique subsets of lymphocytes and other immune effector cells was underway and continues until today.[51,52]

Subtyping of T cells and B cells was greatly facilitated by the discovery of monoclonal antibody formation by hybridoma cell lines in 1975 by Kohler and Milstein.[53] Monoclonal antibodies revolutionized immunology and allowed for specific labeling of cells; the phenotypic description of cell structure and function; an accurate method to assess the ontogeny and trafficking of cells; and along with the advent of fluorescent automated cell sorters, provided the ability to quantitatively monitor cellular immunology. The distinction between T_H1 and T_H2 cells by Mossmann,[54] the role of natural killer cells in innate immunity, the nature of regulatory T cells,[55] T_H17 cells,[56] and the array of B-cell clones that contribute to optimal antibody formation[57] all followed these landmark discoveries. Other major advances in understanding acquired immunity followed including the details of antigen processing,[58] presentation and T-cell signaling by macrophages,[59] the critical interactions between T and B cells,[60] and the discovery and functional role of dendritic cells as antigen-presenting cells.[61]

INNATE IMMUNITY REGAINS ITS PROMINENCE IN THE UNDERSTANDING OF SEPSIS

Despite these historic discoveries in T- and B-cell physiology and basic immunology of adaptive immunity, the importance of the innate immune system in sepsis has become increasingly evident in the last 25 years. Alexander Fleming, the discoverer of penicillin, often considered his greatest discovery to be the isolation of lysozyme from tears and oral secretions. The presence of this and other antimicrobial peptides on mucosal surfaces forms part of the innate barrier defenses against microbial invasion. The discoveries of proinflammatory cytokines, such as tumor necrosis factor (Carswell and Old, 1975) and interleukin-1 (Dinarello and colleagues, 1981), were major milestones in understanding immune cell signaling and response on encountering and endogenous and exogenous danger signals.[62–65] The Janeway hypothesis of innate immune recognition by detection of highly conserved molecular patterns was verified at the molecular level with discovery and description of the toll-like receptors in the early 1990s.[66] The definition of TLR4 as the LPS receptor put an end to a 100-year search for the long awaited receptor for bacterial endotoxin first begun by Pfeiffer and Koch.[67] The discovery of nitric oxidase as the endothelium-derived relaxing factor as the proximate course of hypotension[68] and understanding of myocardial dysfunction in sepsis[69,70] serves as the fundamental treatment strategy of management of sepsis.[71]

SUMMARY

Sepsis is the ultimate clinical expression of the deleterious clash between the host immune response and invasive microorganisms.[72,73] At the beginning of the twentieth century, infections were by far the most common causes of death of Americans. By the beginning of the twenty-first century, the average lifespan of United States citizens had increased by over 30 years, with infections now accounting for a small minority of death.[74,75] Despite advances in public health, sanitation, vaccines, and antituberculosis chemotherapy and other antimicrobial agents, sepsis continues to account for an increasing number of deaths in critically ill patients. Future advances are anticipated when the genomics era and the promise of systems biology and personalized medicine are fully realized in the next few decades. A remarkable history of scientific inquiry into the fundamental nature of microbes and immune defenses preceded much of the current advances in the treatment of infectious diseases. Much work remains before the benefits of these discoveries can be thoughtfully applied to the management of severe sepsis and septic shock worldwide.

REFERENCES

1. Opal SM. The link between coagulation and innate immunity in severe sepsis. Scand J Infect Dis 2003;35:535–44.
2. Funk D, Parrillo JE, Kumar A. Sepsis and septic shock: a history. Crit Care Clin 2009;25(1):83–101, viii.
3. Opal SM. A brief history of microbiology and immunology. In: Artenstein A, editor. The history of vaccines. New York: Springer; 2010.
4. Diamond J. Guns, germs and steel: the fate of human societies. New York: W.W. Norton & Company; 1999. p. 1–32.
5. Kalish ML, Robbins KE, Pieniazek D, et al. Recombinant viruses and early global HIV-1 epidemic. Emerg Infect Dis 2004;10(7):1227–34.
6. Margaret H, Ng L, Lau KM, et al. Association of human-leukocyte antigen class 1 (B*0703) and class 2 (DRB1&0301*) genotypes with susceptibility and resistance to the development of severe acute respiratory syndrome. J Infect Dis 2004;190: 515–8.
7. Sherman IW. Twelve diseases that changed our world. Washington, DC: ASM Press; 2007. p. 83–103.
8. Geroulanos S, Douka ET. Historical perspective of the word sepsis. Intensive Care Med 2006;32:2077.
9. Roush SW, Murphy TV. Historical comparisons in morbidity and mortality for vaccine-preventable disease in the United States. JAMA 2007;298:2155–63.
10. Morgan ES. American slavery, American freedom: the ordeal of colonial Virginia. 1st edition. New York: Norton; 1975. p. 1–454.
11. Corliss JO. A salute to Antony van Leewenhoek of Delft, most versatile 17th century founding father of protistology. Protist 2002;153(2):177–90.
12. Gensini GF, Conti AA. The evolution of the concept of fever in the history of medicine: from pathological picture per se to clinical epiphenomenon (and vice versa). J Infect 2004;49:85–7.
13. Wyklicky H, Skopec M. Ignaz Philipp Semmelweis, the prophet of bacteriology. Infect Control 1983;4(5):367–9.
14. Jones G. The unbalanced reformer. VA Med Mon 1970;97:526–7.
15. Wangesteen ON, Wangesteen SD. The rise of surgery, from a empiric craft to scientific discipline. Minneapolis (MN): University of Minnesota Press; 1978. p. 414–52.
16. Debré P. Louis Pasteur. Baltimore (MD): The Johns Hopkins University Press; 1998. p. 1–473.
17. Brock TD. Robert Koch: a life in medicine and bacteriology. Washington, DC: American Society for Microbiology; 1988. p. 1–353.
18. Kaufmann SHE, Winau F. From bacteriology to immunology: the dualism of specificity. Nat Immunol 2005;6(11):1063–6.
19. Pfeiffer R. Untersuchungen uber das choleragift. Hygeine 1892; 11:939–412.
20. Rietschel ET, Wesphal O. Endotoxin: historical perspectives. In: Braude H, Opal SM, Vogel SN, et al, editors. Endotoxin in health and disease. New York: Marcel Dekker; 1990. p. 1–30.

21. Dubos R, Dubos J. The white plague. Boston: Little Brown; 1956. p. 1–277.
22. Relman DA, Schmidt TN, MacDermott RP, et al. Identification of the uncultured bacillus in Whipple's disease. N Engl J Med 1992;327:293–301.
23. Fredricks DN, Relman DA. Sequence-based identification of microbial pathogens: a reconsideration of Koch's postulates. Clin Microbiol Rev 1996;9: 18–33.
24. Fleming A. Antibacterial action of cultures of a *Penicillium* with special reference to their use in the isolation of *B. influenzae*. Br J Exp Pathol 1929;10:226–32.
25. Lederberg J. The transformation of genetics by DNA: an anniversary celebration if Avery, MacLeod and McCarty (1944). Genetics 1994;136(2):423–6.
26. Watson JD. The double helix: a personal account of the discovery of the structure of DNA. New York: Norton; 1968. p. 1–245.
27. Sanger F, Coulson AR, Hong GF, et al. Nucleotide sequence of bacteriophage λ. J Mol Biol 1982;162:729–73.
28. Fleischmann RD, Adams MD. Whole-genome random sequencing assembly of *Hemophilus influenzae*. Science 1995;269:496–512.
29. Venter JC. The sequence of the human genomes. Science 2001;291:1304–51.
30. Altshuler D. The International Hap Map Consortium. The haplotype map of the human genome. Nature 1995;437:1299–320.
31. Mussap M, Molinari MP, Senna E, et al. New diagnostic tools for neonatal sepsis: the role of a real-time polymerase chain reaction for the early detection and identification of bacterial and fungal species in blood samples. J Chemother 2002; 19(Suppl 2):31–4.
32. Silverstein AM. Darwinism and immunology: from Metchnikoff to Burnet. Nat Immunol 2003;4(1):3–6.
33. Ambrose CT. The Osler slide, a demonstration of phagocytosis from 1876 reports of phagocytosis before Metchnikoff's 1880 paper. Cell Immunol 2006; 240(1):1–4.
34. Jaryal AK. Emil von Behring and the last hundred years of immunology. Indian J Physiol Pharmacol 2001;45(4):389–94.
35. Silverstein AM. Paul Ehrlich, archives and the history of immunology. Nat Immunol 2005;6(7):639.
36. Gensini GF, Conti AA, Lippi D. The contributions of Paul Ehrlich to infectious disease. J Infect 2007;54(3):221–4.
37. Walport MJ. Complement. N Engl J Med 2001;344:1058–66.
38. Pillemer L, Blum L, Lepow IH, et al. The properdin system in immunity: I. Demonstration isolation of a new serum protein, properdin, and its role in immune phenomenon. Science 1956;120(3112):279–85.
39. Super M, Tlthiel S, Lu J. Association of low levels of mannan-binding protein with a common defect in opsonization. Lancet 1989;2:1236–9.
40. Weiser RS, Myrvik QN, Pearsall NN. Fundamentals of immunology. Philadelphia: Lea & Febiger; 1969. p. 87–95.
41. Burnet F. A modification of Jerne's theory of antibody formation using the concept clonal selection. Aust J Sci 1957;20:669–76.
42. Brack C, Hirama M, Lenhard-Schuller R, et al. A complete immunoglobulin gene is created by somatic recombination. Cell 1978;15:1–14.
43. Figl M, Pelinka LE. Karl Landsteiner: discoverer of blood groups. Resuscitation 2004;63(3):251–4.
44. Ribatti D, Crivellato E, Vacca A. The contribution of Bruce Glick to the definition of the role played by the bursa of Fabricius in the development of the B cell lineage. Clin Exp Immunol 2006;145:1–4.

45. Glick B. The bursa of Fabricius and antibody production. PhD dissertation. Columbus (OH): State University, 1955; p. 1–102.
46. Chang TS, Glick B, Winter AR. The significance of the bursa of Fabricius of chickens in antibody production. Poult Sci 1955;34:1187.
47. Ribatti D, Crivellato E, Vacca A. Miller's seminal studies on the role of thymus in immunity. Clin Exp Immunol 1965;139:371–5.
48. Cooper MD, Peterson RDA, South MA, et al. The functions of the thymus system and the bursa system in the chicken. J Exp Med 1966;123:75–102.
49. Stehm ER, Johnston RB. A history of pediatric immunology. Pediatr Res 2005; 57(3):458–67.
50. Peterson RD. Experiments of nature and the new era of immunology: a historical perspective. Immunol Res 2007;38(1–3):55–63.
51. Silverstein AM. The lymphocyte in immunology: from James Murphy to James L. Gowans. Nat Immunol 2001;2(7):569–71.
52. Steinman RM. Dendritic cells: versatile controllers of the immune system. Nat Med 2007;13(10):1155–9.
53. Köhler G, Milstein C. Continuous cultures of fused cells secreting antibody of predefined specificity. Nature 1975;256:495–7.
54. Masopust D, Vezys V, Wherry EJ, et al. A brief history of CD8 T cells. Eur J Immunol 2007;37(Suppl 1):S103–10.
55. Sakaguchi S, Wing K, Miyara M. Regulatory T cells: a brief history and perspective. Eur J Immunol 2007;37(Suppl 1):S116–23.
56. Wynn TA. T_H-17: a giant step from T_H1 and T_H2. Nat Immunol 2005;6(11): 1069–70.
57. Van Epps HL. Bringing order to early B cell chaos. J Exp Med 2006;203(6):1389.
58. Siamon G. The macrophage: past, present and future. Eur J Immunol 2006;37: S9–17.
59. Zinkernagel RM, Doherty PC. Restriction of in vitro T cell-mediated cytotoxicity in lymphocytic choriomeningitis within a syngeneic or semi-allogeneic system. Nature 1974;248:701–2.
60. Claman HN, Chaperon EA. Immunologic complementation between thymus and marrow cells: a model for the two-cell theory of immunocompetence. Transplant Rev 1969;1:92–113.
61. Steinmann RM, Cohn ZA. Identification of a novel cell type in peripheral lymphoid organs of mice. I. Morphology, quantitation, tissue distribution. J Exp Med 1973; 137:1142–62.
62. Cohen S. Cytokine: more than a new word, a new concept proposed by Stanley Cohen thirty years ago. Cytokines 2004;28:242–7.
63. Carswell EA, Old LJ, Kassel RL, et al. An endotoxin-induced serum factor that causes necrosis of tumors. Proc Natl Acad Sci U S A 1975;72:3666–70.
64. Beutler B, Greenwald D, Hulmes JD, et al. Identity of tumour necrosis factor and the macrophage-secreted factor cachectin. Nature 1985;316:552–4.
65. Dinarello CA. Historical insights into cytokines. Eur J Immunol 2007;37(Suppl 1): S34–45.
66. Beutler B, Jiang Z, Georgel P, et al. Genetic analysis of host resistance: toll like receptor signaling and immunity at large. Annu Rev Immunol 2006;24: 353–89.
67. Beutler B, Poltorak A. The search for *Lps*: 1993–1998. J Endotoxin Res 2000;6(4): 269–93.
68. Furchgott R, Zawadski JV. The obligatory role of endothelial cells in the relaxation of arterial smooth muscle by acetylcholine. Nature 1980;288:373–6.

69. Palmer RM, Ferrige AG, Moncada S. Nitric oxide release accounts for the biological activity of endothelium-derived relaxing factor. Nature 1987;327:524–6.
70. Parker MM, Shelhamer JH, Bacharach SL, et al. Profound but reversible myocardial depression in patients with septic shock. Ann Intern Med 1984;100:483–90.
71. Mackensie IMJ. The haemodynamics of human septic shock. Anaesthesia 2001; 56:130–44.
72. Baron RM, Baron MJ, Perrella MA. Pathobiology of sepsis: are we still asking the same questions? Am J Respir Cell Mol Biol 2006;34:129–34.
73. Rosengart MR. Critical care medicine: landmarks and legends. Surg Clin North Am 2006;86:1305–21.
74. Centers for Disease Control. Ten great public health achievements—United States 1900–1999. MMWR 1999;48(12):241–3.
75. Roush SW, Murphy TV. Comparisons in morbidity and mortality for vaccine-preventable disease in the United States. JAMA 2007;298:2155–63.

Evolving Concepts in Sepsis Definitions

Jean-Louis Vincent, MD, PhD[a,*], Eva Ocampos Martinez, MD[a], Eliezer Silva, MD, PhD[b]

KEYWORDS

• Sepsis • Septic shock • PIRO • Diagnosis • Infection

To be able to give a clear name or label to a specific collection of signs and symptoms is important for physicians and patients alike. Having an exact diagnosis helps to identify particular groups of patients, to better understand the underlying disease process, and provides a more defined target for appropriate treatment. However, to be able to reach an accurate diagnosis, and hence, offer optimal medical therapy, a precise definition of the disease process in question is required. Over the years many disease processes have become well defined and are fairly easy to diagnose with the appropriate set of symptoms and test results. For example, acute myocardial infarction is associated with typical symptoms (eg, chest pain), signs (eg, abnormal electrocardiogram), and biomarkers (eg, raised blood troponin levels); patients meeting these criteria can be offered immediate and appropriate therapy. Imprecise definitions of disease limit the ability to form a specific, correct diagnosis and attempts to institute or study therapies in such situations are unlikely to be of benefit and may cause harm.

In sepsis, attempts have also been made to provide clear and accurate definitions, but these efforts have not met with universal support. In 2004, a survey of 1058 physicians, including 529 intensivists, noted that only 17% of those interviewed agreed on any one definition.[1] Sepsis is a complex process that can affect any individual and can originate from multiple sites and be caused by multiple microorganisms. Sepsis can present with a multitude of signs and symptoms, none of which are specific for sepsis and all of which can vary among patients and within the same patient over time. These symptoms can vary in severity from a mild, short-lived fever to fatal septic shock. Faced with such complexity and variation, it may be that a single, simple definition for sepsis will never be possible and we should focus on types of infection rather than on sepsis per se.

Dr Vincent has participated in Eli Lilly and Co sponsored clinical trials, has served as a paid consultant for Eli Lilly and Co, and has been an invited speaker at conferences supported by Eli Lilly and Co

[a] Department of Intensive Care, Erasme University Hospital, Université libre de Bruxelles, 808 route de Lennik, 1070 Brussels, Belgium
[b] Department of Intensive Care, Hospital Israelita Albert Einstein, Sao Paulo, Brazil
* Corresponding author.
E-mail address: jlvincen@ulb.ac.be (J.-L. Vincent).

Crit Care Clin 25 (2009) 665–675
doi:10.1016/j.ccc.2009.07.001
criticalcare.theclinics.com

PREVIOUS AND CURRENT DEFINITIONS OF SEPSIS

Sepsis is derived from "σηψις," the original Greek word for the decomposition of animal or vegetable organic matter.[2] First used more than 2700 years ago by Homer, it was only approximately 100 years ago that the link between bacteria and systemic signs of disease was made;[3] sepsis then became almost synonymous with severe infection. More recently, as the role of the immune response has become clearer, we have realized that what we had called sepsis is in fact a host response to the invading microorganism rather than any specific feature of the microorganism itself. Indeed, sepsis can be initiated by any microorganism, whether it is bacterial, fungal, viral, parasitic, or by microbial products and toxins, and is then propagated by a complex network of inflammatory mediators and cellular dysfunction.

The Sepsis Syndrome

One of the first attempts to establish a set of clinical parameters to define patients who have severe sepsis came in 1989 when Roger Bone and colleagues[4] proposed the term "sepsis syndrome." Sepsis syndrome was defined as hypothermia (less than 96°F [35.5°C]) or hyperthermia (greater than 101°F [38.3°C]); tachycardia (greater than 90 beat/min); tachypnea (greater than 20 breath/min); clinical evidence of an infection site; and the presence of at least one end-organ demonstrating inadequate perfusion or dysfunction expressed as poor or altered cerebral function, hypoxemia (PaO_2 less than 75 torr on room air), elevated plasma lactate, or oliguria (urine output less than 30 mL/h or 0.5 mL/kg body weight/h without corrective therapy). However, although it has been used as an entry criterion for clinical trials,[5,6] sepsis syndrome does not successfully define a homogeneous group of patients.

Systemic Inflammatory Response Syndrome and Multiple Organ Dysfunction Syndrome

Systemic inflammatory response syndrome

Following on from the sepsis syndrome, the American College of Chest Physicians (ACCP) and the Society of Critical Care Medicine (SCCM) convened a Consensus Conference in 1991 in an attempt to create a set of standardized definitions.[7] Thirty-five experts in the field of sepsis were gathered together to provide a framework to define the systemic inflammatory response to infection (ie, sepsis). The end result of this conference was the introduction of the term "systemic inflammatory response syndrome" (SIRS). It had been recognized for some time that the same inflammatory response to infection could also occur in response to other conditions, including acute pancreatitis, trauma, ischemia/reperfusion injury, and burns. SIRS was an attempt to differentiate sepsis from these noninfectious causes.

According to the ACCP-SCCM Consensus Conference,[7] infection was defined as a microbial phenomenon characterized by the invasion of microorganisms or microbial toxins into normally sterile tissues. SIRS was defined, by consensus, as the presence of at least two of four clinical criteria:

- Body temperature >38°C or <36°C
- Heart rate >90 beats/min
- Respiratory rate >20 breaths/min or hyperventilation with a $PaCO_2$ <32 mmHg
- White blood cell count WBC >12,000/mm^3, <4000/mm^3, or with >10% immature neutrophils

SIRS represented a systemic inflammatory response of any etiology, including sepsis, which was therefore defined by the presence of SIRS in association with a confirmed infection. Sepsis associated with organ dysfunction, hypoperfusion abnormality, or sepsis-induced hypotension was called severe sepsis, and septic shock was defined as severe sepsis with sepsis-induced hypotension persisting despite adequate fluid resuscitation.

The SIRS approach was rapidly adopted and has been widely used to define populations of patients in interventional clinical trials. Trzeciak and colleagues[8] reported that 69% of clinical trials in sepsis published between 1993 and 2001 used the Consensus Conference definitions. Similarly, Veloso and colleagues[9] reported that 10 of the 11 multicenter, randomized controlled trials of new therapeutic interventions in adult patients who had severe sepsis published between January 2000 and December 2007, used SIRS as part of the entrance criteria. Nevertheless, in the survey of 1058 physicians, including 529 intensivists, conducted by Poeze and colleagues[1] in 2000, only 5% (22% of the intensivists) gave the ACCP/SCCM definition when asked to define sepsis.

Although the SIRS criteria do have the prognostic value of defining a group of patients who are at an increased risk of developing complications and with increased mortality,[10,11,12] they have been criticized for being too sensitive and nonspecific to be of much clinical use.[13] Most ICU patients and many general ward patients meet the SIRS criteria.[12,14,15,16] In the Sepsis Occurrence in Acutely ill Patients study, 93% of ICU admissions had at least two SIRS criteria at some point during their ICU stay.[12] Moreover, each of the SIRS criteria can be present in many different conditions, so that a label of SIRS provides little or no information about the underlying disease process. For example, fever can be present in sepsis, but also after myocardial infarction, pulmonary embolism, or postoperatively; tachycardia and tachypnea may be present in heart failure, anemia, respiratory failure, hypovolemia, sepsis, and so forth; a raised white blood cell count can be present in many diseases encountered in ICU patients, including trauma, heart failure, pancreatitis, hemorrhage, and pulmonary edema. The use of the SIRS criteria to define septic shock was also unrealistic. Any type of shock is associated with hyperventilation (to compensate for the lactic acidosis), tachycardia (either to compensate for a decreased stroke volume or to achieve a supranormal cardiac output), and an increased white blood cell count (as part of the stress response). The body temperature is often within the normal range in septic shock. Accordingly, the SIRS criteria cannot separate septic from other types of shock. Furthermore, patients who meet the SIRS criteria have a wide range of disease severity, and hence, likely mortality.

Use of the SIRS criteria to identify patients for enrollment in clinical trials has been disappointing, and has likely contributed to the negativity of almost all these trials. Indeed, use of SIRS for entrance into clinical trials generates a very heterogeneous group of patients with multiple underlying pathologies and disease severity; while some patients in such a mixed population may well benefit from the intervention, it is likely that others will not, thus diluting out any beneficial effect.

Multiple organ dysfunction syndrome

With the realization that severe sepsis is frequently associated with the development of multiple organ dysfunction and that multiple organ failure is the most common cause of death in patients who have severe sepsis, the 1991 ACCP-SCCM Consensus Conference also introduced the term "multiple organ dysfunction syndrome" (MODS). MODS was defined as "the presence of altered organ function in an acutely ill patient such that homeostasis cannot be maintained without intervention."[7] Many systems have since been developed to characterize and quantify MODS, including the sequential organ failure assessment,[17] and are increasingly used as measures of morbidity in clinical trials.

2001 Sepsis Definitions Conference

With advances in our understanding of sepsis pathogenesis and pathophysiology and with continued dissatisfaction with available definitions of sepsis, a Consensus Sepsis Definitions Conference of 29 international experts in the field of sepsis was convened in 2001 under the auspices of SCCM, the European Society of Intensive Care Medicine, ACCP, and the Surgical Infection Societies.[18] The conference participants concluded that the definitions of sepsis, severe sepsis, and septic shock, as defined in the 1991 North American Consensus Conference,[7] may still be useful in clinical practice and for research purposes. The key change was in the use of the SIRS criteria, which were considered too sensitive and nonspecific. The participants suggested that other signs and symptoms be added to better reflect the clinical response to infection (**Box 1**). Sepsis is now defined as the presence of infection plus some of the listed signs and symptoms of sepsis. Severe sepsis is now defined as sepsis complicated by organ dysfunction and septic shock is defined as severe sepsis with acute circulatory failure characterized by persistent arterial hypotension unexplained by other causes. Importantly, the list of signs of sepsis is meant as a guide, not all patients who have sepsis will have all the signs and symptoms listed, and many patients who do not have sepsis will have several of them. In addition, the list will change as new biomarkers are identified. These signs of sepsis should be considered as alarm signals that suggest the possibility of an infection and when combined with microbiological results and other evidence of organ involvement, can help in decisions regarding the need for antibiotics (**Fig. 1**).

THE PREDISPOSITION-INFECTION-RESPONSE-ORGAN DYSFUNCTION APPROACH

The inflammatory response to sepsis can vary in course and outcome depending on individual patients characteristics (eg, age, genetic makeup, pre-existing comorbidities) and characteristics of the infecting organism, including virulence, origin, and inoculum (**Fig. 2**). As such, sepsis could be said to be an umbrella term covering a group of diseases rather than being a single disease in its own right. Indeed, the consideration of sepsis as a single entity rather than as a syndrome associated with a complex group of diseases has been given as a key explanation for the apparent failure of most clinical trials in sepsis.[19,20] This assumption has led to the inclusion into clinical trials of heterogeneous groups of patients who are unlikely to respond similarly to the single intervention being trialed.[21] In this context, sepsis has been compared with cancer. Much as sepsis is the inflammatory response to infection but is heterogeneous in its origins, targets, and prognosis, so cancer is the uncontrolled proliferation of abnormal cells that is again heterogeneous in its origins, targets, and prognosis. No oncologist would offer the same treatment to patients who have breast cancer, as to patients who have leukemia or malignant melanoma. Likewise, treatment may depend on the type of cellular proliferation. Yet in sepsis trials, potential new therapies have been expected to work in widely heterogeneous groups of patients. Unlike sepsis, oncologists rapidly took this idea on board and began defining patients not only as having cancer but according to the specific origin, type, and stage of the cancer, enabling homogeneous groups of patients to be identified and effective interventions for each of those groups to be developed and introduced. Recognition that patients who have more severe forms

Box 1
Move from 1991 systemic inflammatory response syndrome criteria to expanded list of signs and symptoms in 2001 Sepsis Definitions Conference

SIRS criteria

- Fever/hypothermia
- Tachycardia
- Tachypnea
- Altered white blood cell count

↓

Sepsis Definitions Conference

General signs and symptoms

- Fever/hypothermia
- Tachypnea/respiratory alkalosis
- Positive fluid balance/edema

General inflammatory reaction

- Altered white blood cell count
- Increased biomarker (C-reactive protein (CRP), IL-6, PCT) concentrations

Hemodynamic alterations

- Arterial hypotension
- Tachycardia
- Increased cardiac output/low systemic vascular resistance (SVR)/high SvO2
- Altered skin perfusion
- Decreased urine output
- Hyperlactatemia (increased base deficit)

Signs of organ dysfunction

- Hypoxemia
- Coagulation abnormalities
- Altered mental status
- Hyperglycemia
- Thrombocytopenia, disseminated intravascular coagulation
- Altered liver function (hyperbilirubinemia)
- Intolerance to feeding (altered gastrointestinal motility)

Abbreviation: PCT, procalcitonin.

of cancer needed different treatments and had different prognoses led to the development of the tumor, nodes, metastases (TNM) grading system to classify patients who have cancer.[22] Patients who have a tumor, therefore, receive a specific classification (eg, T2, N1, M0) for that tumor. The TNM classification is then linked to

Table 2
Components selected for use in PIRO scores in four recent studies

Moreno et al[23]	
P	Age, source of admission, comorbidities (cancer, cirrhosis, AIDS), length of stay before ICU admission, reason for admission (cardiac arrest)
I	Nosocomial, extended, respiratory, fungal
R & O	Organ dysfunction (renal, coagulation), organ failure (cardiovascular, respiratory, central nervous system, coagulation, renal)
Lisboa et al[24]	
P	Chronic obstructive pulmonary disease (COPD), heart failure, immunocompromised, cirrhosis, chronic renal failure
I	Bacteremia
R	Hypotension
O	Acute respiratory distress syndrome (ARDS)
Rello et al[25]	
P	Age, COPD, immunocompromised
I	Bacteremia, multilobar opacities on chest X ray
R	Shock, severe hypoxemia
O	Acute renal failure, ARDS
Rubulotta et al[26]	
P	Age, chronic liver disease, congestive cardiomyopathy
I	Community-acquired urinary tract infection, Gram-positive, Gram-negative, other community-acquired infection, nosocomial infection, fungal nonabdominal infection, fungal abdominal infection
R	Tachycardia, tachypnea
O	Number of organ failures

current literature as being most significant in the prognosis of patients who have CAP or because they were considered to have clinical importance. A score of 1 was given for each variable present giving a total possible score of 8. The mean PIRO score was significantly higher in nonsurvivors than in survivors and mortality rate increased with increasing PIRO score, such that patients who had a PIRO score of 7 had 100% mortality. According to the observed mortality for each PIRO score, patients were stratified into four levels of risk: Low, mild, high, and very high. By Cox regression analysis, mild (hazard ratio [HR] 1.8; 95% CI 1.1–2.9; *P*<.05), high (HR 3.1; 95% CI = 2.0–4.7; *P*<.001) and very high (HR 6.3; 95% CI = 4.2–9.4; *P*<.001) grades of risk were associated with a higher risk of death. Higher PIRO scores were also associated with increased length of ICU stay and duration of mechanical ventilation. The PIRO score again predicted mortality better than the APACHE II score (AUC 0.88 versus 0.75, *P*<.001).

Most recently, Rubulotta and colleagues[26] used two large sepsis databases to generate and validate a version of the PIRO staging model risk stratification in severe sepsis. Using a logistic regression technique, variables were included in the score to give a 0 to 4 point score for each of the PIRO components (0–1 for R) and hence a total score range of 0 to 13 (see **Table 2**). The correlations of the PIRO total score and in-hospital mortality rates were 0.974 (*P*<.0001) and 0.998 (*P*<.0001) in the two databases tested. The AUC was 0.70 compared with 0.69 for the APACHE II score. The authors suggest that although the proposed model should be seen as a "preliminary, hypothesis generating version," it could potentially be used to stratify patients for inclusion into a severe sepsis trial, as a prospectively defined subgroup analysis outcome variable for future clinical trials, and to determine prognosis and individual treatment recommendations for individual patients suffering from severe sepsis.

These studies provide some insight into how the PIRO system could potentially be used in the future to characterize patients who have sepsis. Clearly, further study is needed before this approach can be widely adopted, but even in these early examples, the scores performed better than other predictive models, such as APACHE and SAPS. These studies also demonstrate how the system will need to be adapted to fit specific groups of patients, much as the TNM system is adjusted to specific cancers.[27] Importantly, using the PIRO system for clinical trial inclusion would necessitate a shift from the large heterogeneous studies of today to much smaller studies targeting more specific and clearly defined and characterized groups of patients. Although this could be seen as a threat by the pharmaceutical industry as the potential market would be seen to be smaller and the intervention therefore potentially less lucrative, this approach has been used with success in oncology,[21] and indeed the chances of a positive result would be greater if the intervention were more appropriately targeted.

SUMMARY

Developing effective therapies for any disease process relies on the ability to clearly define the population of patients who will benefit from that intervention. Advances in our understanding of sepsis pathogenesis have made it clear that the global definition or concept of sepsis as a single, homogeneous disease process is inadequate. The idea that all patients who have severe sepsis will respond positively to any single therapeutic intervention is probably too simple, although some interventions may target more general pathways and be globally beneficial. For example, drotrecogin alfa (activated) was shown to be effective at reducing mortality in a clinical trial with a heterogeneous patient population,[28] although even here positive results were restricted to patients who had severe sepsis, highlighting the importance of being able to better characterize patients. Our approach to sepsis and its definition has evolved as we increasingly recognize the complex nature of the process and the importance of targeting treatments according to individual patients' characteristics. Clinical variables are too sensitive and nonspecific and improved biologic and biochemical tools need to be incorporated into current definitions to provide precise and accurate methods of diagnosis. Systems, such as PIRO, that can characterize patients according to their likely prognosis and response to a specific therapy need to be further developed so that treatments can be appropriately directed for individual patients.

REFERENCES

1. Poeze M, Ramsay G, Gerlach H, et al. An international sepsis survey: a study of doctors' knowledge and perception about sepsis. Crit Care 2004;8:R409–13.
2. Geroulanos S, Douka ET. Historical perspective of the word "sepsis" [letter]. Intensive Care Med 2006;32:2077.
3. Schottmueller H. Nature and Management of sepsis. Inn Med 1914;31:257–80.
4. Bone RC, Fisher CJ, Clemmer TP, et al. Sepsis syndrome: a valid clinical entity. Crit Care Med 1989;17:389–93.
5. Bone RC, Fisher CJ, Clemmer TP, et al. The methylprednisolone severe sepsis study group: a controlled clinical trial of high-dose methylprednisolone in the treatment of severe sepsis and septic shock. N Engl J Med 1987;317:653–8.

6. Panacek EA, Marshall JC, Albertson TE, et al. Efficacy and safety of the monoclonal anti-tumor necrosis factor antibody F(ab')2 fragment afelimomab in patients with severe sepsis and elevated interleukin-6 levels. Crit Care Med 2004;32:2173–82.
7. ACCP-SCCM Consensus Conference: definitions of sepsis and multiple organ failure and guidelines for the use of innovative therapies in sepsis. Crit Care Med 1992;20:864–74.
8. Trzeciak S, Zanotti-Cavazzoni S, Parrillo JE, et al. Inclusion criteria for clinical trials in sepsis: did the American College of Chest Physicians/Society of Critical Care Medicine consensus conference definitions of sepsis have an impact? Chest 2005;127:242–5.
9. Veloso T, Neves AP, Vincent JL. Are the concepts of SIRS and MODS useful in sepsis? In: Deutschman CS, Neligan PJ, editors. The evidence based practice of critical care. New York: Elsevier; 2009; in press.
10. Napolitano LM, Ferrer T, McCarter RJ Jr, et al. Systemic inflammatory response syndrome score at admission independently predicts mortality and length of stay in trauma patients. J Trauma 2000;49:647–52.
11. Malone DL, Kuhls D, Napolitano LM, et al. Back to basics: validation of the admission systemic inflammatory response syndrome score in predicting outcome in trauma. J Trauma 2001;51:458–63.
12. Sprung CL, Sakr Y, Vincent JL, et al. An evaluation of systemic inflammatory response syndrome signs in the Sepsis Occurrence in Acutely ill Patients (SOAP) study. Intensive Care Med 2006;32:421–7.
13. Vincent JL. Dear sirs, I'm sorry to say that I don't like you. Crit Care Med 1997;25: 372–4.
14. Pittet D, Rangel-Frausto S, Li N, et al. Systemic inflammatory response syndrome, sepsis, severe sepsis and septic shock: incidence, morbidities and outcomes in surgical ICU patients. Intensive Care Med 1995;21:302–9.
15. Rangel Frausto MS, Pittet D, Costigan M, et al. The natural history of the systemic inflammatory response syndrome (SIRS). A prospective study. JAMA 1995;273: 117–23.
16. Bossink AW, Groeneveld J, Hack CE, et al. Prediction of mortality in febrile medical patients: how useful are systemic inflammatory response syndrome and sepsis criteria? Chest 1998;113:1533–41.
17. Vincent JL, de Mendonca A, Cantraine F, et al. Use of the SOFA score to assess the incidence of organ dysfunction/failure in intensive care units: results of a multicenter, prospective study. Working group on "sepsis-related problems" of the European Society of Intensive Care Medicine. Crit Care Med 1998;26:1793–800.
18. Levy MM, Fink MP, Marshall JC, et al. 2001 SCCM/ESICM/ACCP/ATS/SIS International Sepsis Definitions Conference. Crit Care Med 2003;31:1250–6.
19. Marshall JC. Rethinking sepsis: from concepts to syndromes to diseases. Sepsis 1999;3:5–10.
20. Marshall JC. Sepsis research: where have we gone wrong? Crit Care Resusc 2006;8:241–3.
21. Carlet J, Cohen J, Calandra T, et al. Sepsis: time to reconsider the concept. Crit Care Med 2008;36:964–6.
22. Denoix P. Enquete permanent dans les centres anticancereaux. Bull Inst Natl Hyg 1946;1:70–5.
23. Moreno RP, Metnitz B, Adler L, et al. Sepsis mortality prediction based on predisposition, infection and response. Intensive Care Med 2008;34:496–504.

24. Lisboa T, Diaz E, Sa-Borges M, et al. The ventilator-associated pneumonia PIRO score: a tool for predicting ICU mortality and health-care resources use in ventilator-associated pneumonia. Chest 2008;134:1208–16.
25. Rello J, Rodriguez A, Lisboa T, et al. PIRO score for community-acquired pneumonia: a new prediction rule for assessment of severity in intensive care unit patients with community-acquired pneumonia. Crit Care Med 2009;37:456–62.
26. Rubulotta F, Marshall JC, Ramsay G, et al. Predisposition, insult/infection, response, and organ dysfunction: a new model for staging severe sepsis. Crit Care Med 2009;37:1329–35.
27. Sobin LH, Wittekind C. TNM classification of malignant tumours. 6th edition. Hoboken (NJ): Wiley; 2002.
28. Bernard GR, Vincent JL, Laterre PF, et al. Efficacy and safety of recombinant human activated protein C for severe sepsis. N Engl J Med 2001;344:699–709.

The Pathophysiology of Septic Shock

O. Okorie Nduka, MD[a,b,*], Joseph E. Parrillo, MD[c]

KEYWORDS

- Sepsis • Severe sepsis • Septic shock
- Myocardial depression • Vasodilation

The word "sepsis" comes from the Greek word *sepo* meaning decay or putrefaction, and its original usage described the decomposition of organic matter in a manner that resulted in decay and death.[1] In the Hippocratic model of health and disease, living tissues broke down by 1 of 2 processes. Pepsis was the process through which food was digested, leading to health. Sepsis, however, denoted tissue breakdown that resulted in disease. Hippocrates used this term to describe the process of abnormal tissue breakdown that resulted in a foul odor, pus-formation, and sometimes dead tissue.[2] This usage of the term sepsis persisted for almost 3 millennia, and subsequent work establishing a causal link between microbes and suppurative infections, or systemic symptoms from infection, did not change the use of the term as a description of a constellation of clinical findings, but rather established infection as the underlying cause.[3] The term "shock" comes from the French word *choquer* meaning "to collide with," and aptly describes the body's response to invading microbes and, to a large extent, its disruptive effect on normal physiology. Initially used in the medical literature in the 1700s, its earliest uses connoted a sudden jolt that often led to death (the initial physical injury). This definition evolved to describe widespread circulatory dysfunction following injury.[4]

Sepsis is the systemic maladaptive response of the body to the invasion of normally sterile tissue by pathogenic, or potentially pathogenic, microorganisms. Shock may be defined as a "state in which profound and widespread reduction of effective tissue perfusion leads first to reversible, and then, if prolonged, to irreversible cellular injury."[5] From a clinical standpoint, this progressive cellular dysfunction manifests as a continuum from sepsis, to severe sepsis, and finally to septic shock (**Box 1**).

[a] Division of Critical Care Medicine, Department of Internal Medicine, Cooper University Hospital, Camden, NJ, USA
[b] Altru Hospital, Grand Forks, ND 58206-6003, USA
[c] Robert Wood Johnson Medical School, Department of Medicine, University of Medicine and Dentistry of New Jersey, NJ, USA
* Corresponding author. Division of Critical Care Medicine, Department of Internal Medicine, Cooper University Hospital, Camden, NJ.
E-mail address: Okorie-Okorie@CooperHealth.edu (O.O. Nduka).

Crit Care Clin 25 (2009) 677–702
doi:10.1016/j.ccc.2009.08.002
criticalcare.theclinics.com
0749-0704/09/$ – see front matter

Box 2
Virulence characteristics of bacterial pathogens

Mechanisms of bacterial adherence to host epithelial surfaces

Adhesins: bacterial protein products (integral or secreted) that enable pathogenic organisms to bind onto host tissue elements (eg, collagen fibers)

Flagella, fimbrae, and pili: bacterial appendages whose primary role is mobility, but they enable pathogens to directly attach themselves to host cells and extracellular matrix components

Type III secretion system: functions as a molecular conduit, enabling bacteria to introduce proteins into host cells, altering their function to enhance bacterial survival

Ligand mimicry: by producing proteins similar to host-derived proteins, bacteria are able to bind to relevant ligand receptors

Mechanisms of bacterial invasion following adherence

Bacterial protein secretion systems I, II, III, IV: specialized transporter systems that enable the delivery of bacterial products into the extracellular matrix (I and II) or intracellularly (III and IV), facilitating tissue invasion and intracellular infection

Lipidrafts: avoiding the apical areas of epithelial cells exposed to commensals and resistant to pathogen invasion, pathogenic bacteria bind to the baso-lateral aspects of the host cell plasma membrane. This area is rich in cholesterol and pathogen recognition receptors. Following binding to plasma membrane cholesterol, the pathogens form intracellular vacuoles, rendering them immune to lysosomal endocytosis.

Bacterial host defense evasion mechanisms

Anti-phagocytosis: bacterial pathogens have several mechanisms to avoid phagocytosis: (1) inhibition of opsonization by encapsulation; (2) surface antigenic variation that prevents recognition as pathogens; (3) inhibition of uptake via the release of toxic protein effectors; (4) intracelluar survival and replication in the cytosol and also within lysosomes; (5) induction of immune effector cell apoptosis.

Biofilm formation: a biofilm is a polysaccharide matrix that encapsulates entire bacterial colonies. In addition to being protected from phagocytosis, these bacterial colonies are largely immune to antibiotic drug action by existing in a dormant state. Dead tissue and foreign bodies provide optimal conditions for biofilm formation.

Virulence factor-mediated host immune dysfunction

Discussed in section on immunoinflammatory dysfunction

Virulence factor-induced host tissue injury

Discussed in sections on immunoinflammatory dysfunction and host organ/cellular injury/ dysfunction in septic shock

Quorum-sensing, Cell-to-cell Signaling and Coordinated Gene Expression

Following pathogen adherence to an epithelial surface, specific mucosal defense mechanisms are triggered by the host to suppress pathogen proliferation and prevent invasion of the epithelial barrier. These include secretion of a mucus layer, epithelial cell shedding, and secretion of enzymes such as lysozyme. To establish infection, bacteria must be able not only to evade these additional host defense mechanisms but also to produce virulence factors to facilitate invasion. Expression of virulence factors by a single bacterium is highly unlikely to lead to established infection, much less tissue damage. Therefore the bacterial innoculum or population density to some extent affects the development and severity of infection. The critical bacterial density needed to initiate an infectious process is referred to as a quorum. Bacteria have developed systems of cell-to cell communication that enable them to assess

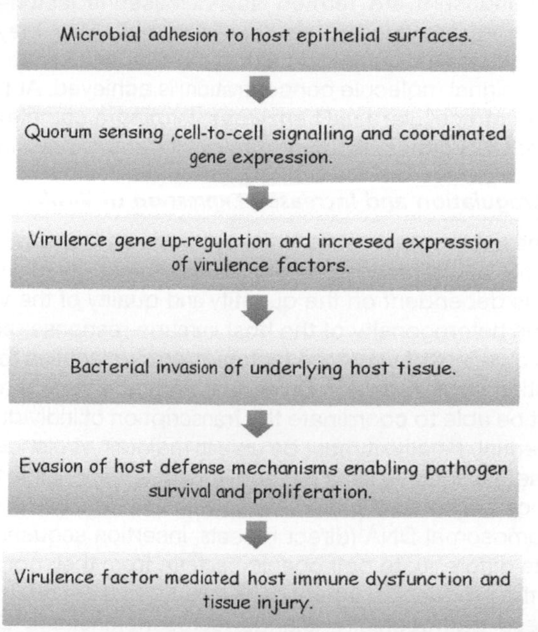

Fig. 2. Sequence of events leading to established infection in human hosts.

their population density and react to their environment as a population, increasing their chances of overwhelming host defense mechanisms and establishing infection.

These bacterial cell-to-cell signaling systems are called quorum-sensing systems (QSSs), and result in coordinated gene activation and expression of high concentrations of extracellular virulence factors by the entire bacterial population. QSSs are described in Gram-positive and Gram-negative bacteria involved in human sepsis, and involve the secretion of signaling molecules called autoinducers, with the autoinducer concentration tightly linked to the regulation of key aspects of genetic expression.[7,8]

Quorum sensing allows both intra- and interspecies bacterial cell-to-cell communication. Animal experiments have demonstrated loss of microbial virulence with deletion of bacterial quorum-sensing genes and restoration of virulence following plasmid insertion. The ability to have virulence gene expression regulated by a global control system (ie, the QSS) prevents virulence factor expression or excessive proliferation when population densities are low, preventing premature pathogen detection. Thus QSSs play a major role in the regulation of biofilm synthesis.[9] Once the critical population density is attained, virulence genes are expressed along with cellular proliferation signals, with swift tissue invasion and establishment of infection.

Recent experiments have shown that QSSs are capable of facilitating host-pathogen communication leading to pathogen-mediated modulation of host immune responses. Some QSSs can recognize and bind to human interferon-γ leading to subsequent expression of QSS genes.[10] This suggests that the critical threshold for QSS gene expression may be somewhat host-dependent, with earlier activation if the host is sensed as being more susceptible.[11]

There are 2 main bacterial QSSs. Gram-positive bacteria synthesize cytosolic autoinducers that are actively transported to the extracellular environment, where they bind to specific receptor proteins on neighboring bacteria, initiating a signaling cascade resulting in QSS control of relevant aspects of cellular function.[12]

Gram-negative autoinducers are termed acyl-homoserine lactones (AHL) and are produced by a different enzyme system (LuxI enzyme). After they are synthesized they diffuse passively between intra- and extracellular environments until critical population density (high signal molecule concentration) is achieved. At this point, the AHL proteins bind to the intracellular LuxR enzymes, forming a complex that acts on the promoter regions of QSS genes, leading to relevant gene expression.

Virulence Gene Upregulation and Increased Expression of Virulence Factors

QSS-regulated gene expression results in the synthesis and release of a variety of virulence factors. Despite coordinated gene expression, the ability of a given pathogen to invade host tissue is dependent on the quantity and quality of the virulence factors it produces. Given the heterogeneity of the host immune response, pathogens need to be able to express a variety of virulence factors in large quantities following QSS activation of transcriptional regulators.[13] Given that virulence factors act synergistically, the pathogen must be able to coordinate the transcription of individual genes to maximize virulence potential. Finally, it must be able to maintain virulence despite changes in the host response. To achieve all of the above, genes responsible for the expression of microbial virulence are housed in discrete genetic units in close proximity to specific sequences of chromosomal DNA (direct repeats, insertion sequences, tRNA genes). These genetic units differentiate pathogenic bacteria from their nonpathogenic counterparts. They are the products of lateral gene transfer and are referred to as pathogenicity islands. These pathogenicity islands represent unstable DNA regions, and changes in their genetic sequences can result in huge clinical consequences. Recently, a genetic alteration involving the pathogenic locus of *Clostridium difficile* resulted in severe cases of *Clostridium difficile*-associated colitis in North America by increasing the strain's toxigenic potential. In addition, these islands may possess gene capture systems (integrons), facilitating the incorporation and dissemination by lateral transfer of antibiotic-resistance genes. A clinically relevant example is the development of a clone of community-acquired methicillin-resistant *Staphylococcus aureus* (MRSA) with genetic alterations leading to increased toxigenic potential and an epidemic of necrotizing soft tissue infections.

With the aid of virulence factors, pathogens penetrate extraepithelial and epithelial barriers and invade host tissue, establishing infection. Further innate immune system activation occurs with recruitment of immune effector cells to the site of infection, with significant host-pathogen interaction. This recruitment represents the initial significant interaction between the host immune cells and the invading pathogen.

IMMUNOINFLAMMATORY DYSFUNCTION IN SEPTIC SHOCK

Although the dysfunctional events that lead to septic shock involve multiple biologic systems, immune response remains central to the development of septic shock.

Normal Immune Response

The immune system includes a structural component consisting of mucosal barriers to host tissue invasion, a nonspecific early response system (the innate immune response) and a more pathogen-specific response system (the adaptive immune response) activated later following the presence of pathogenic stimuli. Normal immune function requires the coordinated action of these components, resulting in early recognition of a potential pathogen and its subsequent elimination with minimal host tissue damage or disruption to physiologic processes. The structural barriers consist of mucocutaneous membranes (including appendages) and the endogenous colonizing flora on these surfaces. Optimal function requires proper appendage function and stability of the endogenous flora population.

The innate immune system must be able to recognize invading pathogens early following tissue invasion and mount a response of sufficient intensity to contain the threat. It must also be able to regulate this intense nonspecific response to protect host tissue from injury and facilitate repair.

The adaptive response is charged with "fine-tuning" the later aspects of the immune response. This fine-tuning ensures that, for any given stimulus, the immune response is focused and measured. To understand the degree of host dysfunction and, thus, the pathophysiology of septic shock, one must appreciate certain features of a normal host immune response to microbial infection.

Temporal variation

The normal immune response may be characterized as an initially nonspecific, highly proinflammatory phase, with a subsequent complementary anti-inflammatory response necessary for the restoration of immune homeostasis and prevention of collateral immune-medicated host tissue injury.

Biologic redundancy

In experimental situations, a single pathogenic stimulus triggers the transcription of proinflammatory genetic material, producing a few proinflammatory mediators. In a 1:1 transmission system, the inactivity of any 1 of these pathways can seriously affect the ability of the host to respond adequately to microbial pathogens. To mount effective immune responses a single stimulus to the mammalian innate immune system results in the transcription of hundreds of proinflammatory genes. In addition, different immune effector pathways exhibit pathogenic cross-reactivity with markedly different types of injury stimulating the same pathways. Furthermore, it is likely that, in the clinical setting, there may be multiple injurious stimuli of different durations. The expression of innate immunity becomes biologically redundant and not prone to dysfunction by the inhibition of a few mediators, which protects the system as a whole from being paralyzed by otherwise trivial subunit dysfunction.

Interaction with other biologic systems (cross talk)

The host response to infection extends beyond the immune system to include other biologic systems (coagulation system, autonomic nervous system [ANS]) that interact with the immune system to reduce the potential for host tissue injury, despite a robust immune response, by maintaining organ perfusion (coagulation system) or by appropriately down-regulating the immune response (ANS).

Heterogeneity (genetic and nongenetic)

The immune response to a given pathogen in a given individual is determined by many factors including, but not limited to, the virulence of the pathogen, the individual's genetic composition, and pre-existing comorbidities. Staphylococcal infection of native cardiac valves should elicit a different host immune response from that in response to the common cold, although they both might be febrile illnesses with a cough. After an invading pathogen triggers an immune response, its severity depends on the degree to which the innate immune system is expressed, which in turn depends on genetic and acquired factors. The physiologic response to ongoing infection in the setting of pre-existing comorbidities differs from the response in the otherwise healthy host. Evidence for genetic differences in the immune response is supported by the observation that, with regard to dying from infection, a strong association exists between adoptees and their natural, but not adoptive, parents.[5] Genetic polymorphisms in septic shock are discussed elsewhere in the issue of the critical care clinics.

Septic shock is often characterized by dysfunction involving all aspects of the immune response. From a structural standpoint, the disruption may be modifiable and transient (intestinal bacterial overgrowth) versus nonmodifiable factors (mucocilliary dysfunction in cystic fibrosis). Immunodysfunction in sepsis may present as an uncontrolled (too intense or too long) early response with subsequent host tissue injury, or as an inadequate response later in the course of the disease. This dysfunction involves cellular and humoral components of the innate and adaptive immune response systems.

Pathogen Recognition

Pattern recognition receptors, pathogen-associated molecular patterns, and danger-associated molecular patterns

The initial event in the innate immune response is the recognition of an invading pathogenic threat. Bacteria and viruses (prokaryotic life forms) have molecular structures that are (largely) not shared with their host, are common to related pathogens, and are invariant. These molecular signatures are also expressed by nonpathogenic and commensal bacteria and, depending on the context, may be referred to as pathogen-associated molecular patterns (PAMPs), or microbial-associated molecular patterns (MAMPs).[14] From a functional standpoint, the endogenous equivalents of these PAMPs are intracellular proteins expressed or released following host tissue injury. These proteins are known as alarmins and, together with PAMPs, are referred to as damage-associated molecular patterns (DAMPs).[15]

Immune cells express a set of receptors known as pattern recognition receptors (PRRs) that can recognize and bind to DAMPs expressed by invading pathogens and injured host tissue. At least 4 families of PRRs are recognized: toll-like receptors (TLRs); nucleotide oligomerization domain leucine-rich repeat (NOD-LRR) proteins; cytoplasmic caspase activation and recruiting domain helicases such as retinoic-acid-inducible gene I (RIG-I)-like helicases (RLHs); and C-type lectin receptors expressed on dendritic and myeloid cells.[16,17] These receptors initiate the innate immune response and regulate the adaptive immune response to infection or tissue injury.

In humans, the TLRs are a family of 10 cell receptors expressed on immune effector cell surfaces and constitute the prototype PRRs; their structure and function illustrate many of the steps involved in initial host-pathogen interaction in sepsis. The TLRs are transmembrane proteins with leucine-rich repeat extracellular domains and an intracellular (cytoplasmic) domain composed of the toll interleukin-1 receptor resistance domain (TIR domain). PAMPs and DAMPs bind to PRRs, such as TLRs, expressed on the surface of host cells. In addition, intracellular PRRs exist and interact with intracellular pathogens, viral particles, and proteins released from damaged tissue (**Fig. 3**, **Table 1**).

In sepsis, there is a full-blown activation of immune responses due to the release of high levels of DAMPs from invading microorganisms or damaged host tissue, which leads to upregulation of TLR expression. This response has been noted in experimental models and in septic patients.[18,19] TLR interaction with DAMPs from host tissue injury primes the innate immune system for enhanced TLR reactivity, resulting in excess lipopolysaccharide (LPS)-induced mortality.[20] Positive feedback loops between DAMPs/PAMPs and their respective receptors may lead to excessive immunoactivation, characterized by a markedly imbalanced cytokine response with resultant tissue injury. In contrast, polymorphisms in the TLRs have been linked to increased risks of infection. This association applies equally to polymorphisms in the downstream signaling cascades. Single nucleotide polymorphisms (SNPs)

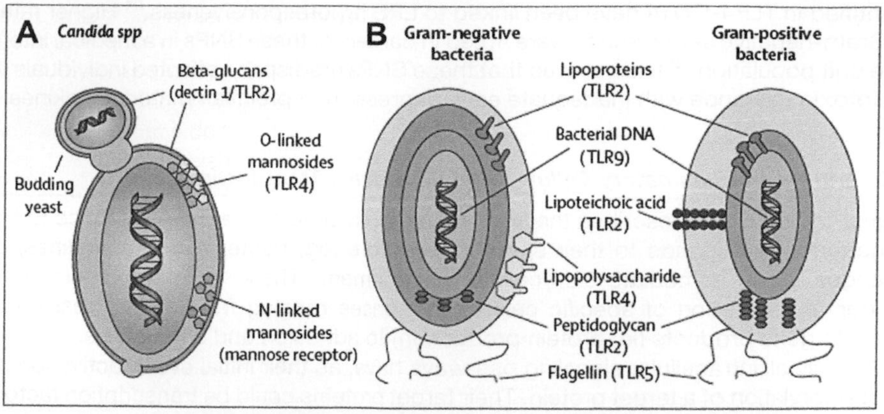

Fig. 3. Innate recognition of pathogens by toll-like (and related) receptors (TLRs). (*A*) The complexity of the interaction between innate immune receptors and fungi. Three distinct components of the cell wall of *Candida albicans* are recognized by 4 different host receptors: N-linked mannosyl residues are detected by the mannose receptor, O-linked mannosyl residues are sensed by TLR4, and B-glucans are recognized by the dectin 1-TLR2 complex. (*B*) Gram-positive and Gram-negative bacteria are recognized by partly overlapping and partly distinct repertoire of TLRs. Gram-positive pathogens exclusively express lipoteichoic acid, Gram-negative pathogens exclusively express LPS; common PAMPs include peptidoglycan, lipoproteins, flagellin, and bacterial DNA. (*Data from* van der Poll T, Opal SM. Host-pathogen interactions in sepsis. Lancet Infect Dis 2008;8:35; with permission.)

Table 1
Role of toll-like and other PRRs in the pathophysiology of sepsis

Pattern Recognition Receptor	Pathogen or Disease State	Relevant PAMPs/DAMPs
TLR 1	Lymedisease Neisseria meningitides	Triacyl lipopeptides
TLR 2	Gram-positive bacteria Mostbacteria Neisseria meningitides *Candida albicans* Hostproteins (DAMPs)	Lipoteiechoic acid Peptidoglycan, triacyl lipopeptides Porins Phospholipomannan, B-glucans HMGB1
TLR-4	Gram-negative bacteria Candida albicans Hostproteins (DAMPs)	Lipopolysaccharide (LPS) D-Mannan, O-linked mannosyl residues Heatshock proteins, fibrinogen, HMGB1
TLR5	Salmonella (flagellated bacteria)	Flagellin
NOD proteins (NOD1 and NOD2)	Gram-negative bacteria	Bacterial peptidoglycan fragmentsdiamino-pimelate (NOD1) and muramyl dipeptide (NOD2)
Cytoplasmic caspase activation and recruiting domain helicases	Viruses	Viral nucleic acids

Data from Dellinger RP, Levy MM, Carlet JM, et al. Surviving Sepsis Campaign: international guidelines for management of severe sepsis and septic shock: 2008. Crit Care Med 2008;36:296–327.

identified in TLR4-CD14 have been linked to LPS hyporesponsiveness.[21] Higher rates of Gram-negative septic shock were noted in carriers of these SNPs in a medical intensive unit population.[22] It is believed that these SNPs predispose affected individuals to endotoxin tolerance with inadequate early expression of proinflammatory cytokines.

Pro- and Anti-inflammatory Cellular Signaling/signal Transduction

Signal transduction describes the sequence of intracellular events in response to the engagement of ligands to their specific receptors (eg, bacterial LPS, cytokines) or changes in the immediate extracellular environment. These molecular interactions trigger the induction of specific cellular responses ranging from the expression of specific gene products (ie, protein production) to adhesion and chemotaxis.

Virtually all intracellular signaling pathways have, as their initial event, activation by phosphorylation of a target protein. Their target proteins could be transcription factors or regulatory (cytoplasmic or nuclear) proteins. This activation is typically accomplished by the binding of an enzyme (a kinase) to the target protein, and can lead to: (1) activation or alteration of its enzymatic activity; (2) changes in the stability of the target protein; (3) subcellular localization of the protein; and (4) interactions with other proteins. Many signaling pathways involve a cascade of 2 or more kinases in series (signaling cascades), involving an upstream kinase involved in enzyme activation and a downstream kinase whose substrate(s) are the protein products of upstream kinase-substrate interaction. Kinase cascades are activated following engagement of ligand-specific receptors (eg, Gram-negative LPS + TLR-4). In addition, certain disruptions of cellular homeostasis (eg, changes in state of oxidation) can lead to activation of kinase cascades.

Kinases are able to phosphorylate other kinases, leading to signal amplification. Thus, a given stimulus may activate multiple kinase cascades, and several kinase cascades may be activated by different stimuli, leading to some measure of redundancy in a cellular signaling pathway. The natural consequence of amplification and redundancy in cellular signaling is a significant degree of overlap and lack of specificity in downstream effects and a requirement for intracellular regulation for effective, host-protective, stimulus-appropriate signal transduction. This negative regulation with resultant transcriptional downregulation is accomplished by dephosphorylation of relevant enzymes leading to a return to baseline levels of activity. Interactions occur between kinase cascades in such a way that increased activity of a given cascade produces suppression of activity in "opposite" cascades. This effect is termed cross talk. In addition, efficient kinase-kinase interaction is facilitated by co-localization of kinases on anchoring or adaptor proteins at relevant intracellular sites. An understanding of the above aspects of cellular signaling is essential to understanding the initial events that occur following host-pathogen interaction in sepsis.

Following the attachment of DAMPs/PAMPs to their specific ligands (TLRS) in severe sepsis, and the subsequent activation of signaling cascades (**Fig. 4**), there is modification of the activity of key intracellular proteins, primarily transcription factors and nuclear and cytoplasmic regulating proteins. For the TLRs, signaling depends primarily on 4 adaptor proteins: the myeloid differentiation primary-response protein 88 (MyD88); and 3 non-MyD88 proteins: (1) toll/interleukin 1 (IL-1) receptor homology (TIR) domain-containing adaptor protein (TIRAP); (2) TIR domain-containing adaptor protein–inducing interferon-β (TRIF); and (3) TRIF-related adaptor molecule (TRAM). These MyD88-dependent and MyD88-independent signal-transduction pathways result in the activation of the prototypical transcription factor, nuclear factor-κB (NFκB). In addition, important enzyme systems regulating several key cellular

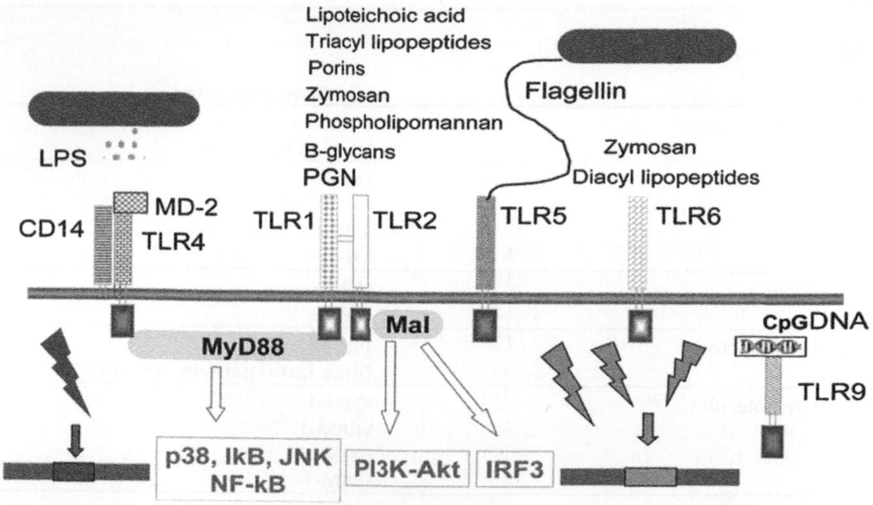

Fig. 4. Binding of toll-like receptors (TLRs) activates intracellular signal-transduction pathways that lead to the activation of transcriptional activators such as interferon regulator factorsp13K/Akt, activator protein-1, and cytosolic nuclear factor-kappa[β] (NF-[κ][β]). Activated NF-[κ][β] moves from the cytoplasm to the nucleus, binds to transcription sites and induces activation of an array of genes for acute phase proteinsiNOS, coagulation factors, proinflammatory cytokinesand enzymatic activation of cellular proteases. TLR9 DNA, TLR 3 dsRNA, and TLR7/8 ssRNA are endosomal. TLR10 ligand is not defined and TLR1 forms heterodimers with TLR2. LPS, lipopolysaccharide; IRF, interferon regulatory factor; JNK; c-Jun N- terminal kinase. (*Adapted from* Cinel I, Opal SM. Molecular biology of inflammation and sepsis: a primer. Crit Care Med 2009;37(1):291–304; with permission.)

functions and aspects of cellular signaling (the caspases, phosphoinositide 3-kinase [PI3K] and Rho GTPases) are activated.

NFκB

NFκB is the prototypical transcription factor involved in modulating the expression of many of the inflammatory responses associated with severe sepsis and septic shock. It exists as homo- or heterogenous dimers composed of members of the Rel family of proteins (P50, P105, P52, P100, P65 [Rel A], C-Rel). The Rel family of proteins plays pivotal roles in inflammation, and various combinations of NFκB differ in their degree of transcriptional activity (NFκB1-P50 + P105, NFKB2-P52 + P100, Rel A [P65]).

In the absence of cellular activation, NFκB exists in the cytoplasm maintained in a latent form by interacting with inhibitors of the IkB family (IkB-α, IkB-β, IkB-γ, IkB-ε, Bcl-3, p100, p105). MyD88-dependent and MyD88-independent kinase pathways activate NFκB following TLR ligation by diverse stimuli, including bacterial products (LPS, peptidoglycans), cytokines (tumor necrosis factor-α [TNF-α], IL-8, IL-1β), reactive oxygen species, and changes in the cellular environment, such as ischemia. Regardless of the nature of the stimuli, activation occurs by phosphorylation of IkB molecules followed by their degradation by the 26S proteosome. This step results in nuclear translocation of NFκB, its binding to specific gene promoter regions, and gene transcription. NFκB is involved in the induction of several predominantly proinflammatory gene products (**Table 2**).

The degree of NFκB activation in septic patients seems to correlate with patient survival and outcome in septic shock.[23–25] In addition to the pathophysiologic

Table 2
NFkB-inducible genes involved in sepsis

Class	NFkB-Dependent Genes
Acute phase proteins	C-reactive protein LPS-binding protein
Cytokines	TNF-α G-CSF, GM-CSF IL-1a, IL-1B, IL-2, IL-6, IL-12 IFN-β
Chemokines	MIP-1α MIP-2
Coagulation factors	Tissue factor Tissue factor pathway inhibitor
Adhesion molecules	ICAM-1 VCAM-1 E-selectin ELAM-1
Enzymes	Inducible nitric oxide synthase Cyclo-oxygenase-2 C3 complement Phospholipase A2 Matrix metalloproteinases
Immunoreceptors	IL-2 receptor-a Major histocompatibility complex class 1

consequences of excessive NFκB activation, inadequate stimulation can also lead to increased morbidity in septic shock. Studies support the observation that defective NFκB signaling leads to immunosuppression in sepsis, favoring apoptosis in immune effector cells with undesirable consequences.[26,27] Thus, excessive activation, especially early in the disease course, or excessive negative regulation in sepsis may produce either excess inflammation with collateral host tissue damage or immunoparalysis and consequent direct tissue damage.

The caspases

Caspases are a family of cysteine proteases synthesized as proenzymes and activated by proteolysis. They are further subdivided into initiator caspases, activated by autocleavage, and executioner caspases, activated by cleavage induced by their initiator counterparts. The caspases play important roles in the cellular processes of inflammation and apoptosis following PAMP/DAMP-PRRs interaction. Following cleavage, caspases produce many of the phenotypic changes seen in apoptosis, including cytoskeletal disintegration, DNA fragmentation, and disruption of cellular DNA repair molecular machinery. Although the TLRs are the most studied PRPs, the cytoplasmic NOD-like receptors (NLRs) are the most ubiquitous. Three members of the NLR family (NALP3, ICE protease-activating factor [IPAF], and apoptosis-associated speck-like protein [ASC]) are involved in caspase activation. It is believed that, following pathogen recognition by TLRs, a signal is communicated intracellularly that is recognized by the nucleotide-binding domains of the NLRs. This recognition results in the activation of a multiprotein complex termed an inflammasome. The inflammasomes are multienzyme complexes (>70 KDa) that serve as molecular platforms for the activation of caspases 1 and 5, resulting in caspase-mediated activation and secretion of the proinflammatory cytokines IL-1β and IL-18. The signals and mechanisms leading to inflammasome assembly/activation are in general still poorly understood. The inflammasome complexes assembled in sepsis are well characterized and consist of 2 different multiprotein complexes, the NALP1 and NALP3 inflammasomes (**Fig. 5**). IL-1β is a highly potent proinflammatory cytokine, requiring inflammasome complex assembly as a prerequisite for caspase-1 activation before its precursor, pro-IL-1β (p35), released following TLR ligation, can be converted to its active form, which represents a mechanism to prevent uncontrolled expression of IL-1β. In addition to the release of proinflammatory cytokines, the caspases target the enzyme, caspase-activated DNase (CAD). CAD activation induces DNA fragmentation leading to apoptosis. Cytoskeletal caspase targets include spectrin, nuclear lamin, and the enzyme gelosin, which cleaves actin.[28,29] All these play roles in cytoskeletal disintegration. Inflammation-mediated caspase activation contributes to the host response in septic shock. Experiments in murine sepsis models show that the deletion of caspase-1 genes prevents the development of sepsis in affected mice.[30]

Phosphoinositide 3-kinases

Phosphatidylinositol 3-kinases (PI3Ks) are a group of enzymes that, when activated, catalyze the production of membrane phosphatidylinositol triphosphate (PIP3). PI3K

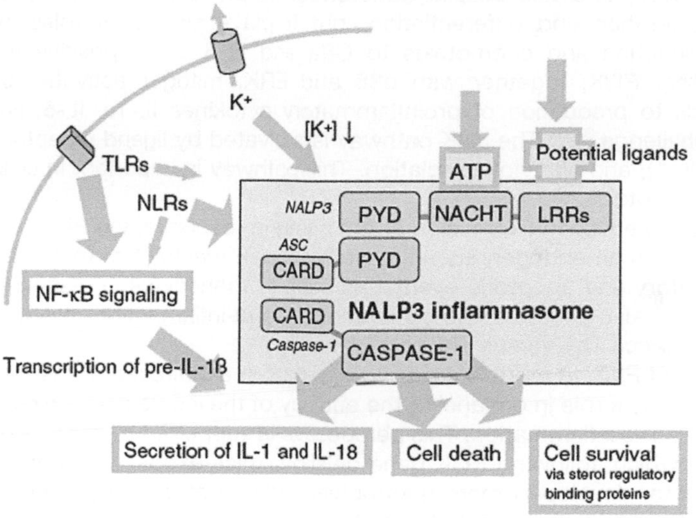

Fig. 5. The NALP3 inflammasome complex. The NLAP3 inflammasome is composed of NALP3, ASC, and caspase-1 (a second adaptor protein CADD is present in NALP 3 but lacking in NALP). ASC interacts with 1 of the NALP proteins through Cognate pyrin domain (PYD) interactions and with procaspase-1 through homotypic caspase recruitment domain (CARD) interactions. The human inflammasome complex brings 2 molecules of procaspase-1 (the second via CARDINAL) into close proximity, leading to autocatalysis and the subsequent release of the active catalytic p20 and p10 domains of caspase-1. NALP3 binds ATP via the NACHT (nucleoside triphosphatase [NTPase] domain), is a precursor of IL-1B into its biologically active fragment, and a potent mediator of fever and inflammation. There is no CARDINAL homolog in the mouse and, hence, murine NALP3 is believed to recruit only a single caspase-1 molecule. (TLRs, toll-like receptors; ATP, adenosine triphosphate; NLRs, nucleotide-binding oligomerization domain (NOD)-like receptors; ASC, apoptosis-associated specklike protein containing a CARD; NALP, NACHT-, LRR-, and PYD-containing protein; LRRs, leucine-rich repeats). (*From* Trendelenburg G. Acute neurodegeneration and the inflammasome: central processor for danger signals and the inflammatory response? J Cereb Blood Flow Metab 2008;28:867–81; with permission).

is activated by a variety of growth factor, hormonal, and chemokine receptors and, together with its downstream counterpart, the serine/threonine kinase Akt (protein kinase B), regulates key aspects of cell proliferation and survival. The downstream targets of PI3K/Akt signaling include direct regulators of neutrophil functioning, including chemotaxis, adhesion, and apoptosis.[26] Three isoforms of PI3Ks exist (PI3K-a, PI3K-b, and PI3K-y) with PI3K-y found exclusively in leukocytes. PI3K can function either as a positive or negative regulator of TLR signaling and, depending on the cell type or specific TLR involved, activate either the NFKB or mitogen-activated protein kinase (MAPK) signaling pathways.[31] The NFKB signaling pathway has already been reviewed. The MAPK signaling pathway consists of 3 distinct pathways described in leukocytes: p38, extracellular signal-regulated kinase (ERK), and c-jun NH_2-terminal kinase (JNK). These are serine/threonine enzymes that act as the final kinase in a 3-kinase cascade.

The p38 pathway is activated by a broad range of PAMPs (LPS, peptidoglycan) and inflammatory cytokines (tumor necrosis factor [TNF], IL-1, platelet-activating factor), and plays a role in neutrophil cytokine production, adhesion, chemotaxis, respiratory burst, and apoptosis.[32,33] The ERK pathway is activated by several mitogens (platelet-derived growth factor, insulin, epidermal growth factor, angiotensin II), and in monocyte LPS and cellular adherence. Its primary role is as a regulator of cellular proliferation and differentiation, but it plays significant roles in cytokine (TNF-a) production and chemotaxis to C6a and IL-8. As a positive mediator of TLR signaling, PI3K, together with p38 and ERK, mitogen-activated phosphokinases, leads to production of proinflammatory cytokines IL-1a, IL-6, and IL-8 on microbial challenge.[34,35] The JNK pathway is activated by ligand receptor GTPases, cytokines (IL-1), and ultraviolet radiation. This pathway is important in cellular proliferation and apotosis.

In addition to enabling expression of the immune response, the PI3K/Akt signaling pathway acts as an endogenous negative feedback mechanism that serves to limit proinflammatory and apoptotic events, as seen in monocytes in response to endotoxin.[36] It can also promote the generation of anti-inflammatory cytokine IL-10,[37] and helps balance Th1 versus Th2 responses.[38]

The ability of PI3K to modulate events in sepsis in a bidirectional fashion suggests that it could play a role in enhancing the efficacy of the innate immune response and limiting excessive inflammation. This perspective is supported by recent experimental evidence in which, following PI3K gene deletion, mice exposed to a pneumococcal virulence factor developed more neutrophil-mediated alveolar injury despite inadequate alveolar macrophage recruitment.[39]

Rho GTPases

Cell surface ligand receptors consist of an extracellular ligand-binding domain connected by a single transmembrane region to an intracellular domain that possesses either intrinsic enzyme activity or enzyme activation capabilities. The G-protein–linked family of receptors are the most ubiquitous and are referred to as GTPases (GTP hydrolysis is required for receptor activation and signal transduction). The Rho and Rac subfamilies of GTPases play a central role in the regulation of cell motility by controlling actin cytoskeleton rearrangement following the binding of specific proteases to the cell surface. Following DAMP-PRP interaction, Rho- and Rac-GTPases help regulate the mechanical aspects of the cellular response by the innate immune system. These include cellular migration, pathogen uptake, phagocytosis, and maintenance of endothelial integrity.[40,41] Rac1 activation is required for PI3K activation on TLR stimulation.[42]

Release of Pro- and Anti-Inflammatory Mediators

One of the immediate consequences of cellular signaling in severe sepsis and septic shock is the synthesis and release of increased amounts of mediators into the systemic circulation in an attempt to activate more immune effector cells and recruit them to the site of infection. These highly potent molecules are normally present in the circulation in low concentrations, but in high concentrations, or with prolonged exposure, they can exert potentially harmful biologic effects. Over-expression of inflammatory mediators early in the course of sepsis plays a significant role in the eventual development of septic shock. This sequential release of mediators has been termed the cytokine cascade. The availability of precise molecular tools, and the ability to measure cytokine levels, has shed light on the patterns of cytokine release in sepsis, with the earliest cytokines, highly proinflammatory TNF-a and IL-1β, being responsible for the earliest clinical events in sepsis. The subsequent, and sometimes concomitant, release of counterinflammatory mediators has also been observed. In addition, a clearer understanding of the source, structure, and actions of specific cytokines in the development of septic shock has emerged (**Table 3**), and novel mediators have been discovered. Selected novel cytokine mediators and new ideas regarding the role of otherwise well-known mediators are reviewed below.

High-mobility group box 1 protein

High-mobility group box 1 protein (HMGB1) is a nuclear and cytoplasmic protein originally discovered 3 decades ago as a nuclear binding protein, and was so named because of its rapid mobility on electrophoresis gels. HMGB1 is amongst the most ubiquitous, abundant proteins in eukaryotes, and plays a major role in facilitating gene transcription by stabilizing nucleosome formation. More recent findings suggest that HMGB1 is active in DNA recombination, repair, replication, and gene transcription, facilitated by internal repeats of positively charged domains of the N terminus (HMG boxes). HMGB1 is released passively by necrotic (but not apoptotic) cells, and from macrophages, dendritic cells, and natural killer cells, on activation by microbial pathogens.

The known biologic effects of HMGB1 are based on data obtained from cell cultures. HMGB1 stimulates the release of proinflammatory cytokines, including TNF and IL-8, in macrophages/monocytes and endothelial cells. HMGB1 can also bind to and induce the expression of the cellular receptor for advanced glycation end products (RAGE) and adhesion molecules (vascular cell adhesion molecule-1 [VCAM-1], intercellular adhesion molecule-1 [ICAM-1]) in human endothelial cells. The induced expression of RAGE facilitates activation of the transcription factor NFKB and MAPKs. These observations suggest a role for HMGB1 as a proinflammatory cytokine, with significant adverse effects on gut barrier function, and as a regulator of the coagulation system.

At present, HMGB1 does not seem to contribute significantly to the development of septic shock.

Macrophage migration inhibitory factor

Originally described as a T cell product, macrophage migration inhibitory factor (MMIF) is a cytokine produced by various cell types including other immune effector and neuroendocrine cells. MMIF is capable of activating T cells and inducing proinflammatory cytokine production in macrophages. Serum MMIF concentrations are increased in septic patients and, in severe sepsis, elevated MMIF concentrations seem to be an early indicator of poor outcome of septic patients in intensive care.

Table 3
Cytokine and noncytokine mediators of septic shock

Class	Mediator	Source	Role in Septic Shock
Proinflammatory Cytokines	Interleukin-1β	Monocytes Macrophages Lymphocytes Endothelial cells	Fever, hypotension, T cell and macrophage activation, myocardial suppression
	Tumor necrosis factor-α	Activated macrophages	Fever, hypotension, myocardial depression (myocytes in culture), neutrophil and endothelial cell activation
	Interleukin-6	T cells B cells Endothelial cells	Induction of lymphocyte (B and T cell) proliferation
	Interleukin-8	Activated macrophages and monocytes Kupffer cells	Chemotactic for neutrophils and T cells
	Interleukin-17	Activated T cells	Induces the synthesis of other cytokines IL-6, G-CSF, GM-CSF, IL-1β, TGF-β, TNF-α and chemokines
	Interleukin-18	Activated macrophages	Alongwith IL-12, initiates the cell-mediated immune response. Increased secretion of interferon-γ
	Interferon-γ	Natural killer cells	Defense against viral and intracellular bacterial pathogens
	Macrophage inhibitory factor/macrophage migration inhibitory factor (MIF)	Activated macrophages	Increased TNF expression Increased TLR4 expression

Anti-inflammatory cytokines	Interleukin-10	Epithelial cells Monocytes Lymphocytes	Downregulation of macrophage function leading to decreased TNF-a
	IL-4	?	Induces differentiation of naive helper T cells to Th2 cells
	IL-1Ra	Monocytes	Block IL-1 activity
	TGF-B	Various host cells	Interferes with phagocytic activation
Endothelial Factors	Nitric oxide		Increased microvascular permeability Lossof vasomotor tone Myocardial depression Peripheral venous pooling
Hormones	Vasopressin Glucocorticoids	Posterior pituitary gland Hypothamic-pituitary axis	Relative deficiency may cause or worsen circulatory failure
Arachidonic acid metabolites	Prostaglandins Leukotrienes Thromboxanes	Immune effector cells Pancreas	Airway reactivity Vasoconstriction Platelet aggregation Increased vascular permeability
Others	Platelet-activating factor	Endothelial cells Macrophages Neutrophils	Histamine release from platelets Activation of endothelial cells
	Complement proteins C3a-C5a		Histamine release, Increased capillary permeability, vasodilation
	Myocardial depressant factors	Pancreas	Negative inotropy Impaired phagocytosis

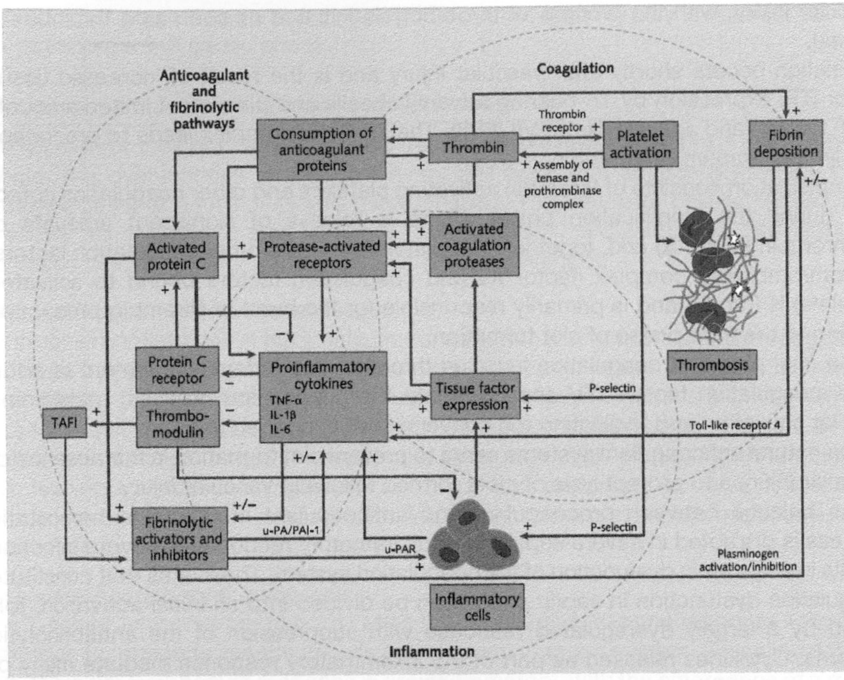

Fig. 6. Schematic overview of the major pathways involved in the interrelation between coagulation, anticoagulant pathways, and fibrinolysis and inflammation. +, stimulatory effect; –, inhibitory effect; IL, interleukin; PAI-1, plasminogen activator inhibitor-1; TAFI, thrombin activatable fibrinolysis inhibitor; TNF, tumor necrosis factor; u-PA, urinary plasminogen activator; u-PAR, urokirlase-type plasminogen activator receptor. (*From* Levi M, van der Poll T. The central role of the endothelium in the crosstalk between coagulation and inflammation in sepsis. Adv Sepsis 2004;3:93; with permission).

observations supporting the existence of central autonomic interaction with the immunoinflammatory response involved a serendipitous finding that, with central administration of a TNF inhibitor, efferent vagal activity was stimulated with systemic anti-inflammatory action.[48]

Subsequent work in animal sepsis models demonstrated significant inhibition of TNF expression following vagal stimulation and improved disease end points in these models.[49,50] In addition, rendering these animals immune to vagal stimulation either by genetic manipulation or vagotomy led to an exaggerated proinflammatory cytokine response.[51] It is now understood that these cytokine-suppressive effects of vagal stimulation are mediated by the release of its neurotransmitter acetylcholine (ACh) and its subsequent interaction with ACh receptors expressed by macrophages and other immune effector cells.[52,53] The best characterized of these cholinergic receptors that suppress cytokines is the α7 subunit of the nicotinic acetylcholine receptor (α7 nAChR).

This autonomic parasympathetic-mediated immune modulation system has been termed the inflammatory reflex (**Fig. 7**), with an immunosensing afferent arm (cytokine stimulation of vagal afferents) and an efferent immunosuppressing arm (the cholinergic anti-inflammatory pathway).[54] Recent studies suggest that the spleen plays a significant role as an effector organ for this pathway.

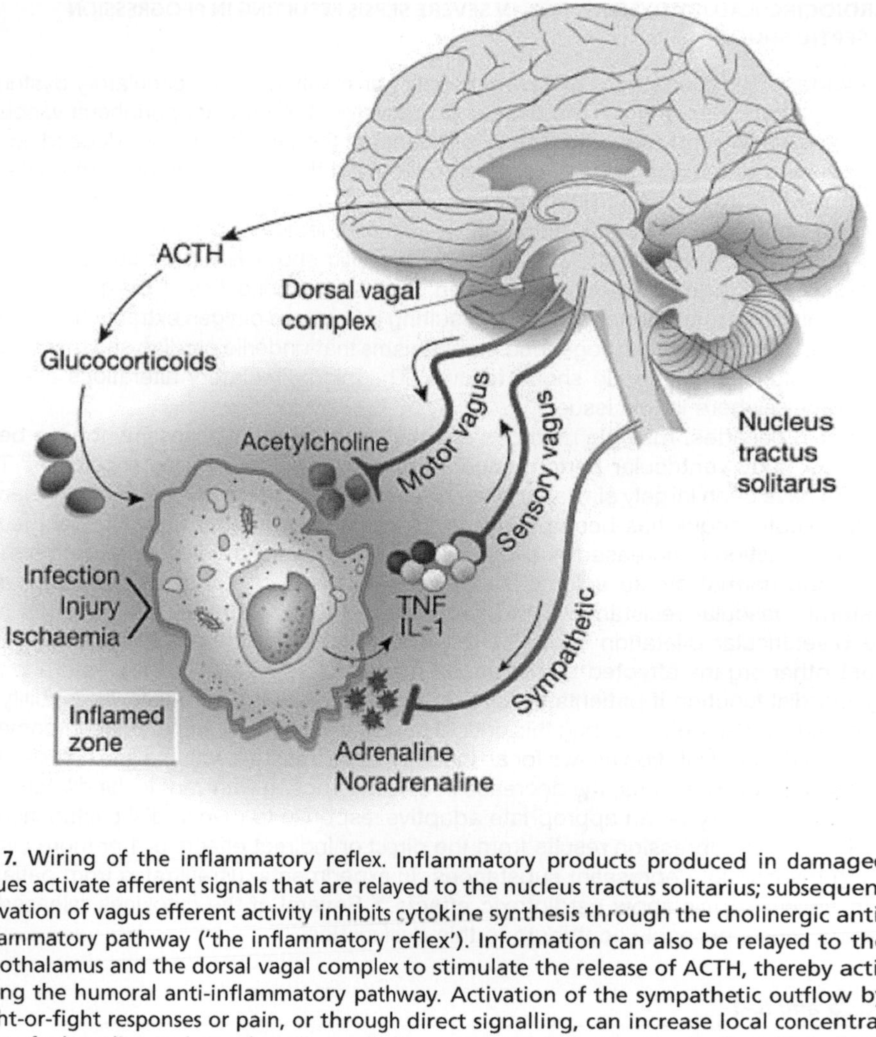

Fig. 7. Wiring of the inflammatory reflex. Inflammatory products produced in damaged tissues activate afferent signals that are relayed to the nucleus tractus solitarius; subsequent activation of vagus efferent activity inhibits cytokine synthesis through the cholinergic anti-inflammatory pathway ('the inflammatory reflex'). Information can also be relayed to the hypothalamus and the dorsal vagal complex to stimulate the release of ACTH, thereby activating the humoral anti-inflammatory pathway. Activation of the sympathetic outflow by flight-or-fight responses or pain, or through direct signalling, can increase local concentrations of adrenaline and noradrenaline, which can suppress inflammation further. (*Data from* Tracey KJ. The inflammatory reflex. Nature 2002;420:857).

The sympathetic ANS consists of sympathetic neurons and the adrenal medulla, with catecholamines as the neurotransmitter. In addition to the adrenal medulla and sympathetic neurons, immune effector cells are also a source of catecholamines in severe sepsis.[55] Early uncomplicated sepsis is characterized by high circulating catecholamine levels with significant metabolic (catabolic state), immunomodulaory (excessive inflammation), and cardiocirculatory (increased cardiac output) consequences. Prolonged elevation of circulating catecholamines is toxic to host cells, predisposing the patient to cardiocirculatory failure with hypotension resulting from peripheral vasodilatation and compromised myocardial contractility.[56] Septic shock is more often characterized by depletion of endogenous catecholamine stores and, possibly, catecholamine resistance.

CARDIOCIRCULATORY DYSFUNCTION IN SEVERE SEPSIS RESULTING IN PROGRESSION TO SEPTIC SHOCK

The widespread disruptions in severe sepsis can result in cardio-circulatory dysfunction manifesting as shock. The dysfunction involves the cardiac, peripheral vascular (macrovascular) and microcirculatory elements of the circulation and, depending on the degrees of cardiac or vascular dysfunction and the volume status of the patient, a clinical picture ranging from cold, clammy and under-perfused to one of hyperdynamic shock, may be seen, although, in clinical medicine, hyperdynamic shock is seen much more frequently. The situation in septic shock is further complicated by widespread microcirculatory dysfunction, further impairing tissue oxygen delivery, and diminished mitochondrial activity resulting in impaired oxygen extraction. A review of characteristics and pathogenetic mechanisms that underlie cardiac and macrovascular dysfunction in septic shock follows. The microcirculatory alterations are discussed elsewhere in this issue.

Over 5 decades, multiple methods of myocardial function assessment have been used to study ventricular performance in severe sepsis and septic shock.[57–60] The results have been largely similar and the characteristic pattern of cardiac performance during septic shock has been proved to be one of reduced left and right ventricular ejection fractions, increased end-diastolic and end-systolic volumes of both ventricles, and normal stroke volume; heart rate and cardiac output are elevated, and systemic vascular resistance is reduced. The reduction in the ejection fraction and the biventricular dilatation occur 24 to 48 hours after the onset of sepsis and, like most other organs affected by the septic process, it is reversible with restoration of myocardial function if patients survive up to 10 days after their onset. An inability to maintain cardiac output during this critical period is associated with a poor outcome,[61] and ventricular dilatation allows for an increased end-diastolic volume and helps maintain cardiac output. Thus, the decrease in ejection fraction with ventricular dilatation in septic shock may be an appropriate adaptive response to myocardial dysfunction.

Myocardial depression results from the direct or indirect effects of 1 or more circulating myocardial depressant substances. In experiments, ultrafiltrates from patients with severe sepsis show cardiotoxic effects.[62] Several of the cytokines released in severe sepsis probably contribute to this dysfunction.

TNF-a and IL-1

TNF-a and IL-1 are associated with myocyte dysfunction and may explain the early myocardial depression seen in sepsis. In one series of studies using in vitro myocardial cells and human septic shock serum, TNF and IL-1 were shown to be responsible for the myocardial depressant activity present in human sera.[63] These cytokines are potent inducible nitric oxide synthase (iNOS) inducers, and this probably represents one of the direct mechanisms for myocardial depression.

Nitric Oxide

Severe sepsis is associated with increased expression of iNOS and increased nitric oxide production. NO interferes with myocyte calcium metabolism and may impair contractile function. In addition, reactive nitrogen species such as peroxynitrite, produced by NO interacting with superoxide ions, are directly toxic to myocytes. Experimental observations support a role for NO-mediated myocardial depression in sepsis. Cardiac function was preserved following LPS challenge in iNOS-deficient mice.[64]

Vascular Dysfunction

Vascular alterations in septic shock are mainly due to the effects of mediators on vascular smooth muscle and endothelial dysfunction.

The NO released seems to be primarily responsible for vascular smooth muscle dysfunction in sepsis. NO causes a hyperpolarization of smooth muscle plasma membranes, rendering them unresponsive to catecholamines and causing a vasodilatory state. In addition to the above, these patients may have relative vasopressin or cortisol deficiencies, leading to further catecholamine unresponsiveness and refractory shock.

Endothelial dysfunction leads to an inability of the endothelial cells to maintain vascular tone with loss of blood pressure. In addition, endothelial damage leads to capillary leak with intravascular volume depletion and edema formation in involved organs.

SUMMARY

Septic shock remains a significant challenge for clinicians. Recent advances in cellular and molecular biology have significantly improved our understanding of its pathogenetic mechanisms. These improvements in understanding should translate to better care and improved outcomes for these patients.

REFERENCES

1. Geroulanos S, Douka ET. Historical perspective of the word “sepsis.” Intensive Care Med 2006;32:2077.
2. Vincent JL, Abraham E. The last 100 years of sepsis. Am J Respir Crit Care Med 2006;173:256–63.
3. Schottmueller H. Wesen und Behandlung der Sepsis [The nature and therapy of sepsis]. Inn Med 1914;31:257–80 [in German].
4. Cannon WB. Traumatic shock. New York: D Appleton and Co; 1923.
5. Kumar A, Parrillo J. Shock: classification, pathophysiology, and approach to management. In: Parillo JE, Dellinger RP, editors. Critical care medicine: principles of diagnosis and management in the adult. 3rd edition. Philadelphia: Mosby Elsevier; 2008. p. 377–422.
6. Campisi Laura, Brau Frédéric, Glaichenhaus Nicolas. Imaging host–pathogen interactions. Immunol Rev 2008;221(1):188–99.
7. Bassler BL. Small talk. Cell-to-cell communication in bacteria. Cell 2002;109: 421–4.
8. Taga ME, Bassler BL. Chemical communication among bacteria. Proc Natl Acad Sci U S A 2003;100(Suppl 2):14549–54.
9. Davies DG, Parsek MR, Pearson JP, et al. The involvement of cell-to-cell signals in the development of a bacterial biofilm. Science 1998;280:295–8.
10. Shiner EK, Rumbaugh KP, Williams SC. Inter-kingdom signaling: deciphering the language of acyl homoserine lactones. FEMS Microbiol Rev 2005;29:935–47.
11. Hooi DS, Bycroft BW, Chhabra SR, et al. Differential immune modulatory activity of *Pseudomonas aeruginosa* quorum-sensing signal molecules. Infect Immun 2004;72:6463–70.
12. Miller MB, Bassler BL. Quorum sensing in bacteria. Annu Rev Microbiol 2001;55: 165–99.

13. Whiteley M, Lee KM, Greenberg EP. Identification of genes controlled by quorum sensing in *Pseudomonas aeruginosa*. Proc Natl Acad Sci U S A 1999;96: 13904–9.
14. Cinel I, Dellinger RP. Advances in pathogenesis and management of sepsis. Curr Opin Infect Dis 2007;20:345–52.
15. van der Poll T, Opal SM. Host-pathogen interactions in sepsis. Lancet Infect Dis 2008;8:32–43.
16. Creagh EM, O'Neill LA. TLRs, NLRs and RLRs: a trinity of pathogen sensors that co-operate in innate immunity. Trends Immunol 2006;27:352–7.
17. Granucci F, Foti M, Ricciardi-Castagnoli P. Dendritic cell biology. Adv Immunol 2005;88:193–233.
18. Uematsu S, Akira S. Toll-like receptors and innate immunity. J Mol Med 2007;84: 712–25.
19. Mollen KP, Anand RJ, Tsung A, et al. Emerging paradigm: toll-like receptor 4-sentinel for the detection of tissue damage. Shock 2006;26:430–7.
20. Paterson HM, Murphy TJ, Purcell EJ, et al. Injury primes the innate immune system for enhanced toll-like receptor reactivity. J Immunol 2003;171: 1473–83.
21. Arcaroli J, Fessler MB, Abraham E. Genetic polymorphisms and sepsis. Shock 2005;24:300–12.
22. Gibot S, Cariou A, Drouet L, et al. Association between a genomic polymorphism within the CD14 locus and septic shock susceptibility and mortality rate. Crit Care Med 2002;30:969–73.
23. Arcaroli J, Silva E, Maloney JP, et al. Variant IRAK-1 haplotype is associated with increased nuclear factor-kappaB activation and worse outcomes in sepsis. Am J Respir Crit Care Med 2006;173:1335–41.
24. Zaph C, Troy AE, Taylor BC, et al. Epithelial cell-intrinsic IKK-beta expression regulates intestinal immune homeostasis. Nature 2007;446:552–6.
25. Liu YJ, Soumelis V, Watanabe N, et al. TSLP: an epithelial cell cytokine that regulates T cell differentiation by conditioning dendritic cell maturation. Annu Rev Immunol 2007;25:193–219.
26. Peck-Palmer OM, Unsinger J, Chang KC, et al. Deletion of MyD88 markedly attenuates sepsis-induced T and B lymphocyte apoptosis but worsens survival. J Leukoc Biol 2008;83:1009–18.
27. Adib-Conquy M, Moine P, Asehnoune K, et al. Toll-like receptor-mediated tumor necrosis factor and interleukin-10 production differ during systemic inflammation. Am J Respir Crit Care Med 2003;168:158–64.
28. Ayscough KR, Gourlay CW. The actin cytoskeleton: a key regulator of apoptosis and aging. Nat Rev Mol Cell Biol 2005;6:583–9.
29. Fischer U, Jänicke RU, Schulze-Osthoff K. Many cuts to ruin: a comprehensive update of caspase substrates. Cell Death Differ 2003;10(1):76–100.
30. Sarkar A, Hall MW, Exline M, et al. Caspase-1 regulates *E. coli* sepsis and splenic B cell apoptosis independently of IL-1[beta] and IL-18. Am J Respir Crit Care Med 2006;174:1003–10.
31. Cantley LC. The phosphoinositide 3-kinase pathway. Science 2002;296:1655–7.
32. Nick JA, Young SK, Arndt PG, et al. Selective suppression of neutrophil accumulation in ongoing pulmonary inflammation by systemic inhibition of p38 MAP kinase. J Immunol 2002;169(9):5260–9.
33. Yum HK, Arcaroli J, Kupfner J, et al. Involvement of phosphoinositide 3-kinases in neutrophil activation and the development of acute lung injury. J Immunol 2001; 167(11):6601–8.

34. Ojaniemi M, Glumoff V, Harju K, et al. Phosphatidylinositol kinase is involved in Toll-like receptor 4-mediated cytokine expression in mouse macrophages. Eur J Immunol 2003;335:597–605.
35. Guillot L, Le Goffic R, Bloch S, et al. Involvement of toll-like receptor 3 in the immune response of lung epithelial cells to double-stranded RNA and influenza A virus. J Biol Chem 2005;280:5571–80.
36. Guha M, Mackman N. The PI3K-Akt pathway limits LPS activation of signaling pathways and expression of inflammatory mediators in human monocytic cells. J Biol Chem 2002;277:32124–32.
37. Pengal RA, Ganesan LP, Wei G, et al. Lipopolysaccharide-induced production of interleukin-10 is promoted by the serin threonine kinase Akt. Mol Immunol 2006; 43:1557–64.
38. Fukao T, Koyasu S. PI3K and negative regulation of TLR signaling. Trends Immunol 2003;24:358–63.
39. Maus UA, Backi M, Winter C, et al. Importance of phosphoinositide 3-kinase gamma in the host defense against pneumococcal infection. Am J Respir Crit Care Med 2007;175(9):958–66.
40. Hall A, Rho GT. Pases and the actin cytoskeleton. Science 1998;279:509–14.
41. Ruse M, Knaus UG. New players in TLR-mediated innate immunity. Immunol Res 2006;34:33–48.
42. Arbibe L, Mira JP, Teusch N, et al. Toll-like receptor 2-mediated NF-kappa B activation requires a RacI dependent pathway. Nat Immunol 2000;1:533–54.
43. Hotchkiss RS, Karl IE. The pathophysiology and treatment of sepsis. N Engl J Med 2003;348:138–50.
44. Rapaport SI, Tatter D, Coeur-Baron N. *Pseudomonas* septicemia with intravascular clotting leading to the generalized Shwartzman reaction. N Engl J Med 1964;271:80.
45. Corrigan JJ, Ray WL, May N. Changes in the blood coagulation system associated with septicemia. N Engl J Med 1968;279:851–6.
46. Beller FK. The role of endotoxin in disseminated intravascular coagulation. Thromb Diath Haemorrh Suppl 1969;36:125–49.
47. Corrigan JJ, Jordan CM. Heparin therapy in septicemia with disseminated intravascular coagulation. N Engl J Med Shock 1970;283:778–82.
48. Bernik TR, Friedman SG, Ochani M, et al. Pharmacological stimulation of the cholinergic antiinflammatory pathway. J Exp Med 2002;195:781–8.
49. Borovikova LV, Ivanova S, Zhang M, et al. Vagus nerve stimulation attenuates the systemic inflammatory response to endotoxin. Nature 2000;405:458–62.
50. Altavilla D, Guarini S, Bitto A, et al. Activation of the cholinergic anti-inflammatory pathway reduces NF-kappab activation, blunts TNF-alpha production, and protects against splanchic artery occlusion shock. Shock 2006;25:500–6.
51. Huston JM, Ochani M, Rosas-Ballina M, et al. Splenectomy inactivates the cholinergic antiinflammatory pathway during lethal endotoxemia and polymicrobial sepsis. J Exp Med 2006;203:1623–8.
52. Wang H, Yu M, Ochani M, et al. Nicotinic acetylcholine receptor alpha7 subunit is an essential regulator of inflammation. Nature 2003;421:384–8.
53. Wang H, Liao H, Ochani M, et al. Cholinergic agonists inhibit HMGB1 release and improve survival in experimental sepsis. Nat Med 2004;10:1216–21.
54. Tracey KJ. Physiology and immunology of the cholinergic antiinflammatory pathway. J Clin Invest 2007;117:289–96.
55. Flierl MA, Rittirsch D, Nadeau BA, et al. Phagocyte-derived catecholamines enhance acute inflammatory injury. Nature 2007;449:721–5.

56. Annane D, de la Grandmaison G, Brouland JP, et al. Inappropriate sympathetic activation at onset of septic shock: a spectral analysis approach. Am J Respir Crit Care Med 1999;160:458–65.
57. Calvin JE, Driedger AA, Sibbald WJ. An assessment of myocardial function in human sepsis utilizing ECG gated cardiac scintigraphy. Chest 1981;80:579–86.
58. Parker MM, McCarthy KE, Ognibene FP, et al. Right ventricular dysfunction and dilatation, similar to left ventricular changes, characterize the cardiac depression of septic shock in humans. Chest 1990;97:126–31.
59. Munt B, Jue J, Gin K, et al. Diastolic filling in human severe sepsis: an echocardiographic study. Crit Care Med 1998;26:1829–33.
60. Poelaert J, Declerck C, Vogelaers D, et al. Left ventricular systolic and diastolic function in septic shock. Intensive Care Med 1997;23:553–60.
61. Parker MM, Shelhamer JH, Natanson C, et al. Serial cardiovascular variables in survivors and nonsurvivors of human septic shock: heart rate as an early predictor of prognosis. Crit Care Med 1987;15:923–9.
62. Parrillo JE, Burch C, Shelhamer JH, et al. A circulating myocardial depressant substance in humans with septic shock: septic shock patients with a reduced ejection fraction have a circulating factor that depresses in vitro myocardial cell performance. J Clin Invest 1985;76:1539–53.
63. Kumar A, Thota V, Dee L, et al. Tumor necrosis factor-alpha and interleukin-1 beta are responsible for depression of in vitro myocardial cell contractility induced by serum from humans with septic shock. J Exp Med 1996;183:949–58.
64. Ullrich R, Scherrer-Crosbie M, Bloch KD, et al. Congenital deficiency of nitric oxide synthase 2 protects against endotoxin-induced myocardial dysfunction in mice. Circulation 2000;102:1440–6.

Animal Models of Sepsis

Sergio L. Zanotti-Cavazzoni, MD, FCCM[a,*], Roy D. Goldfarb, PhD, FAPS[b]

KEYWORDS

- Sepsis • Septic shock • Animal models • Severe sepsis
- Drug development

Sepsis is a complex and heterogeneous syndrome defined by the systemic inflammatory response to infection.[1] Development of organ failure leads to severe sepsis. Septic shock is hypotension not responsive to intravenous fluids.[2] Severe sepsis and septic shock are among the most important causes of morbidity and mortality in patients admitted to intensive care units. The incidence of severe sepsis in the United States is estimated around 750,000 cases per year, with over 210,000 annual deaths.[3] The resources required to care for critically ill patients with sepsis create an enormous burden on the health care system. According to estimates, the yearly cost of caring for patients with sepsis in the United States is more than $16 billion.[3] When one considers the impact this disease has on our society, it is evident that efforts to develop novel therapies to treat sepsis would be of great value. Over the last 3 decades, important advances in our understanding of the underlying mechanisms of severe sepsis and septic shock have been made. However, translating these findings to effective novel therapies has proven difficult. Despite a significant amount of basic research and multiple clinical trials, to date, only one drug, activated protein C (drotrecogin alpha), has received regulatory approval for use in sepsis and the mortality of severe sepsis and septic shock remains elevated.[4–6]

Clearly the need to advance our understanding of this complex disease and to develop new therapies that can improve patient outcomes remains a priority within the field of critical care medicine. Studying sepsis in humans is difficult for many reasons, including the complexity of the disease, the heterogeneous nature of the population, the lack of clearly defined biomarkers to make a diagnosis, and other factors associated with clinical research.[7] In view of these difficulties, the use of animal models has been proposed as a valuable tool in the study of sepsis.[8] Animal models of

Financial disclosures: none.

[a] Division of Critical Care Medicine, Cooper University Hospital, University of Medicine and Dentistry of New Jersey—Robert Wood Johnson Medical School, One Cooper Plaza, Dorrance 360, Camden, NJ 08103, USA
[b] Division of Cardiology, Cooper University Hospital, University of Medicine and Dentistry of New Jersey—Robert Wood Johnson Medical School, One Cooper Plaza, Dorrance 360, Camden, NJ 08103, USA
* Corresponding author.
E-mail address: zanotti-sergio@cooperhealth.edu (S.L. Zanotti-Cavazzoni).

Crit Care Clin 25 (2009) 703–719
doi:10.1016/j.ccc.2009.08.005 **criticalcare.theclinics.com**

sepsis present unique features that make them ideal to further elucidate mechanisms of disease and to identify pathways that could become potential targets for therapy.[9] Furthermore, animal models have become an important part of the novel drug discovery and development process.[10–12] However, the growing list of failed sepsis drugs, many of which initially were tested successfully in animal models, has raised concerns over the value and clinical relevance of animal models in sepsis.[13–15] In this review, we start with a general discussion of relevant factors that can determine the validity of a sepsis animal model. We briefly review some of the currently used animal models of sepsis (small animal models and large animal models) and discuss the clinical relevance of animal models in sepsis research today. Finally, we address potential reasons for the apparent underperformance of animal models in predicting therapeutic success of novel drugs in clinical trials.

GENERAL CONSIDERATIONS: IMPORTANT FACTORS TO CONSIDER IN ANIMAL MODELS OF SEPSIS

It is difficult for preclinical animal models of sepsis to completely replicate the complexity of clinical human sepsis. In humans, sepsis develops over hours to days, often results in a prolonged clinical course, and often leads to multiorgan failure. Animal models of sepsis, by contrast, usually result in very acute and short clinical courses, raising the question of potential different pathophysiological circumstances. Animal models of sepsis vary significantly in their complexity and clinical relevance. There are factors that have an important impact on determining a particular animal model's clinical relevance and translational power (**Table 1**). In this section we will discuss the role some of these factors play in animal models of sepsis.

Method of Inducing Sepsis

Perhaps the most critical factor in relation to the clinical relevance and the ability to translate findings to humans from an animal model is the method used to induce experimental sepsis. Early models of sepsis used the administration of toxins, such

Table 1
Factors that affect clinical relevance of an animal model of sepsis

Factor	Comments
Method of inducing sepsis	Endotoxin may not replicate clinical sepsis. Peritonitis models, such as cecal ligation and puncture, are likely more relevant to human disease.
Adjuvant therapy	Models in which animals do not receive supportive care (fluids, antibiotics) are likely to have mortality rates in excess of what is seen in human sepsis. These models may not be as relevant for testing novel therapies.
Species	Significant interspecies differences in response to septic insult may exist.
Age	Sepsis in humans is more prevalent in older patients. Most animal models use young animals (age equivalent to humans <18 years old).
Gender	Animal models use predominantly male animals. In humans, at least 50% of patients are females. Hormonal differences may confer better outcomes in sepsis for females.
Severity/mortality	Mortality of model should parallel mortality of human sepsis.

as endotoxin or lipopolysacharide (LPS), to replicate the clinical picture of human sepsis. Endotoxin can be administered through different routes and models have used intravenous, intraperitoneal, and intratracheal routes. Advantages of using endotoxin include technical ease to perform and homogenous response to insult, which make it straightforward to replicate. However, critics have pointed out that this toxic insult does not replicate human clinical sepsis.[16,17] A bolus injection of endotoxin quickly causes a pronounced increase in proinflammatory cytokines; this elevation is transient and has been described in animals and in human volunteers.[17–20] By comparison, the rise in proinflammatory cytokines is significantly lower in patients with sepsis who develop a host response to infection (bacteria). Also, this rise takes place over a longer period than that produced by endotoxin administration. Furthermore, the cardiovascular changes described in animal models of endotoxemia do not replicate what is commonly seen in patients with sepsis. The administration of endotoxin as a continuous infusion with concomitant fluid resuscitation has been used to correct this problem.[21] Although multiple studies have been published using endotoxin, its short-term effects on the inflammatory cascade and lack of an active nidus of infection make them less attractive today. Administration of live bacteria through multiple routes replicates many of the characteristics seen in clinical sepsis. Administration of bacteria cultured in vitro at predefined doses of colony forming units can cause reproducible clinical alterations and mortality. In addition, this model can allow investigators to target particular types of sepsis (ie, gram-negative vs gram-positive). Unfortunately, injection of bacteria usually does not lead to colonization and replication of bacteria essential in development of a focus of infection. This has led to criticism similar to that directed at endotoxin models. According to this criticism, a focus of infection is needed to create a more protracted host response. Without that focus, the clinical changes observed are a result of one acute and transient insult.[16] The response observed in animals is likely due to acute immune reaction and lysis of bacteria creating a toxic model as opposed to a true sepsis model.[16,22] In an attempt to overcome this problem, several models mimicking fecal peritonitis have been developed. Among these models, cecal ligation and puncture (CLP) has gained widespread use and is considered by some experts as the gold standard for animal models of sepsis.[13]

CLP will produce a polymicrobial infection with a resultant immune, hemodynamic, and biochemical response in animals that replicates that seen in patients with sepsis.[23–25] Other models of sepsis caused by peritonitis require implantation of infected clots, injection of fecal content into the peritoneum, or invasive procedures.[26–28] Studies comparing CLP models to endotoxin models have shown different cytokine responses, different hemodynamic profiles, and, perhaps most significant, different effects on mortality in response to various experimental treatments.[19,29] Downsides to models that induce sepsis by peritonitis include the potential for abscess formation (changing the model from sepsis to an intra-abdominal abscess model) and the lack of surgical intervention with removal of devitalized tissue (a common procedure in patients with peritonitis caused by a perforated viscus). Despite its limitations, septic peritonitis models are frequently used and considered clinically relevant to human sepsis.[16]

Adjuvant Therapy

Current clinical guidelines emphasize the importance of aggressive and standardized critical care support when treating patients with sepsis.[30,31] The current therapeutic approach of patients with sepsis is based on early administration of appropriate antibiotics and goal-directed hemodynamic resuscitation.[32,33] Unfortunately, the level of support and the types of adjuvant therapy used in different models of sepsis are extremely variable. Studies in mice have shown that as in humans, delays in starting antibiotics increases mortality.[34] Hemodynamic support, an essential component of clinical treatment in sepsis, poses several challenges in animals. Which route should be used for administration of fluids? What is the best way to monitor adequate cardiovascular resuscitation? In models where no hemodynamic support is provided, do animals die from sepsis or from circulatory collapse? Several studies highlight the importance of adequate hemodynamic support. These studies show improved survival in animals treated with fluid resuscitation.[35,36] Other therapeutic modalities commonly used in patients with severe sepsis, such as mechanical ventilation, vasopresors, and metabolic control, are even more difficult to incorporate into animal models. Why is this an important factor? One could highlight the importance of incorporating adjuvant therapies commonly used in clinical practice with a hypothetical example. In this example, suppose that a novel drug has been evaluated in a preclinical model that does not incorporate basic adjuvant therapy (antibiotics and fluid resuscitation), and this drug is found to reduce mortality. How can an investigator know if the beneficial effect is due to antibiotic properties of this novel compound or its effect on a specific pathway? Will this benefit in mortality disappear once the drug is tested in a clinical trial that incorporates such therapies as antibiotics and hemodynamic support? Studies have shown an incremental and additive benefit on survival as the level of adjuvant therapy is increased in animal models of sepsis (**Fig. 1**).[37] Finally, there are also important pathophysiological implications for models that do not include adjuvant therapy. In a study with serial echocardiography, we have shown that early and aggressive fluid resuscitation is needed in a CLP murine model of sepsis to replicate the hemodynamic profile seen in fluid-resuscitated patients with severe sepsis and septic shock.[36] Animal models with underresuscitated animals may not replicate the cardiovascular and hemodynamic abnormalities seen in clinical sepsis.

Species

If the goal of an animal model is to replicate human disease as closely as possible, it is obvious we should seek animals that closest resemble human beings. However, using

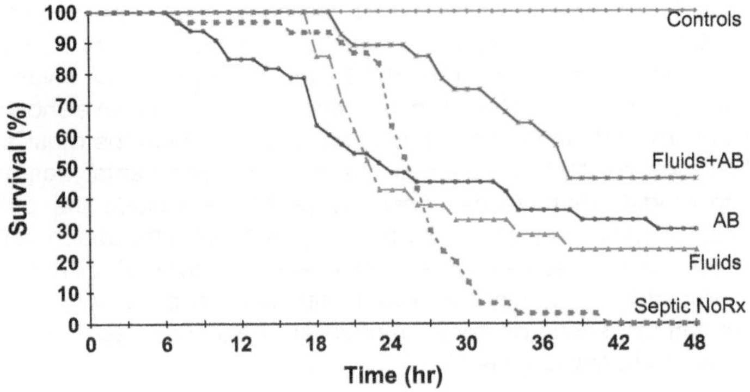

Fig. 1. Effect of adjuvant therapy on survival in a murine model of sepsis. In a CLP model of sepsis, survival at 48 hours was significantly affected by the level of supportive therapy provided to the animals post-CLP. Septic animals with no treatment (Septic NoRx) had 0% survival at 48 hours; with fluids-only (Fluids), survival improved to 22%; with antibiotics only (AB), survival was 30%; and the combination of antibiotics and fluids (Fluids + AB) improved survival to 46%. Control animals (sham CLP) had 100% survival.

nonhuman primates is fraught with ethical, social, and financial challenges. Rats and mice are the most commonly used species in great part because of their low cost and ease to breed. Larger animals, such as pigs, dogs, and sheep, are also used in sepsis models, but in smaller numbers, probably because of higher costs. Although many species share common pathways of disease with humans, there are interspecies differences particular to sepsis that may be significant. For example, rodents and dogs are particularly resistant to endotoxin, where as humans and sheep are very sensitive to its effects.[38] In a study in which the amount of endotoxin was titrated to a given cytokine response (IL-6 level), it was shown that rodents required a 250-fold larger dose administered intraperitoneally to achieve a similar response as humans receiving intravenous endotoxin.[39] Furthermore, interspecies organ failure development in response to sepsis may vary.

Age and Gender

Sepsis predominantly affects the elderly. Most epidemiologic studies show that patients over 65 years old are more likely to develop sepsis.[3,40,41] Older patients are also more likely to develop complications and die from sepsis.[42] However, almost universally, animal models of sepsis use young animals with physiologic ages equivalent to humans less than 18 years old. An important reason for this is cost, as aged animals are more expensive. Recent studies have addressed the impact of age on animal models of sepsis. Turnbull and colleagues[43] have shown that, in a murine CLP model of sepsis, aged animals had higher mortality than young animals (75% vs 20%). In this study, the response to treatment with antibiotics was also decreased in aged mice.[43] Subsequent studies from the same group have shown decreased immune function in older septic mice.[44] Aged mice also have demonstrated increased sensitivity to endotoxin.[45,46] The importance of considering age in our preclinical models is further reflected in a subgroup analysis of the PROWESS (Recombinant Human Activated Protein C Worldwide Evaluation in Severe Sepsis) study for activated protein C that reported a significant difference in the absolute risk reduction in mortality for patients treated with the drug over 65 years old (8.6%) as compared with those under 65 years old (2.7%).[47] Gender may also be an important factor to consider in our preclinical models of sepsis. In clinical practice, at least 50% of patients are female.[40] Even so, most preclinical models use male animals. This becomes particularly important when one considers a growing body of literature suggesting that hormonal differences may account for improved outcomes in females with sepsis (animal models and clinical sepsis).[48–50]

Comorbidity

Lastly, we will discuss the role of comorbid diseases in animal models of sepsis. Comorbidity represents perhaps the biggest dichotomy between animal models and clinical reality. In patients with sepsis, comorbid conditions are common.[40] One large clinical study has shown that patients with sepsis have on average 1.07 comorbid conditions and that at least 15% of patients with sepsis have diabetes or cancer.[5] In contrast, animal models are almost exclusively done in healthy and often young animals.[14] The lack of comorbid conditions in animal models of sepsis likely represents a shortcoming. If one considers that the clinical course of healthy patients with sepsis (a rare event in clinical practice) is very different from that of patients with multiple comorbidities, it is easy to presume that studying healthy animals probably does not accurately replicate what happens in clinical practice. As we try to improve our animal models of sepsis, it is likely worthwhile to study animals with comorbid conditions known to play important roles in human sepsis (eg, diabetes, cardiovascular disease, and cancer).

SMALL ANIMAL MODELS OF SEPSIS

Small animal models of sepsis have been widely used in research. Major advantages of small animals, in particular rodents (rats and mice), include low cost, ease to breed and house, and the low level of resistance from the lay community for the use of such animals in research. Rodents conserve many biologic features common to mammals. However, they have distinct differences from humans in response to disease. These differences may be more pronounced than those seen in larger animal models (eg, baboons) using species phylogentically closer to humans. However, one clear scientific advantage of mice is the availability of genetically modified animals or knockouts. Knockout mice, animals in which a specific gene has been deleted, have proved extremely useful in studying mechanisms of disease. Small animal models also present disadvantages. Because mice are so small, the same mouse cannot be used for the serial acquisition of blood or tissue samples to evaluate time-dependant pathways of pathology. To acquire this data, scientists must perform tests on separate groups of mice and then obtain blood and tissue samples after euthanasia. For example, murine total blood volume is 2 mL, so that sufficient blood sampling can often lead to hypovolemic shock, altering the model from one of sepsis to one of sepsis plus hemorrhagic shock. Furthermore, acquisition of core tissue samples is impossible in a time-serial fashion. Finally, technical limitations are imposed by the small size of the animals, making invasive procedures for monitoring (especially hemodynamics) and other forms of critical care support very challenging. However, rodent models are still the most commonly used models for sepsis research. In this section, we will discuss the model of CLP and a more recently described model with colon ascendens stent peritonitis (CASP).

CLP in rodents, the most commonly used model of experimental sepsis, is considered by many the most suitable model for sepsis research.[16,19,23,51,52] CLP was developed almost 30 years ago and is still considered a relevant model for the induction of sepsis due to polymicrobial peritonitis.[25] The relevance of CLP in today's sepsis research is highlighted by recent reviews of this technique.[53,54] CLP is performed by ligation of the cecum below the ileocecal valve after a midline laparotomy, followed by needle puncture of the cecum. Perforation of the cecum leads to a polymicrobial peritonitis, followed by translocation of bacteria into the blood. Bacteremia triggers an inflammatory response that leads to hemodynamic instability, septic shock, multiorgan failure, and finally death. When used in rodents, CLP will replicate many of the clinical features seen in sepsis (hypothermia, tachypnea, tachycardia, hypotension). An important concern related to the widespread use of CLP is the lack of consistency in technical aspects among different CLP models. The lack of consistency is of particular significance because it most often involves aspects that directly affect the severity of the model. Severity in the CLP model is influenced by three important factors: length of cecum ligated, size of needle used for perforation, and post-CLP supportive therapy. The length of the cecum ligated is a major determinant of mortality and increased levels of proinflammatory cytokines have been described with increasing length of cecum ligation.[55] Other key determinants of severity in CLP are the needle size used for puncture of the cecum and the number of punctures.[56] The importance of the severity in a CLP model is illustrated by a recent study in which animals with different severity grades of CLP-induced sepsis were used to study the functional roles of C5a receptors.[57] In this study, both the underlying pathophysiology and the response to therapeutic intervention were based on severity. Therapeutic interventions that were highly effective in midgrade-severity sepsis were not effective in a more severe grade of sepsis.[57] Finally, a very important determinant of severity/mortality in CLP is post-CLP supportive care. There is a great degree of variability among different CLP models with respect to the treatment animals receive after induction of sepsis. The role of antibiotics on CLP-induced mortality is well established.[58] Fluids have also been shown to affect mortality in CLP models.[36,37] The amount of fluid not only modulated mortality, but also has been shown to have significant implications on the cardiovascular response. This becomes especially important when one is trying to study sepsis hemodynamics and replicate what we see in humans.[36] Therefore, it is important to consider these factors when evaluating CLP models. Perhaps more important yet, investigators should report all these factors in their models so the scientific community can fully appraise their results within the context of a given model.

One problem that can arise with CLP-induced sepsis is the formation of a walled-off abscess, thus producing more of an intra-abdominal abscess model than a true sepsis model. One proposed solution to this concern has been the introduction of the CASP model of sepsis. In CASP, a stent is inserted into the colon ascendens of the rodent, this leads to persistent leakage of fecal material into the peritoneal cavity, causing a polymicrobial sepsis and peritonitis.[59] The procedure involves a laparotomy, insertion and fixation of the stent, and fluid resuscitation. CASP is associated with bacteremia and elevated circulating endotoxin (LPS) levels.[59,60] Bacteremia is detected as early as 12 hours post–stent implantation and increased serum LPS is seen as early as 2 hours post–stent implantation.[59,60] CASP produces a robust inflammatory response similar to that seen in clinical human sepsis.[59–61] The severity (measured by mortality rate) can be titrated based on the diameter of the stent.[59] In addition, the stent can be removed at predefined time points, replicating source control procedures that would occur in patients with abdominal sepsis due to peritonitis. It has been shown that early removal of stents (at 3 hours) will rescue mice but removal of stent (at 9 hours) will not decrease mortality.[59] CASP mortality is associated with multiple-organ failure.[62] A direct comparison between the CLP and CASP models has shown stronger induction of cytokines and higher bacterial counts in blood with the CASP model.[60] It has been proposed that this occurs because CASP produces a more consistent diffuse peritonitis with persistent systemic inflammation, as opposed to CLP, which can lead to a walled-off abscess with less systemic inflammation. Potential disadvantages of the CASP model include a less-characterized hemodynamic response and less experience to identify possible confounding variables.

LARGE ANIMAL MODELS OF SEPSIS

Large animals have long been used as models to study the fundamental mechanisms of sepsis and to test novel therapeutic agents and modalities.[27,63] To model humans, scientists have used numerous species, such as rabbits, cats, dogs, sheep, and pigs, leading to subhuman primates.[63] Larger animals address many of the deficiencies of rodent models. For example, the larger size allows for serial sampling of blood, other fluids, and tissues. Also, detailed hemodynamic, cardiodynamic, and other organ function evaluations can be made in serial fashion in the same animal. Furthermore, in contrast to rodent models, the ability to obtain vast amounts of time-dependant data for a wide variety of variables allows for great statistical power and ability to derive correlations with relatively few animals.

Despite these advantages, challenges remain in applying large animal models in the study of human sepsis. Experimental therapies for large animal models require at least 100 to 1000 times more compound than mice because the large sizes make each experiment more expensive. The animal housing regulations for large animals is quite rigorous, detailed, and expensive, as are monitoring regulations, especially when experiments are conducted overnight. Use of species more closely related to humans, such as primates, presents extraordinary difficulties: These animals are extremely difficult to handle, being two to three times stronger than humans per pound; they a present biohazard to the work staff, as they carry many diseases transmittable to humans (eg, herpes B infection); and the availability of these animals is very low. These factors present daunting obstacles to using primates in research on new therapies, which is why few laboratories conduct these studies.

Despite the many difficulties of studying sepsis in large animal models, two features support the employment of these models. First, Food and Drug Administration (FDA) guidelines suggest that all new drug applications include data from two species, one of which must be nonrodent. Second, large animals accommodate serial samples of data, blood, and tissue. This lowers the number of animals required to complete a full study. For example, two groups of eight pigs or sheep can be used to test a novel therapeutic in which continuous organ function data and frequent blood samples can be obtained over 24, 48, or 72 hours. The collection of 5 mL of blood from a sheep or pig every 6 hours for 72 hours would yield six experimental and one or two basal samples. To replicate this protocol in mice, experimenters would have to bleed and euthanize eight groups of 10 mice in two treatment groups, totaling 160 mice. Suddenly, sheep or pigs don't look that expensive any more.

Canine models of shock and sepsis have not been as prevalent as in the past. Two scientific considerations have reduced their use. Canine models of hemorrhagic shock, endotoxemia, bacteremia, and other acute shock states induce a significant splanchnic injury, which is expressed as pooling of splanchnic blood with concomitant bleeding in the intestine.[64,65] This feature makes these models too much of a gut injury model for utility toward human responses. In addition, dogs, along with rodents and cats, are among several species that show a relative resistance to the effects of endotoxin.[24] Pigs, rabbits, sheep, nonhuman primates, and humans show an enhanced response.[66] Despite this difference in endotoxin sensitivity, most studies have continued to use high-endotoxin doses in resistant species. However, the main reason for the decline in use of dogs for study of all types is the high visibility this species has in the community at large. While there are many valid reasons not to study canines, cats and dogs are generally not used in scientific experiments mainly because of society's antipathy to their use for such purposes.

Sheep have been used for septic studies.[67] This model is relevant because sheep replicate human cardiopulmonary changes in sepsis and septic shock. The hyperdynamic situation described by Dr Pittet and colleagues,[20,67] with the lower dosage of endotoxin, mimics the commonly observed situation with endotoxin doses that resemble those that induce sepsis-like changes in volunteers. This model and similar ones have demonstrated cytokine release in models of sepsis using sheep.[68] Sheep models have also been used to evaluate pulmonary transvascular fluid flux during sepsis.[69] Fischer and colleagues[70,71] demonstrated in a sheep model that hypoxic pulmonary vasoconstriction is lost during sepsis. It has also been shown that myocardial contractile force is depressed even in milder forms of sepsis in sheep, which is similar to what happens in porcine models and in human sepsis.[72] A prime rationale for the use of sheep as experimental subjects in many studies is that this species presents a unique model for the study of transvascular fluid flux. Sheep are unique in that they have a single lymphatic that drains the lung.[71] Multiple small afferent lymphatics drain the lung and then pass across the pulmonary ligament and enter the caudal mediastinal lymph node, which is drained by a single efferent. Relatively pure lung lymph can be obtained by tying off the caudal end of the node and cauterizing the surface of the diaphragm. Preparation of chronic lung lymphatic allows the measure of pulmonary transvascular fluid flux over several weeks. For this purpose, the sheep model is unique.

Porcine models of sepsis have been used extensively because pigs are readily available, large, and have a low profile in the community. Pigs are much better suited for studies of sepsis and shock compared with canine models because dogs, but not pigs, have a sphincter around the hepatic vein that is sensitive to adrenergic stimulation.[65] In response to adrenergic stimulation, such as that after the onset of shock, this sphincter constricts in canine models, raising intestinal venous pressure, injuring the mucosal barrier, and promoting translation of gut flora.[65] The pig is very sensitive to sepsis-induced capillary leak, promoting the development of pulmonary edema. Therefore, volume resuscitation must be done with caution in this model. A fluid resuscitation quantity of approximately 2 L on day 1 and 1 L on subsequent days can be administered with minimal risk for clinically significant pulmonary edema.[27] In the pig, a significant rise in pulmonary vascular resistance also exacerbates the pulmonary leak. The coagulation changes in porcine sepsis are similar to those seen in human sepsis.[73] The typical hemodynamic profile of lethal porcine septic shock is a decrease in cardiac output concomitant with tachycardia. Mean arterial pressure, stroke volume, and ejection fraction all decrease, while mean pulmonary artery pressure and pulmonary vascular resistance increase.[74]

Sepsis has been modeled by endotoxin infusion, bacterial infusion, and peritonitis as infection stimulus. (See **Table 1**) demonstrates endotoxin infusion amounts and time ranges in previous experimentation.[75,76] Murphey and Traber[77] and Vassilev and colleagues[76] used a novel approach for endotoxin infusion titration to mean pulmonary artery pressure. Murphey and Traber[77] held endotoxin infusion after the initial rise of mean pulmonary artery pressure above 45 mm Hg and then restarted the infusion at a fixed dose when the mean pulmonary artery pressure dropped to less than 40 mm Hg. The potential benefit of such an approach is to counter the profound rise in pulmonary vascular resistance that may occur in the pig after *Escherichia coli* infection and may be the determining factor for survival. Lee and colleagues[78] allowed up to 18 hours to elapse after surgery to implant an osmotic pump before starting continuous intraperitoneal infusion of *Salmonella enteritidis* endotoxin. This allowed for complete recovery from surgical stress and its accompanying stress hormones and anesthesia. Intravenous bacterial infusion models have used *E coli*, *Pseudomonas aeruginosa*, or group A streptococcus.[24,27,79–81] Peritonitis models have used peritoneal injection of diluted cecal content or diluted cecal content plus *E coli*, direct installation of *E coli*, open gastrotomy with subsequent closure, or a bacteria-impregnated autologous clot.[27]

To avoid many limitations inherent in other animal models, the use of nonhuman primates has been proposed.[63] Hinshaw's group pioneered baboon models.[64] These models have been further developed.[63] The baboon offers all the advantages of a large animal: It is comparable to the human in nearly all physiologic and immunologic aspects, and it is available for acute and chronic studies (including survival). Cross-reactivity with human therapeutic and diagnostic reagents allows, on the one hand, testing of new species-specific therapies, such as antihuman antibodies, and, on the other hand, monitoring with available human analytical procedures.

CLINICAL RELEVANCE OF ANIMAL MODELS IN SEPSIS RESEARCH TODAY

Despite huge expenditure of time and resources on the evaluation of new drugs for the treatment of sepsis and septic shock, little success has been achieved. As of today, only one drug, activated protein C (drotrecogin alpha) has been approved by the FDA for the treatment of sepsis.[4] Activated protein C has not been widely accepted and its efficacy and proper use are still debated.[82–84] A common pathway to all the failed drugs studied in sepsis has been the use of animal models. Preclinical studies in these models have revealed that hundreds of biologic interventions can improve outcomes in any of dozens of animal models of sepsis; yet, with very few exceptions, these have not translated into effective treatments for human sepsis. This has prompted a reevaluation of the process of developing new therapies of sepsis, including initial in vitro testing, animal models, and the design of clinical trials.[12,66,85] The use of animal models, in particular, has been questioned and reevaluated.[6,13,15,51] The classic approach is to insist that further advances can be made only after careful experimentation in established animal models, while a new school of thought has arisen that insists that these studies may be misleading if not irrelevant.

We believe that animal models remain clinically relevant in sepsis both for further elucidation of potential mechanisms of disease and as part of novel drug discovery. Many potential reasons have been discussed in the literature as to why so many therapeutic agents that showed benefit in animal models later failed to show the same benefit in clinical trials. We have discussed some factors that play a role in animal models and might explain this phenomenon. Another proposed explanation has centered on the severity (mortality rate) of animal models in which drugs showed benefit and the severity (mortality of placebo group) in clinical trials. The severity of the septic insult has varied significantly between animal models and clinical populations with sepsis, severe sepsis, and septic shock. Eichacker and colleagues[86] performed a meta-analysis of trials involving immunomodulatory drugs for sepsis. In this study, they showed that the mortality in control groups (untreated patients/animals) was 88% for animals but only 39% for humans.[86] Furthermore, regardless of multiple factors (timing, dosing, and duration of insult) the benefit from these therapeutic agents increased as the risk of death increased. This benefit was consistent in different types of sepsis animal models. Similar trends were seen in a subgroup analysis of the PROWESS study that evaluated activated protein C in patients with severe sepsis.[47] Benefit from the drug was increased in patients with higher risk of death as measured by Acute Physiology and Chronic Health Evaluation (APACHE) II scores and number of organ failures.[47] These findings suggest that we should pair the severity of our animal models to the severity expected in the eventual clinical trial.

The classic paradigm of discovery therapeutics has been successful in many other disease states. This process proceeds smoothly from molecular discovery (now using "high through-put screening" directed toward a prediscovered "therapeutic target," to increasingly complex nonclinical (animal) models up the phylogenetic path to eventual phase I, II, and III clinical studies. In sepsis and critical care, this pathway is littered with false starts, failed clinical trials, dead ends, and clinical studies whose overall results were dismal, but whose subgroup analysis has yielded surprisingly effective results in selected populations of subjects. Relative failure may logically relate to failures at several steps—failure to properly identify the key "drug target" for the disease under study (in our case, sepsis), failure to design and use appropriate preclinical models, and failure to adequately design and conduct appropriate clinical trials—or, less often considered, failure may stem from failure of the fundamental drug discovery paradigm.

The current central dogma for drug and therapeutic discovery process relies on Paul Ehrlich's "magic bullet" concept: one disease, one target. Translated for the genetic era, this means: one gene, one target, one agent, one disease.[87] This underlying assumption implies effective and safe agents will be discovered because of selectivity of agents to define targets, inducing defined and designed biologic effects.

The recent application of many new technologies in molecular biology has made apparent that the host response to pathogen invasion (sepsis) is not linear, but rather network based.[88,89] Calvano and colleagues,[88] on behalf of a large-scale collaborative research program, analyzed changes in blood leukocyte gene expression patterns in human subjects receiving an inflammatory stimulus (bacterial endotoxin) and in subjects who were critically ill.[90] They reported genome-wide expression varied significantly among different subjects and leukocyte subpopulations. As expected, traumatic injury induced dramatic changes in apparent gene expression that were greater in magnitude than the analytical noise and interindividual variance. Many biologic pathways affect the progression of infectious disease, and distinct biologic pathways are inhibited or activated during different stages and by different types of infectious disease. SABiosciences (www.sabiosciences.com) lists 25 distinct biologic pathways recommended for infectious disease research, including those related to chemokines and their receptors, cytokines, adhesion molecules, interferon and its receptor, NFkβ signaling, Toll-like receptor signaling, and tumor necrosis factor α ligand and its receptors.

We have discovered similar widespread gene activation in myocardium of infected pigs.[89] Myocardial samples were taken at basal (before) and hourly after implantation of an *E coli*–infected clot intra-peritoneal. Gene transcription (Affymetrix) was determined to be differentially regulated at a greater than or less than twofold change ($P<.05$). Peritonitis significantly increased gene expression changes over time. A comparison of sham versus infected animals at 2, 3, 4, and 6 hours after clot implant revealed that 32, 74, 189, and 601 genes were significantly dysregulated, respectively. One important biologically associated network is the Toll-like receptor signaling pathway; its changes between basal and 4 hours of peritonitis is illustrated in **Fig. 2**. The green boxes indicate which gene transcripts were significantly dysregulated. Clearly illustrated in this figure is the complex interrelationship among so many important inflammatory mediators. The wide distribution of the green boxes (significant dysregulation) demonstrates the complexity of the host response to peritonitis. These data demonstrate extreme complexity of response and suggest that the underlying assumption of "one target, one disease" may indeed be an intellectual construct no longer supportable by available data. As we have reviewed above, the notable lack of success in development of new therapeutic agents for sepsis poses a severe challenge to this paradigm of drug development.

The logic of using of animal models to help in developing new and more successful therapies for treatment of sepsis and shock cannot be dismissed, despite numerous failures and weaknesses of previous studies. Such experimentation is mandated by the ethical rules for the conduct of research. For example, a recent draft from the FDA of guidelines for development of new anticancer drugs lists numerous nonclinical (animal) data as requirements for a new drug application.[10,15] In this published *Guidance for Industry*, nonclinical (animal) pharmacology and toxicology is a mandated section that includes animal studies on general pharmacology (definition of mechanism of action), safety pharmacology, pharmacokinetics, general toxicology, reproduction toxicology, genotoxicity, carcinogenicity, and immunotoxicity. Therefore, the use of animal models for developing new therapeutics for sepsis will

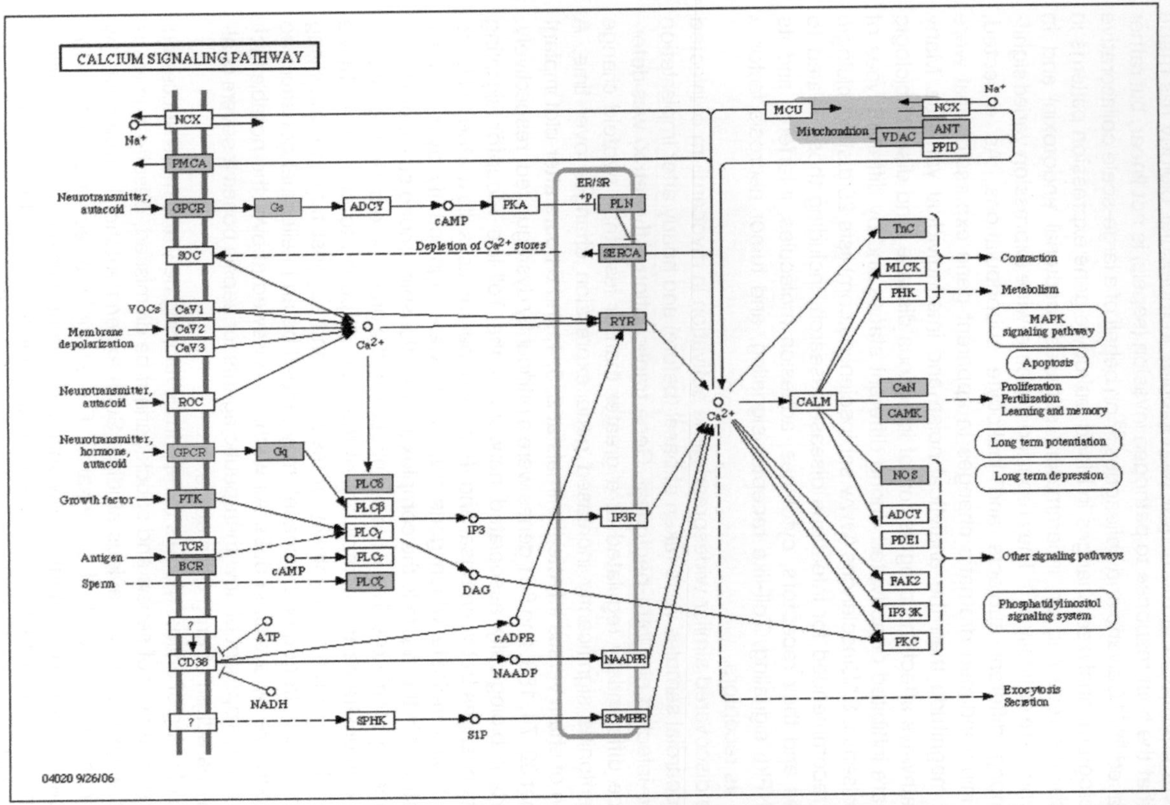

Fig. 2. Alterations in Toll-like receptor signaling pathway induced by peritonitis. This figure is based on data obtained by biopsy of hearts of pigs subjected to near lethal *E coli* peritonitis.[75,90] Gene transcription was evaluated following mRNA isolation by Affymetrix porcine chips. The relationship between gene products was analyzed by GeneSifter, Inc Green boxes indicate transcripts significantly altered by peritonitis.

continue. So, our challenge is to ensure that animal experimentation is as useful as it can be in the development of novel therapeutics.

SUMMARY

We have reviewed important factors that determine clinical relevance of animal models of sepsis and have discussed in further detail specific models as they relate to small and large animals. Finally, we have discussed some of the current concerns and potential explanations related to the role of animal models in sepsis, especially as they relate to their poor performance in predicting successful novel therapeutics. It is apparent that animal models of sepsis will continue to be an important part of ongoing sepsis research. We should pay more attention to factors that will increase the relevance of our animal models. Furthermore, we should seek to understand the advantages and limitations of each individual animal model. It is hoped that this will lead to a better use of this tool and will allow us to obtain valuable information from our animal models of sepsis.

REFERENCES

1. Abraham E, Matthay MA, Dinarello CA, et al. Consensus conference definitions for sepsis, septic shock, acute lung injury, and acute respiratory distress syndrome: time for a reevaluation. Crit Care Med 2000;28:232.
2. Bone RC, Balk RA, Cerra FB, et al. The ACCP/SCCM Consensus Conference Committee, American College of Chest Physicians/Society of Critical Care Medicine. Definitions for sepsis and organ failure and guidelines for the use of innovative therapies in sepsis. Chest 1992;101:1644.
3. Angus DC, Linde-Zwirble WT, Lidicker J, et al. Epidemiology of severe sepsis in the United States: analysis of incidence, outcome, and associated costs of care. Crit Care Med 2001;29:1303.
4. Bernard GR, Vincent JL, Laterre PF, et al. Efficacy and safety of recombinant human activated protein C for severe sepsis. N Engl J Med 2001;344:699.
5. Esper AM, Moss M, Lewis CA, et al. The role of infection and comorbidity: factors that influence disparities in sepsis. Crit Care Med 2006;34:2576.
6. Marshall JC, Deitch E, Moldawer LL, et al. Preclinical models of shock and sepsis: what can they tell us? Shock 2005;24(Suppl 1):1.
7. Cohen J, Guyatt G, Bernard GR, et al. New strategies for clinical trials in patients with sepsis and septic shock. Crit Care Med 2001;29:880.
8. Fink MP, Heard SO. Laboratory models of sepsis and septic shock. J Surg Res 1990;49:186.
9. Bockamp E, Maringer M, Spangenberg C, et al. Of mice and models: improved animal models for biomedical research. Physiol Genomics 2002;11:115.
10. Food and Drug Administration. Nonclinical evaluation for anticancer pharmaceuticals. 2009.
11. Guidance for industry; providing regulatory submissions in electronic format—NDAs. US Dept Health, Center for drug Evaluation and Research; 1999.
12. Marshall JC. Such stuff as dreams are made on: mediator-directed therapy in sepsis. Nat Rev Drug Discov 2003;2:391.
13. Dyson A, Singer M. Animal models of sepsis: why does preclinical efficacy fail to translate to the clinical setting? Crit Care Med 2009;37:S30.
14. Esmon CT. Why do animal models (sometimes) fail to mimic human sepsis? Crit Care Med 2004;32:S219.

away from tissues, thereby leading to inadequate oxygen extraction required for normal cellular metabolism, even in the context of normal hemodynamic parameters.[8,10–12]

The arterioles, capillaries, and venules of the microcirculation are the architecture on which complex and integrated homeostatic, hemostatic, and immune functions occur. Sepsis results in dysfunction of all these systems via dysregulation of vasomotor control, endothelial injury, coagulation activation, and disordered leukocyte trafficking (**Fig. 1**).

Central to the functions of the microcirculation is the endothelium. The endothelium is an intricate organ composed of almost 10^{13} cells and covering 4000 to 7000 m^2 in an adult and is responsible for regulation of microvessel thrombosis, profibrinolysis, leukocyte adherence, microvascular tone, permeability, and blood flow.[13] Under normal circumstances, the endothelium will regulate blood flow by recruiting microvessels with endogenous vasodilators. Nitric oxide (NO) seems to be the key molecule in the regulation of the microvasculature as determined by the endothelium.[14] Systemic inflammatory mediators and endotoxins disrupt the intracellular coupling and signaling pathways used by endothelial cells to act as a unified system. This disruption may result in the maldistribution of blood flow in tissue beds.[15]

In addition to controlling local blood flow via modulation of vascular tone, the endothelium is critical to the maintenance of hemostasis by expressing anti- and procoagulant proteins. Endothelial cells in a healthy state have primarily anticoagulant properties through their production of thrombomodulin (which activates protein C), tissue factor pathway inhibitor, heparin (which potentiates the action of antithrombin III), and tissue plasminogen activator. In sepsis, endothelial dysfunction may lead to activation of the extrinsic coagulation pathway and promulgation of the intrinsic coagulation pathway and dampened anticoagulation activity, resulting in a heterogeneous imbalance of hemostasis and, ultimately, microvascular flow.[16] Specifically, there is increased endothelial cell tissue factor release, decreased thrombomodulin

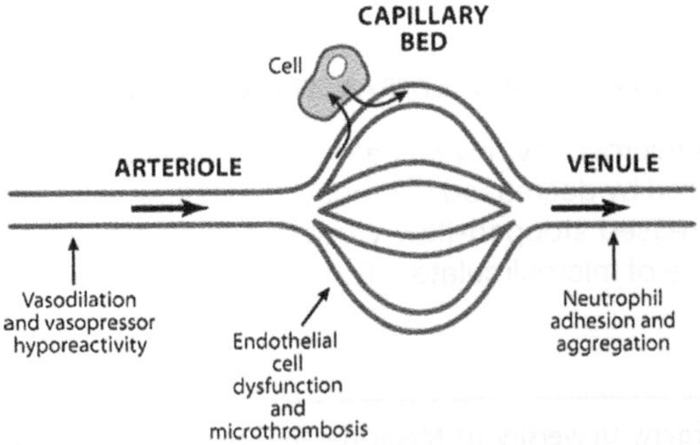

Fig. 1. Sepsis is a disorder of the microcirculation. Much of the pathophysiology of sepsis can be explained within the microcirculatory unit—the terminal arteriole, the capillary bed, and the postcapillary venule. The arteriole is where the characteristic vasodilation and vasopressor hyporesponsiveness of sepsis occurs. The capillary bed is where the effects of endothelial cell activation/dysfunction are most pronounced and microvascular thromboses are formed. The postcapillary venule is where leukocyte trafficking is most disordered—leukocytes adhere to the vessel wall, aggregate, and further impair flow through the microcirculation. (*From* Trzeciak S, Cinel I, Phillip Dellinger R, et al. Resuscitating the microcirculation in sepsis: the central role of nitric oxide, emerging concepts for novel therapies, and challenges for clinical trials. Acad Emerg Med 2008;15:399–413; with permission.)

expression, and, therefore, decreased protein C activation. Low levels of protein C have been related to poor outcomes in septic patients.[17]

Endothelial cells are constantly reacting to and participating in the dynamic milieu of biochemical actions. In this way, they help tissues adapt to second-to-second changes in metabolic needs and insults. However, at times, endothelial response may be maladaptive and harmful to the surrounding tissue. In the presence of proinflammatory stimuli, such as interleukin-1, interleukin-6, tumor necrosis factor-α, or oxidative stress,[18] endothelial "activation" occurs, leading to a procoagulant environment, proadhesive cell surfaces, dysregulation of vasomotor tone, and compromised barrier function. This inflammatory environment is further propagated by the release of additional cytokines directly from endothelial cells, which leads to further local microvascular damage, disrupted tight junctions, edema, and tissue hypoxia. Under these conditions, the upregulation of the gene for hypoxia-inducible factor-1 will increase the expression of vascular endothelial growth factor (VEGF). Studies have shown VEGF to be associated with disease severity, organ failure, and death in septic patients.[19,20]

Sepsis also affects the function of cellular components of blood as they pass through the microcirculatory vessels. In a complex, multistep adhesion cascade involving E-selectin and intracellular adhesion molecule-1, activated endothelial cells mediate leukocyte trafficking and firm adhesion to the endothelium. Furthermore, red blood cells exhibit an impaired ability to deform and pass easily through microvessels,[21,22] leading to aggregation, adherence,[23] and further decreased oxygen availability to tissues.

In summary, sepsis induces many changes in the microvascular environment, many of which are mediated by the activation and dysfunction of endothelial cells. The common end result of these effects is decreased oxygen transport to cells, which, if left uncorrected, may lead to organ failure and death.[24]

NITRIC OXIDE AND MICROCIRCULATION

Modulation of NO is central in the pathophysiology of sepsis. NO has a fundamental role in maintaining the flow in microvessels by mediating vascular tone, leukocyte adhesion, platelet aggregation, microthrombi formation, and microvascular permeability.[25–32] Although systemic NO production is upregulated in sepsis, in specific tissues,[33] NO production may be heterogeneous (ie, relatively deficient) because of several factors. Variation in the extent of expression of inducible nitric oxide synthase (iNOS)[33,34] and consumption of NO by reactive oxygen radicals in ischemic tissues may lead to a relative paucity of NO in microcirculatory beds despite a total body excess.[34,35] In turn, this may lead to the known pathologic shunting of oxygenated blood from susceptible tissues, which characterizes the heterogeneous tissue perfusion of sepsis.[8,10,36] One mechanism affecting this diversion is the opening of arteriovenous shunts in capillary beds.[35]

EVALUATION OF MICROCIRCULATION IN SEPTIC PATIENTS

Historically, global hemodynamic parameters have been the primary focus of clinical investigations and management strategies for patients with sepsis. However, evaluation of the microcirculation is important to fully understand the pathophysiology of circulatory derangements in sepsis and organ failure. In vivo visualization of microcirculatory beds was formerly only available in animal models, but new technology has made it possible in the clinical arena. In patients with sepsis, microcirculatory failure in the early phase of therapy and persistence of these

SUMMARY

Septic shock is a common and deadly disease that traditionally has been diagnosed and treated by evaluation and optimization of global hemodynamic indices. However, microcirculatory dysfunction is a critically important element in the pathophysiology of this disease. New techniques of in vivo video microscopy permit the assessment of microcirculatory function in human subjects. With the advent of these techniques, the microcirculation may represent a new frontier for developing novel therapies for sepsis.

REFERENCES

1. Angus DC, Linde-Zwirble WT, Lidicker J, et al. Epidemiology of severe sepsis in the United States: analysis of incidence, outcome, and associated costs of care. Crit Care Med 2001;29(7):1303–10.
2. Hotchkiss RS, Karl IE. The pathophysiology and treatment of sepsis. N Engl J Med 2003;348(2):138–50.
3. Rivers E, Nguyen B, Havstad S, et al. Early goal-directed therapy in the treatment of severe sepsis and septic shock. N Engl J Med 2001;345(19):1368–77.
4. Lin SM, Huang CD, Lin HC, et al. A modified goal-directed protocol improves clinical outcomes in intensive care unit patients with septic shock: a randomized controlled trial. Shock 2006;26(6):551–7.
5. Jones AE, Brown MD, Trzeciak S, et al. The effect of a quantitative resuscitation strategy on mortality in patients with sepsis: a meta-analysis. Crit Care Med 2008;36(10):2734–9.
6. Otero RM, Nguyen HB, Huang DT, et al. Early goal-directed therapy in severe sepsis and septic shock revisited: concepts, controversies, and contemporary findings. Chest 2006;130(5):1579–95.
7. Ellis CG, Bateman RM, Sharpe MD, et al. Effect of a maldistribution of microvascular blood flow on capillary O(2) extraction in sepsis. Am J Physiol Heart Circ Physiol 2002;282(1):H156–64.
8. Farquhar I, Martin CM, Lam C, et al. Decreased capillary density in vivo in bowel mucosa of rats with normotensive sepsis. J Surg Res 1996;61(1):190–6.
9. Fries M, Weil MH, Sun S, et al. Increases in tissue Pco2 during circulatory shock reflect selective decreases in capillary blood flow. Crit Care Med 2006;34(2): 446–52.
10. Lam C, Tyml K, Martin C, et al. Microvascular perfusion is impaired in a rat model of normotensive sepsis. J Clin Invest 1994;94(5):2077–83.
11. De Backer D, Creteur J, Preiser JC, et al. Microvascular blood flow is altered in patients with sepsis. Am J Respir Crit Care Med 2002;166(1):98–104.
12. Sakr Y, Dubois MJ, De Backer D, et al. Persistent microcirculatory alterations are associated with organ failure and death in patients with septic shock. Crit Care Med 2004;32(9):1825–31.
13. Aird WC. Endothelium as an organ system. Crit Care Med 2004;32(5 Suppl): s271–9.
14. Palmer RM, Ferrige AG, Moncada S. Nitric oxide release accounts for the biological activity of endothelium-derived relaxing factor. Nature 1987;327(6122): 524–6.
15. Tyml K, Wang X, Lidington D, et al. Lipopolysaccharide reduces intercellular coupling in vitro and arteriolar conducted response in vivo. Am J Physiol Heart Circ Physiol 2001;281(3):H1397–406.
16. Aird WC. Vascular bed-specific hemostasis: role of endothelium in sepsis pathogenesis. Crit Care Med 2001;29(7 Suppl):s28–34 [discussion: s34–5].

17. Yan SB, Helterbrand JD, Hartman DL, et al. Low levels of protein C are associated with poor outcome in severe sepsis. Chest 2001;120(3):915–22.
18. Terada LS, Hybertson BM, Connelly KG, et al. XO increases neutrophil adherence to endothelial cells by a dual ICAM-1 and P-selectin-mediated mechanism. J Appl Physiol 1997;82(3):866–73.
19. Shapiro NI, Yano K, Okada H, et al. A prospective, observational study of soluble Flt-1 and vascular endothelial growth factor in sepsis. Shock 2008; 29(4):452–7.
20. Yano K, Liaw PC, Mullington JM, et al. Vascular endothelial growth factor is an important determinant of sepsis morbidity and mortality. J Exp Med 2006; 203(6):1447–58.
21. Bateman RM, Jagger JE, Sharpe MD, et al. Erythrocyte deformability is a nitric oxide-mediated factor in decreased capillary density during sepsis. Am J Physiol Heart Circ Physiol 2001;280(6):H2848–56.
22. Condon MR, Kim JE, Deitch EA, et al. Appearance of an erythrocyte population with decreased deformability and hemoglobin content following sepsis. Am J Physiol Heart Circ Physiol 2003;284(6):H2177–84.
23. Kempe DS, Akel A, Lang PA, et al. Suicidal erythrocyte death in sepsis. J Mol Med 2007;85(3):273–81.
24. Aird WC. The role of the endothelium in severe sepsis and multiple organ dysfunction syndrome. Blood 2003;101(10):3765–77.
25. Azuma H, Ishikawa M, Sekizaki S. Endothelium-dependent inhibition of platelet aggregation. Br J Pharmacol 1986;88(2):411–5.
26. Cambien B, Bergmeier W, Saffaripour S, et al. Antithrombotic activity of TNF-alpha. J Clin Invest 2003;112(10):1589–96.
27. Hutcheson IR, Whittle BJ, Boughton-Smith NK. Role of nitric oxide in maintaining vascular integrity in endotoxin-induced acute intestinal damage in the rat. Br J Pharmacol 1990;101(4):815–20.
28. Kubes P, Suzuki M, Granger DN. Nitric oxide: an endogenous modulator of leukocyte adhesion. Proc Natl Acad Sci U S A 1991;88(11):4651–5.
29. Mendelsohn ME, O'Neill S, George D, et al. Inhibition of fibrinogen binding to human platelets by S-nitroso-N-acetylcysteine. J Biol Chem 1990;265(31):19028–34.
30. Radomski MW, Palmer RM, Moncada S. Endogenous nitric oxide inhibits human platelet adhesion to vascular endothelium. Lancet 1987;2(8567):1057–8.
31. Radomski MW, Vallance P, Whitley G, et al. Platelet adhesion to human vascular endothelium is modulated by constitutive and cytokine induced nitric oxide. Cardiovasc Res 1993;27(7):1380–2.
32. Shultz PJ, Raij L. Endogenously synthesized nitric oxide prevents endotoxin-induced glomerular thrombosis. J Clin Invest 1992;90(5):1718–25.
33. Cunha FQ, Assreuy J, Moss DW, et al. Differential induction of nitric oxide synthase in various organs of the mouse during endotoxaemia: role of TNF-alpha and IL-1-beta. Immunology 1994;81(2):211–5.
34. Morin MJ, Unno N, Hodin RA, et al. Differential expression of inducible nitric oxide synthase messenger RNA along the longitudinal and crypt-villus axes of the intestine in endotoxemic rats. Crit Care Med 1998;26(7):1258–64.
35. Ince C, Sinaasappel M. Microcirculatory oxygenation and shunting in sepsis and shock. Crit Care Med 1999;27(7):1369–77.
36. Trzeciak S, Dellinger RP, Parrillo JE, et al. Early microcirculatory perfusion derangements in patients with severe sepsis and septic shock: relationship to hemodynamics, oxygen transport, and survival. Ann Emerg Med 2007;49(1): 88–98, 98, e1–2.

37. Doerschug KC, Delsing AS, Schmidt GA, et al. Impairments in microvascular reactivity are related to organ failure in human sepsis. Am J Physiol Heart Circ Physiol 2007;293(2):H1065–71.
38. Vincent JL, De Backer D. Microvascular dysfunction as a cause of organ dysfunction in severe sepsis. Crit Care 2005;9(Suppl 4):s9–12.
39. Levy MM, Macias WL, Vincent JL, et al. Early changes in organ function predict eventual survival in severe sepsis. Crit Care Med 2005;33(10):2194–201.
40. Shapiro N, Howell MD, Bates DW, et al. The association of sepsis syndrome and organ dysfunction with mortality in emergency department patients with suspected infection. Ann Emerg Med 2006;48(5):583–90, 590, e1.
41. Trzeciak S, McCoy JV, Phillip Dellinger R, et al. Early increases in microcirculatory perfusion during protocol-directed resuscitation are associated with reduced multi-organ failure at 24 h in patients with sepsis. Intensive Care Med 2008;34(12):2210–7.
42. Goedhart PT, Khalilzada M, Bezemer R, et al. Sidestream Dark Field (SDF) imaging: a novel stroboscopic LED ring-based imaging modality for clinical assessment of the microcirculation. Opt Express 2007;15:15101–14.
43. Groner W, Winkelman JW, Harris AG, et al. Orthogonal polarization spectral imaging: a new method for study of the microcirculation. Nat Med 1999;5(10): 1209–12.
44. Harris AG, Sinitsina I, Messmer K. The Cytoscan Model E-II, a new reflectance microscope for intravital microscopy: comparison with the standard fluorescence method. J Vasc Res 2000;37(6):469–76.
45. Mathura KR, Vollebregt KC, Boer K, et al. Comparison of OPS imaging and conventional capillary microscopy to study the human microcirculation. J Appl Physiol 2001;91(1):74–8.
46. Mazzarelli J, Guglielmi M, Ross F, et al. Leukocyte dynamics measured by orthogonal polarization spectral imaging correlate with video microscopy [abstract]. Shock 2005;23(Suppl 3):122.
47. Creteur J, De Backer D, Sakr Y, et al. Sublingual capnometry tracks microcirculatory changes in septic patients. Intensive Care Med 2006;32(4): 516–23.
48. Marik PE. Sublingual capnography: a clinical validation study. Chest 2001; 120(3):923–7.
49. Nakagawa Y, Weil MH, Tang W, et al. Sublingual capnometry for diagnosis and quantitation of circulatory shock. Am J Respir Crit Care Med 1998;157(6 Pt 1): 1838–43.
50. Weil MH, Nakagawa Y, Tang W, et al. Sublingual capnometry: a new noninvasive measurement for diagnosis and quantitation of severity of circulatory shock. Crit Care Med 1999;27(7):1225–9.
51. Jin X, Weil MH, Sun S, et al. Decreases in organ blood flows associated with increases in sublingual PCO2 during hemorrhagic shock. J Appl Physiol 1998; 85(6):2360–4.
52. Povoas HP, Weil MH, Tang W, et al. Comparisons between sublingual and gastric tonometry during hemorrhagic shock. Chest 2000;118(4):1127–32.
53. Povoas HP, Weil MH, Tang W, et al. Decreases in mesenteric blood flow associated with increases in sublingual PCO2 during hemorrhagic shock. Shock 2001; 15(5):398–402.
54. De Backer D, Creteur J, Noordally O, et al. Does hepato-splanchnic VO2/DO2 dependency exist in critically ill septic patients? Am J Respir Crit Care Med 1998;157(4 Pt 1):1219–25.

55. Guzman JA, Lacoma FJ, Kruse JA. Relationship between systemic oxygen supply dependency and gastric intramucosal PCO2 during progressive hemorrhage. J Trauma 1998;44(4):696–700.
56. Nelson DP, Beyer C, Samsel RW, et al. Pathological supply dependence of O2 uptake during bacteremia in dogs. J Appl Physiol 1987;63(4):1487–92.
57. Boerma EC, Van der Voort PH, Spronk PE, et al. Relationship between sublingual and intestinal microcirculatory perfusion in patients with abdominal sepsis. Crit Care Med 2007;35(4):1055–60.
58. De Backer D, Hollenberg S, Boerma C, et al. How to evaluate the microcirculation: report of a round table conference. Crit Care 2007;11(5):R101.
59. Bihari D, Smithies M, Gimson A, et al. The effects of vasodilation with prostacyclin on oxygen delivery and uptake in critically ill patients. N Engl J Med 1987; 317(7):397–403.
60. Shoemaker WC, Appel PL, Kram HB, et al. Prospective trial of supranormal values of survivors as therapeutic goals in high-risk surgical patients. Chest 1988;94(6):1176–86.
61. De Backer D, Creteur J, Dubois MJ, et al. The effects of dobutamine on microcirculatory alterations in patients with septic shock are independent of its systemic effects. Crit Care Med 2006;34(2):403–8.
62. De Backer D, Verdant C, Chierego M, et al. Effects of drotrecogin alfa activated on microcirculatory alterations in patients with severe sepsis. Crit Care Med 2006;34(7):1918–24.
63. Hoffmann JN, Vollmar B, Laschke MW, et al. Microcirculatory alterations in ischemia-reperfusion injury and sepsis: effects of activated protein C and thrombin inhibition. Crit Care 2005;9(Suppl 4):s33–7.
64. Iba T, Kidokoro A, Fukunaga M, et al. Activated protein C improves the visceral microcirculation by attenuating the leukocyte-endothelial interaction in a rat lipopolysaccharide model. Crit Care Med 2005;33(2):368–72.
65. Baker CH, Wilmoth FR. Microvascular responses to E. coli endotoxin with altered adrenergic activity. Circ Shock 1984;12(3):165–76.
66. Hollenberg SM, Broussard M, Osman J, et al. Increased microvascular reactivity and improved mortality in septic mice lacking inducible nitric oxide synthase. Circ Res 2000;86(7):774–8.
67. Hollenberg SM, Tangora JJ, Piotrowski MJ, et al. Impaired microvascular vasoconstrictive responses to vasopressin in septic rats. Crit Care Med 1997;25(5):869–73.
68. Price SA, Spain DA, Wilson MA, et al. Subacute sepsis impairs vascular smooth muscle contractile machinery and alters vasoconstrictor and dilator mechanisms. J Surg Res 1999;83(1):75–80.
69. Bakker J, Grover R, McLuckie A, et al. Administration of the nitric oxide synthase inhibitor NG-methyl-L-arginine hydrochloride (546C88) by intravenous infusion for up to 72 hours can promote the resolution of shock in patients with severe sepsis: results of a randomized, double-blind, placebo-controlled multicenter study (study no. 144-002). Crit Care Med 2004;32(1):1–12.
70. Hollenberg SM, Cunnion RE, Zimmerberg J. Nitric oxide synthase inhibition reverses arteriolar hyporesponsiveness to catecholamines in septic rats. Am J Physiol 1993;264(2 Pt 2):H660–3.
71. Hollenberg SM, Easington CR, Osman J, et al. Effects of nitric oxide synthase inhibition on microvascular reactivity in septic mice. Shock 1999;12(4):262–7.
72. Hollenberg SM, Piotrowski MJ, Parrillo JE. Nitric oxide synthase inhibition reverses arteriolar hyporesponsiveness to endothelin-1 in septic rats. Am J Physiol 1997;272(3 Pt 2):R969–74.

73. Watson D, Grover R, Anzueto A, et al. Cardiovascular effects of the nitric oxide synthase inhibitor NG-methyl-L-arginine hydrochloride (546C88) in patients with septic shock: results of a randomized, double-blind, placebo-controlled multicenter study (study no. 144-002). Crit Care Med 2004;32(1):13–20.
74. Anning PB, Sair M, Winlove CP, et al. Abnormal tissue oxygenation and cardiovascular changes in endotoxemia. Am J Respir Crit Care Med 1999;159(6): 1710–5.
75. Avontuur JA, Bruining HA, Ince C. Inhibition of nitric oxide synthesis causes myocardial ischemia in endotoxemic rats. Circ Res 1995;76(3):418–25.
76. Corso CO, Gundersen Y, Dorger M, et al. Effects of the nitric oxide synthase inhibitors N(G)-nitro-L-arginine methyl ester and aminoethyl-isothiourea on the liver microcirculation in rat endotoxemia. J Hepatol 1998;28(1):61–9.
77. Kubes P, Granger DN. Nitric oxide modulates microvascular permeability. Am J Physiol 1992;262(2 Pt 2):H611–5.
78. Nishida J, McCuskey RS, McDonnell D, et al. Protective role of NO in hepatic microcirculatory dysfunction during endotoxemia. Am J Physiol 1994;267(6 Pt 1): G1135–41.
79. Spain DA, Wilson MA, Bar-Natan MF, et al. Nitric oxide synthase inhibition aggravates intestinal microvascular vasoconstriction and hypoperfusion of bacteremia. J Trauma 1994;36(5):720–5.
80. Spain DA, Wilson MA, Bloom IT, et al. Renal microvascular responses to sepsis are dependent on nitric oxide. J Surg Res 1994;56(6):524–9.
81. Spain DA, Wilson MA, Garrison RN. Nitric oxide synthase inhibition exacerbates sepsis-induced renal hypoperfusion. Surgery 1994;116(2):322–30 [discussion: 330–1].
82. Tribl B, Bateman RM, Milkovich S, et al. Effect of nitric oxide on capillary hemodynamics and cell injury in the pancreas during *Pseudomonas* pneumonia-induced sepsis. Am J Physiol Heart Circ Physiol 2004;286(1):H340–5.
83. Binion DG, Fu S, Ramanujam KS, et al. iNOS expression in human intestinal microvascular endothelial cells inhibits leukocyte adhesion. Am J Physiol 1998;275(3 Pt 1):G592–603.
84. Sundrani R, Easington CR, Mattoo A, et al. Nitric oxide synthase inhibition increases venular leukocyte rolling and adhesion in septic rats. Crit Care Med 2000;28(8):2898–903.
85. Hickey MJ, Granger DN, Kubes P. Inducible nitric oxide synthase (iNOS) and regulation of leucocyte/endothelial cell interactions: studies in iNOS-deficient mice. Acta Physiol Scand 2001;173(1):119–26.
86. Hickey MJ, Sharkey KA, Sihota EG, et al. Inducible nitric oxide synthase-deficient mice have enhanced leukocyte-endothelium interactions in endotoxemia. FASEB J 1997;11(12):955–64.
87. Lush CW, Cepinskas G, Sibbald WJ, et al. Endothelial E- and P-selectin expression in iNOS-deficient mice exposed to polymicrobial sepsis. Am J Physiol Gastrointest Liver Physiol 2001;280(2):G291–7.
88. Dellinger RP, Parrillo JE. Mediator modulation therapy of severe sepsis and septic shock: does it work? Crit Care Med 2004;32(1):282–6.
89. Lopez A, Lorente JA, Steingrub J, et al. Multiple-center, randomized, placebo-controlled, double-blind study of the nitric oxide synthase inhibitor 546C88: effect on survival in patients with septic shock. Crit Care Med 2004;32(1): 21–30.
90. De Caterina R, Libby P, Peng HB, et al. Nitric oxide decreases cytokine-induced endothelial activation. Nitric oxide selectively reduces endothelial expression of

adhesion molecules and proinflammatory cytokines. J Clin Invest 1995;96(1):60–8.
91. Boughton-Smith NK, Hutcheson IR, Deakin AM, et al. Protective effect of S-nitroso-N-acetyl-penicillamine in endotoxin-induced acute intestinal damage in the rat. Eur J Pharmacol 1990;191(3):485–8.
92. Gundersen Y, Corso CO, Leiderer R, et al. The nitric oxide donor sodium nitroprusside protects against hepatic microcirculatory dysfunction in early endotoxaemia. Intensive Care Med 1998;24(12):1257–63.
93. Siegemund M, van Bommel J, Vollebrecht K, et al. Influence of nitric oxide donor SIN-1 on the gut oxygenation in a normodynamic, porcine model of low-dose endotoxemia [abstract]. Intensive Care Med 2000;26:S362.
94. Zhang H, Rogiers P, Smail N, et al. Effects of nitric oxide on blood flow distribution and O2 extraction capabilities during endotoxic shock. J Appl Physiol 1997;83(4):1164–73.
95. Spronk PE, Ince C, Gardien MJ, et al. Nitroglycerin in septic shock after intravascular volume resuscitation. Lancet 2002;360(9343):1395–6.
96. Spronk P, Ince C, Gardien M, et al. Nitroglycerin for septic shock. Lancet 2003;361(9360):880.
97. Randomized Trial of Inhaled Nitric Oxide to Augment Tissue Perfusion in Sepsis (NCT00608322). Available at: http://www.ClinicalTrials.gov. National Library of Medicine, Bethesda. Accessed May, 2009.
98. The Effect of Nitroglycerine on Microcirculatory Abnormalities During Sepsis (NCT00493415). Available at: http://www.ClinicalTrials.gov. National Library of Medicine, Bethesda. Accessed May, 2009.
99. Abraham E, Singer M. Mechanisms of sepsis-induced organ dysfunction. Crit Care Med 2007;35(10):2408–16.
100. Cinel I, Dellinger RP. Advances in pathogenesis and management of sepsis. Curr Opin Infect Dis 2007;20(4):345–52.
101. Fink MP. Bench-to-bedside review: cytopathic hypoxia. Crit Care 2002;6(6):491–9.
102. Hotchkiss RS, Karl IE. Reevaluation of the role of cellular hypoxia and bioenergetic failure in sepsis. JAMA 1992;267(11):1503–10.
103. Watts JA, Kline JA. Bench to bedside: the role of mitochondrial medicine in the pathogenesis and treatment of cellular injury. Acad Emerg Med 2003;10(9):985–97.
104. Singer M, De Santis V, Vitale D, et al. Multiorgan failure is an adaptive, endocrine-mediated, metabolic response to overwhelming systemic inflammation. Lancet 2004;364(9433):545–8.

suggest a doubling of total United States cases by 2050 with an increase in population of only 33%.[1] Despite major advances in technology and constant refinement of our understanding of sepsis pathophysiology, numerous clinical trials have failed until recently to produce any new drugs with consistent beneficial effects on this patient population. Nonetheless, the last 50 years have seen a gradual improvement in mortality. This improvement is perhaps related to improvements in supportive care.[5,7]

Historically, critically ill patients with overwhelming infection have not been considered a unique subgroup comparable to neutropenic patients for purposes of selection of antimicrobial therapy. However, critically ill patients with severe sepsis and septic shock, like neutropenics, are characterized by distinct differences from the typical infected patient. These differences affect management strategy.

These differences include:

Marked alterations in antibiotic pharmacokinetics

- An increased frequency of hepatic and renal dysfunction
- A high prevalence of unrecognized immune dysfunction
- A predisposition to infection with resistant organisms
- A marked increase in frequency of adverse outcome if there is a failure to rapidly initiate effective antibiotic therapy

Critical management decisions in this patient group must often be made emergently in the absence of definitive data regarding the infecting organism, its sensitivity pattern, patient immune status, and organ function. The speed in which an appropriate antimicrobial regimen is administered at first presentation strongly influences outcomes in severe sepsis and septic shock. For this reason, a particularly thoughtful and judicious approach to initial empiric antimicrobial therapy is required.[4,8–11]

Understanding of basic pharmacologic principles of antimicrobial therapy is crucial for its appropriate use in critically ill patients with sepsis and septic shock. This article reviews principles in the rational use of antibiotics in sepsis and presents evidence-based recommendations for optimal antibiotic therapy.

RATIONAL USE OF ANTIBIOTICS IN SEPSIS

Along with appropriate resuscitation, optimal use of antibiotic regimens is the critical determinant of survival in sepsis and septic shock.[8,12] Beyond the issues related to the infecting organisms and their sensitivity profile, optimal antimicrobial therapy includes assessment of host factors (eg, immune status, organ function, site of infection), pharmacokinetics (eg, drug absorption, distribution, elimination), and pharmacodynamics (eg, mode of action, bacteriocidal vs bacteriostatic characteristics, rate of killing).[13–17] In many circumstances in the critically ill, standard antimicrobial regimens require modification (**Table 1**). Because the infecting organism is not known at the time of antibiotic initiation, empiric antibiotic therapy is based on clinical presentation and epidemiologic factors, including local flora, resistance patterns and previous antibiotic exposure. Other patient factors that may affect antibiotic choice include specific susceptibilities (eg, encapsulated organisms in splenectomized patients, *Pseudomonas* in neutropenics), antibiotic toxicity (anaphylaxis, angioneurotic edema, Stevens-Johnson syndrome, allergic interstitial nephritis), and organ dysfunction (selection and dosing of antibiotics). The metabolic and immunologic derangements in critically ill patients and simultaneous use of many other pharmacologic agents can substantially affect the pharmacokinetics and pharmacodynamics of antimicrobial therapy. An inappropriate antibiotic prescription in critically ill septic patients can

Table 1
Indication for extended empiric antibiotic therapy of severe sepsis/septic shock

Therapy	Indication
Gram-negative coverage	1. Nosocomial infection 2. Neutropenic or immunosuppressed 3. Immunocompromised due to chronic organ failure (eg, liver, kidneys, lung, heart)
Gram-positive coverage (vancomycin or alternative novel gram-positive agent)	1. High-level endemic methicillin-resistant *Staphylococcus aureus* (community-acquired or nosocomial) 2. Neutropenic patient 3. Intravascular catheter infection 4. Nosocomial pneumonia
Fungal/yeast coverage (triazole, echinocandin, amphotericin B)	1. Neutropenic fever or other immunosuppressed patient unresponsive to standard antibiotic therapy 2. Prolonged broad-spectrum antibiotic therapy 3. Positive relevant fungal cultures 4. Consider empiric therapy if high-risk patient with severe shock

substantially increase mortality (septic shock, nosocomial pneumonia) and morbidity (seeding of prosthetic valves, vascular grafts, artificial joints).

CLINICAL PHARMACOLOGY OF ANTIBIOTICS

Effective treatment of an established infection requires delivery of a sufficient amount of drugs to the local site of infection for adequate time to affect a cure. Because this cannot be directly measured, substitute in vitro parameters reflecting probability of success of antimicrobial therapy have been established (antibiotic susceptibility testing).

Susceptibility testing involves serially diluting antibiotic solutions overnight until the growth of the specific pathogen occurs. An organism is deemed susceptible to the antibiotic if the minimum inhibitory concentration (MIC) is one sixteenth to one fourth of the peak achievable serum concentration (or urine concentration if a urinary pathogen). Despite a satisfactory MIC, failure of antibiotic therapy may occur if the antibiotic concentrations at the target site (cerebrospinal fluid, bile, prostatic tissue, pancreas, necrotic avascular tissue) are not well equilibrated with serum. Another cause of antibiotic failure is the highly protein-bound compound (ceftriaxone) or failure of the drug to penetrate the bacterial cell wall (beta-lactam therapy in *Legionella*). Conversely, an antibiotic considered modestly effective through in vitro susceptibility testing may be highly effective clinically if concentrated well at the target site (aminoglycosides for urosepsis, macrolides for intracellular *Legionella*).

The use of the MIC as the sole factor while deciding antibiotic therapy is problematic. With certain antibiotics (aminoglycosides, fluoroquinolones), a substantial proportion of the bacteria may be inhibited or killed when the MIC is subtherapeutic (post-antibiotic effect). A similar effect occurs because of impaired resistance to phagocytosis by the pathogens recently exposed to therapeutic antibiotic concentrations. MIC testing has another reason for a limited association with clinical response: The test evaluates a pathogen's response to a constant concentration of antibiotic, whereas the standard dosing actually is intermittent, resulting in varying concentrations at the target site. Furthermore, MIC does not distinguish between bacterial killing and inhibition of bacterial growth.

Pharmacokinetics

The goal of antibiotic therapy is to deliver an appropriate drug at a high enough concentration to the infectious site to kill the pathogenic organism. In serious infections, the local drug concentration must exceed the MIC for the best cure rates. Many factors can affect the local drug concentration (pharmacokinetics) by influencing drug absorption, distribution, and elimination. In contrast to impaired absorption from the gastrointestinal tract in critically ill patients who develop poor gut perfusion, bowel edema, and ileus, intravenous administration results in consistently predictable peak levels crucial for the efficacy of many antimicrobial agents.

Overall, antimicrobial distribution is affected by the patient's size, percentage of body fat, and degree of edema; each significantly affects drug concentration at the target site. Drug volume of distribution, which equals the amount of drug administered divided by the plasma drug concentration, describes the relative distribution of the drug within the body compartments. Extracellular volume is markedly increased in states of total body fluid overload (cirrhosis, renal failure, congestive heart failure, sepsis with fluid resuscitation, trauma, and anasarca) commonly seen in the intensive care unit. In these circumstances, the serum level of drugs that primarily distribute to the extracellular fluid are markedly low (eg, aminoglycosides).[18] Decreased serum proteins and albumin can substantially increase free-drug levels and should be factored in when performing dosage calculations.

Local factors determining antibiotic concentration at the site of infection are also important. The vascularity index of a site (vascular endothelial area divided by the tissue volume) can be important in infections of bone or limbs with impaired blood flow. Thus, for antibiotics to be effective, debridement of necrotic tissue, vascular repair, or both is required. Because of the high vascularity index, adequate drug levels are easily achieved in joint, pleural, and peritoneal space infections. Nonfenestrated capillaries that limit the movement of larger molecules, including antibiotics, often perfuse organs such as the brain, the eyes, and the prostate. The antibiotic must diffuse through the endothelial membrane (depending on its lipid solubility, the pharmacokinetics of the drug, and the fluid pH) or be instilled directly. Abscesses present a series of barriers to effective therapy; antimicrobials cannot be effectively delivered into the avascular core of abscesses or other necrotic tissue (depending on size). Furthermore, aminoglycosides and erythromycin show decreased activity at the acid pHs that exist in abscesses. Aminoglycosides and vancomycin are also bound to and inactivated by DNA that exists in abundance in pus. Finally, because beta-lactams work best on rapidly growing cell populations, slow-growing organisms in abscesses require longer duration of therapy.

In intensive care unit patients, an abnormal clearance rate of the drug will usually prolong the half-life of antibiotics; in some cases, elimination may be more rapid. In either case, close attention must be paid to dosage adjustments and dosing intervals. Many antibiotics (aminoglycosides, quinolones, tetracyclines, vancomycin, sulfonamides, and amphotericin) are primarily eliminated through glomerular filtration. Shock states will substantially lower the glomerular filtration rate, whereas the hyperdynamic phase of burn injury and sepsis (without shock) can be associated with an increased glomerular filtration rate. Although renal injury will impair drug clearance, dosage adjustment is generally not required for most drugs until the creatinine clearance falls under 30% of normal. Drug dosing in septic shock must anticipate that serum creatinine may inaccurately reflect true renal function as reflected by creatinine clearance, and is better reflected by the urine output. No good measure exists for estimation of altered liver clearance. Antibiotics that may require dosage adjustment with liver failure include erythromycin, nafcillin, mezlocillin, rifampin, tetracycline, isonicotinic acid hydrazide, clindamycin, chloramphenicol, and metronidazole.

Pharmacodynamics

The goal of antibiotic therapy is to maximize efficacy while minimizing toxicity. Pharmacodynamics include microbiologic activity, pharmacokinetic properties, and interactions among the drug, the host, and the organism. Whether a drug is bacteriostatic or bacteriocidal is basically a pharmacodynamic property of a drug. Bacteriostatic antibiotics inhibit growth of organisms, whereas bacteriocidal antibiotics kill the organisms. A bacteriocidal drug has a minimal bactericidal concentration that is only two to four times of the MIC, as opposed to a bacteriostatic drug with a minimal bactericidal concentration more than 16 times higher than its MIC. An alternative approach defines a bacteriocidal antimicrobial as one that yields 3-log bacterial kill (1000-fold reduction in organisms) over 24 hours. Some drugs can be bacteriostatic for one group of organisms but bacteriocidal for another. Because host immune defenses augment antibiotic efficacy in vivo, bacteriocidal activity of antibiotic regimens is only definitively required for clinical cure in limited circumstances. These include those circumstances involving endovascular infections, particularly endocarditis, meningitis, and cerebral abscess; infections in neutropenics; and osteomyelitis (particularly *Staphylococcus aureus* osteomyelitis). Septic shock probably also represents a condition where cidal therapy is optimal, although this possibility is still not widely accepted. For most other infections, exceeding the MIC of the target organism by several factors (even without cidality ie, bacteriostatic activity) is sufficient to bring about cure.

The use of multiple antibiotics is common in the intensive care unit for many reasons. Treatment of life-threatening infections is commenced on an empiric basis. Missing a causative organism will reduce the probability of survival. Although broad-spectrum agents have become available, only rarely are all possible likely pathogens effectively covered with a single antimicrobial agent. Multicenter trials have shown the importance of initiation of empiric broad-spectrum therapy on presentation rather than waiting until an infection is identified (**Fig. 1**).[10,19] Outcome in such patients is clearly improved if the causative organism is included in the initial empiric regimen and is substantially degraded if it is not. In neutropenic patients, a successful empiric regimen should be continued until resolution of neutropenia, whereas narrowing the regimen to a single agent following identification of the organism is reasonable in other cases.

Use of multiple antimicrobial agents remains contentious in nonneutropenic patients as many of the newer compounds (meropenem, imipenem-cilastatin, piperacillin-tazobactam, moxifloxacin) achieve similar breadth of coverage as single drugs and it may be unnecessary to cover every organism present in an infection.[20] Multi-antibiotic therapy might also be used to prevent emergence of resistance, an application that has only been demonstrated for treatment of tuberculosis and is otherwise speculative. Many clinical and animal studies demonstrate that *Pseudomonas aeruginosa* can develop resistance to beta-lactam antibiotics during therapy.[21] The addition of aminoglycosides to prevent resistance is one basis for recommending double therapy in serious *Pseudomonas* infections. However, the effectiveness of this therapy in such cases has not been proven.

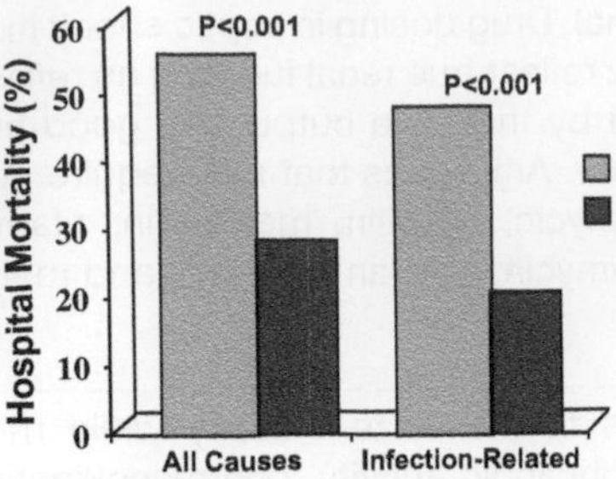

Fig. 1. Mortality and adequacy of empiric antimicrobial therapy. In a series of bacteremic patients admitted to intensive care units, initiation of inappropriate antibiotic therapy (ie, antibiotics to which organisms were resistant) was associated with a doubling of risk of death. (*Data from* Kollef MH, Sherman G, Ward S, et al. Inadequate antimicrobial treatment of infections: a risk factor for hospital mortality among critically ill patients. Chest 1999;115:462–74.)

The argument that use of multiple agents routinely results in synergistic or additive effects with a concomitant decrease in toxicity is unproven with limited exceptions (amphotericin plus flucytosine). The combination of beta-lactams with aminoglycosides is commonly prescribed. Both of these drugs demonstrate bacteriocidal activity: The beta-lactam is thought to cause cell-wall injury in such a way that the aminoglycoside can enter and kill the organism. Clinically, the combination of vancomycin or penicillin/ampicillin with an aminoglycoside results in higher cure rates of enterococcal endocarditis than those from either drug individually.[22–24] Although the required duration of therapy of *S aureus* and streptococcal endocarditis is shortened, overall cure rates with combination therapy are not improved.[22,24]

Older analyses suggest that an antipseudomonal penicillin with an antipseudomonal aminoglycoside is more effective than either alone in the treatment of neutropenic gram-negative sepsis,[25] although more recent analyses that include studies using modern cephalosporins and carbapenems are more equivocal on this question.[26] There is also some evidence of increased efficacy with combination therapy of serious pseudomonal infections.[27] Thus, no definitive evidence exists for efficacy of combination antibiotic therapy other than endocarditis or, arguably, neutropenic patients with gram-negative sepsis. The most accepted reason to use a combination of drugs may be to maximally broaden the breadth of antimicrobial coverage in conditions where suboptimal initial coverage may result in increased mortality.

Dosing Strategies for Antibiotics

Bacteriocidal antibiotics belong to two major groups according to whether the dominant mechanism for bacterial killing is concentration-dependent or time-dependent. These mechanisms significantly affect dosing strategies.

Aminoglycosides and fluoroquinolones exhibit concentration-dependent killing.[17,28,29] Optimal dosing for maximum bacterial killing and, in the case of aminoglycoside, minimum toxicity can be achieved using a schedule that emphasizes large doses administered infrequently. Achievement of a peak concentration of 10 to 12 times the MIC is associated with optimal outcome for both agents. Many studies and meta-analyses support once-daily dosing for aminoglycoside antibiotics. Less frequent dosing with these agents is possible due to a post-antibiotic effect, during which persistent suppression of bacterial growth occurs even when antibiotic concentrations are subtherapeutic. An intact immune system is likely required to continue bacterial killing to take advantage of the post-antibiotic effect phase.

Beta-lactams fall into a second category of antibacterial agents that exert bacteriocidal effects independent of the peak concentration.[17,28,29] For this class, bacterial kill is related to the proportional duration of time of the dosing interval that the organism is exposed to an antibiotic in excess of the MIC (time-dependent killing). In general, intermittent dosing regimens that achieve a serum concentration of two to four times the MIC (approximately two times maximal bactericidal concentration) for 40% to 60% of the dosing interval yield satisfactory results for beta-lactams. However, limited human and animal studies demonstrate that optimal (and improved) results can be seen with continuous or extended infusion of beta-lactams resulting in time above the MIC values of 100%.[30–33]

Antibiotic Resistance

Resistance to multiple antibiotics has become a major problem in critically ill patients.[34–37] Methicillin-resistant *S aureus* (MRSA) and vancomycin-resistant enterococci (VRE) are rapidly advancing problems in the nosocomial setting. Although MRSA can still be treated with vancomycin, vancomycin-resistant strains have recently been described. At present, VRE and potential vancomycin- and methicillin-resistant species can be treated with the newer antibacterial compounds, including quinipristin-dalfopristin, linezolid, and daptomycin. Plasmid-mediated beta-lactamases produced by some gram-negative bacilli mediate resistance to ampicillin, amoxicillin, ticarcillin, piperacillin, mezlocillin, and many cephalosporins. These organisms can be effectively treated with more advanced cephalosporins, beta-lactam/beta-lactamase inhibitor combinations, and carbapenems. Carbapenems and cefoxitin are potent inducers of chromosomal beta-lactamase in some gram-negative bacilli. This is rarely an issue for carbapenems due to their potent activity. However, cefoxitin may render concomitantly administered penicillins ineffective by this mechanism. Many third-generation cephalosporins produce chromosomal beta-lactamase in *Enterobacter* spp although carbapenems and fourth-generation cephalosporins still remain active. Metallo-beta-lactamases that render gram negatives resistant to even carbapenems are increasingly seen. In treatment of serious gram-negative infections, many intensive care units with a high frequency of multiresistant organisms continue two-drug empiric therapy pending identification of the organism's sensitivity pattern. Virtually pan-resistant gram-negative bacilli requiring treatment with marginal agents, such as colistin, are causing serious infections with increasing frequency.

FAILURE OF ANTIBIOTIC THERAPY

Clinical deterioration or failure to improve and persistence of fever and high white blood cell counts in an otherwise improved patient are often incorrectly considered a failure of antibiotic therapy.[38] Once severe sepsis has developed, sepsis-associated symptoms can progress independent of eradication of inciting organisms. Additionally, disease other than infection (eg, liver failure, drug or malignancy-related fever, salicylate toxicity, pancreatitis, adrenal insufficiency) can frequently cause infectious-appearing clinical symptomatology in the critically ill. The causes of antibiotic failure are varied. They include overly delayed administration of appropriate therapy, inappropriate spectrum of activity of the antimicrobial regimen, inadequate antimicrobial blood levels, inadequate penetration of the antimicrobial to the target site, antimicrobial neutralization or antagonism, superinfection or unsuspected secondary bacterial infection, unusual bacterial or nonbacterial infection, and noninfectious source of illness or fever with or without colonization.

In the critically ill patient, inadequate blood levels of antibiotics most commonly arise because of a lack of appreciation of increased volume of distribution as a consequence of expanded extracellular volume (saline resuscitation fluids remain in the extracellular space).[28,29] In addition, many antibiotics have a significant gradient between serum and the tissue target site, even in well-perfused organs. For that reason, maximal recommended dosing should be used in all life-threatening infections, particularly those involving relatively protected or poorly perfused sites. One of the most common causes of apparent failure of antibiotic therapy is inadequate antibiotic penetration. Impaired vascularity of an infected tissue can substantially impede delivery of the antibiotic. Abscesses are an extreme example of this, as they have no intrinsic blood supply. Most abscesses require surgical drainage for cure. However, small abscesses (with a decreased area to penetrate), anaerobic lung abscesses, small/multiple brain abscesses, and, occasionally, renal abscesses can be cured with prolonged antibiotic therapy. Chronic vascular insufficiency (eg, infected diabetic foot ulcer) requires either revascularization or a more penetrant drug (fluoroquinolones, clindamycin, metronidazole, or rifampin). An infecting organism or its toxins may also impair the vascular supply (eg, *Aspergillus*, *Rhizopus*, *Mucor*, necrotizing fasciitis, or clostridial gangrene), thus requiring aggressive surgical debridement with an appropriate antimicrobial therapy.

Although antibiotic antagonism is an unusual cause of antibiotic failure therapy, it should always be considered.[39–42] It may be better to use single agents with broad activity rather than multiple agents with potentially antagonistic activity. Concurrent unrecognized bacterial infection in a critically ill patient is another possible cause of antibiotic failure. Therefore, each patient should be carefully assessed initially at admission. In a critically ill patient on prolonged therapy with broad-spectrum antibiotics, superinfections, such as decubitus ulcers, bacterial sinusitis, line sepsis, and *Clostridium difficile* colitis, may occur, and should be carefully monitored as possible infectious complications of an intensive care unit stay.

ANTIBIOTIC THERAPY AND SOURCE CONTROL

Empiric Antibiotic Regimens Should Approach 100% Coverage of Pathogens for the Suspected Source of Infection

Initial administration of inappropriate antimicrobials increases morbidity in a wide range of infections. One study found that, in 17.1% of community-acquired bacteremia cases and in 34.3% of nosocomial bacteremia cases admitted to the intensive care unit, the antimicrobial therapy initiated was inadequate.[11] Similarly, in another large study, 18.8% and 28.4% of community acquired and nosocomial septic shock cases were initially treated with inadequate antimicrobial therapy.[43] Retrospective studies have shown that the risk of death, which is 30% to 60% in intensive care unit bacteremia (see **Fig. 1**),[4,10] increases to 70% to 100% in gram-negative shock[4] when the initial empiric regimen fails to cover the inciting pathogen. More recent data suggest that survival of septic shock with inappropriate initial antimicrobial therapy is reduced approximately 5-fold (range 2.5- to 10-fold in selected subgroups) from 50% to about 10%.[43] These findings of sharply increased mortality risk with initial inadequate antimicrobial therapy apply to serious infections caused by gram-negative and gram-positive bacteria as well as *Candida* spp.[4,43–48]

As a consequence, empiric regimens should err on the side of overinclusiveness. The most common reason for initiation of inappropriate antimicrobial therapy is a failure of the clinician to appreciate the risk of infection with antibiotic-resistant organisms (either otherwise uncommon organisms with increased native resistance or antibiotic-resistant isolates of common organisms). Selection of an optimal antimicrobial regimen requires knowledge of the probable anatomic site of infection; the patient's immune status, risk factors, and physical environment; and the local microbiologic flora and organism-resistance patterns. Risk factors for infection with resistant organisms include prolonged hospital stay, prior hospitalization, and prior colonization or infection with multiresistant organisms.

Superior empiric coverage can be obtained through the use of a local antibiogram or infectious diseases consultation.[49,50] Although not routinely required, extended-spectrum gram-negative regimens, vancomycin, and/or antifungal therapy may be appropriate in specific, high-risk cases with severe sepsis (see **Table 1**). In addition, given that 90% to 95% of patients with septic shock have comorbidities or other factors that make them high risk for resistant organisms, it may be appropriate to treat all patients with septic shock using a combination of antimicrobials that result in a broadly expanded spectrum of coverage for the first few days. This approach should yield improved initial adequacy of antimicrobial coverage while ensuring that high-risk patients are not inappropriately categorized as low risk.

Intravenous Administration of Broad-spectrum Antimicrobial Should be Initiated Immediately (Preferably <30 minutes) Following the Clinical Diagnosis of Septic Shock

Appropriate, intravenous, empiric broad-spectrum therapy should be initiated as rapidly as possible in response to clinical suspicion of infection in the presence of hypotension (ie, presumptive septic shock). An assumption that hypotension is caused by anything other than sepsis in the setting of documented or suspected infection should be avoided in the absence of strong data indicating a specific alternative etiology. Retrospective studies of human bacteremia, pneumonia, and meningitis with sepsis suggest that mortality in sepsis increases with delays in antimicrobial administration.[9,47,51–53] One major retrospective analysis of septic shock has suggested that the delay to initial administration of effective antimicrobial therapy is the single strongest predictor of survival.[8] Initiation of effective antimicrobial therapy within the first hour following onset of septic shock–related hypotension was associated with 79.9% survival to hospital discharge (**Fig. 2**). For every additional hour to effective antimicrobial initiation in the first 6 hours post-hypotension onset, survival dropped an average of 7.6%. With effective antimicrobial initiation between the first and second hour post-hypotension onset, survival had already dropped to 70.5%. With effective antimicrobial therapy delay to 5 to 6 hours after hypotension onset, survival was just 42.0% and, by 9 to 12 hours, 25.4%. The adjusted odds ratio of death was already significantly increased by the second hour post-hypotension onset and the ratio continued to climb with longer delays.

Substantial delays before initiation of effective therapy have been shown in several studies of serious infections.[9,53–55] In septic shock, the median time to delivery of effective antimicrobial therapy following initial onset of recurrent/persistent hypotension was 6 hours.[8] Only 14.5% of all patients who had not received effective antimicrobials before shock received them within the first hour of documentation of onset of recurrent or persistent hypotension (see **Fig. 2**). Only 32.5% had received them by 3 hours post-hypotension onset and 51.4% by 6 hours postonset. Even 12 hours after the first occurrence of recurrent or sustained hypotension, 29.8% of patients had not received effective antimicrobial therapy.

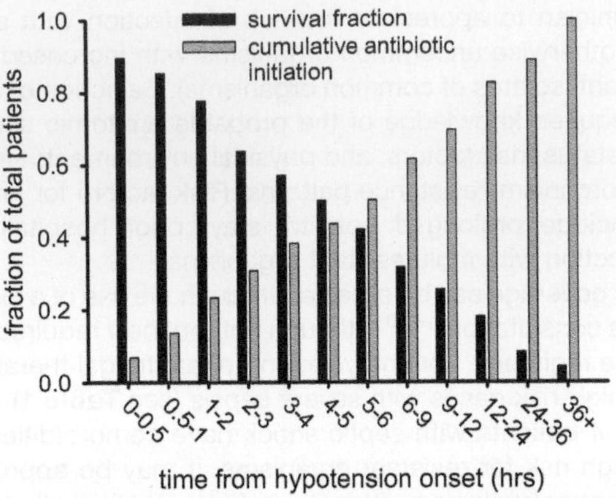

Fig. 2. Cumulative initiation of effective antimicrobial therapy and survival in septic shock. In a large retrospective study of septic shock, Kumar and colleagues demonstrated that median time to effective/appropriate antimicrobial therapy was 6 hours and that for every hour delay over the first 6 hours, the projected mortality increased by 7.6%. The x-axis represents time (hours) following first documentation of septic shock–associated hypotension. Black bars represent the fraction of patients surviving to hospital discharge and the gray bars represent the cumulative fraction of patients having received effective antimicrobials at any given time. (*From* Kumar A, Roberts D, Wood KE, et al. Duration of hypotension before initiation of effective antimicrobial therapy is the critical determinant of survival in human septic shock. Crit Care Med 2006;34:1589–96; with permission.)

A potential survival advantage may exist if a pathogenic organism can be isolated in severe infections, including septic shock. Every effort should be made to obtain appropriate site-specific cultures to allow identification and susceptibility testing of the pathogenic organism; however, such efforts should not delay antimicrobial therapy.

Antimicrobial Therapy Should be Initiated with Dosing at the High End of the Therapeutic Range in all Patients with Life-threatening Infection

Early optimization of antimicrobial pharmacokinetics can improve outcome of patients with severe infection, including septic shock. This is most easily achieved by initiating antibiotic therapy with high-end dosing regimens.

Early in sepsis, before the onset of hepatic or renal dysfunction, cardiac output is increased in many patients. In association with increased free-drug levels due to decreased albumin levels, drug clearance can be transiently increased.[14] As the illness progresses, intensive care unit patients with sepsis or septic shock exhibit substantially increased volumes of distribution and decreased clearance rates. Consequently, suboptimal dosing of antibiotics is common in these conditions.[18,56–60] Data are most well developed in reference to aminoglycosides but also exist for fluoroquinolones, beta-lactams, and carbapenems.[18,56–60] Failure to achieve targets on initial dosing has been associated with clinical failure with aminoglycosides.[61,62] Similarly, clinical success rate for treatment of serious infections tracks with higher peak blood levels of fluoroquinolones (nosocomial pneumonia and other serious infections)[63–65] and aminoglycosides (gram-negative nosocomial pneumonia and other serious infections).[66,67] Although there are extensive data in experimental animals and in less serious human infections, data for optimization of outcomes in critically ill, infected patients using beta-lactams are relatively limited.[17,68]

Achievement of optimal serum concentrations of aminoglycosides (peak antibiotic serum concentration:pathogen MIC ratio of $\geq$12) and longer periods of bactericidal beta-lactam and carbapenem serum concentrations (minimum time above MIC in serum of 60% of dosing interval) are appropriate targets.[32,63,69] This can most easily be attained with once-daily dosing with aminoglycosides (**Fig. 3**).[70] For beta-lactams and related antibiotics, increased frequency of dosing (given identical total daily dose) is recommended (**Fig. 4**). For example, piperacillin/tazobactam can be dosed at either 4.5 g every 8 hours or 3.375 g every 6 hours for serious infections; all things being equal, the latter would achieve a higher time above MIC and should be the preferred dosing option. A similar dosing approach should be used for other beta-lactams in critically ill patients with life-threatening infections. Limited data suggest that continuous-infusion beta-lactams and related drugs may be even more effective, particularly for relatively resistant organisms.[33,71–74]

Multidrug Antimicrobial Therapy is Preferred for the Initial Empiric Therapy of Septic Shock

Probable pathogens should be covered by at least two antimicrobials with different bacteriocidal mechanisms. Given that highly resistant organisms are endemic in the critical care environment, multidrug antimicrobial therapy reduces the probability of failure to cover these organisms. In addition, most patients with septic shock (even those without specific preexisting immune defects) exhibit significant deficits of neutrophil and monocyte function during the course of their illness.[75–81] Furthermore, malnutrition and organ dysfunction (eg, renal or hepatic failure), which are common in intensive care unit patients, suppress cell-mediated immunity. Based on these data, septic shock patients likely have reduced ability to clear infection and may be best managed with multidrug therapy similar to that recommended for patients with neutropenic sepsis.[82,83]

No prospective, controlled study has specifically compared multiple versus single antimicrobial therapy in a broad range of severe sepsis or septic shock patients. Most infectious disease physicians and other experts suggest that there is no advantage to multidrug therapy in serious infections, including bacteremia.[27,84] However, subgroup analyses of the sickest subset of patients with gram-negative bacteremia with or without shock have tended to suggest improved survival with the use of two or more antibiotics to which the causative organism is sensitive.[85–88] Similarly, at least

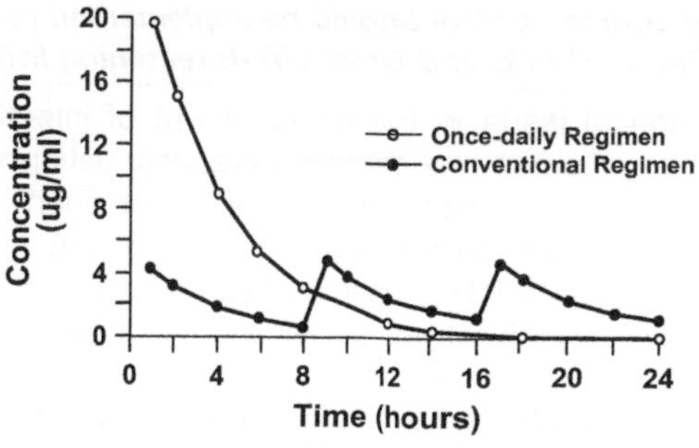

Fig. 3. Conventional versus daily aminoglycoside dosing. Once-daily regimens of aminoglycosides yield substantially higher peak concentrations and area under the concentration curve. (*Courtesy of* David Nicolau.)

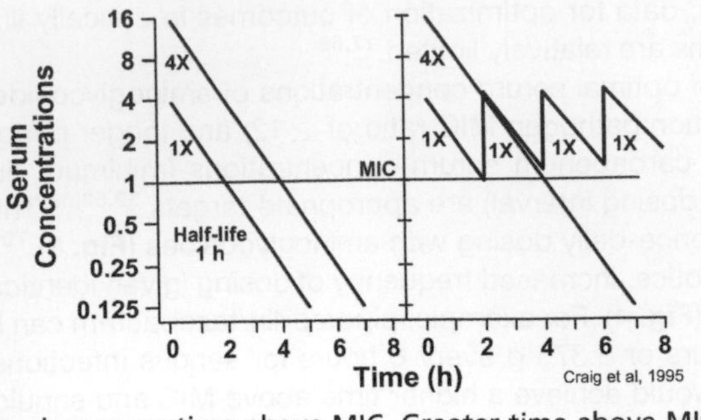

Fig. 4. Effect of dose change on time above MIC. Greater time above MIC for beta-lactams can be achieved by more frequent administration than by increasing the size of the dose (for an equivalent increase in total daily dose). This concept can be extended to continuous or extended infusion of beta-lactams. (*Courtesy of* William Craig.)

two retrospective and one prospective analyses of the most severe, critically ill patients with bacteremic pneumococcal pneumonia suggested improvement in outcome if two or more effective agents were used.[89–91] This occurred even as patients with pneumococcal bacteremia with a lower severity of illness demonstrated no such benefit.[89] A recent secondary analysis of a prospective study of community-acquired pneumonia has shown benefit with multidrug therapy compared with monotherapy but only in the subset of septic shock.[92]

Empiric Antimicrobial Therapy Should be Adjusted to a Narrower Regimen Within 48 to 72 Hours if a Plausible Pathogen is Identified or if the Patient Stabilizes Clinically (ie, Resolution of Shock)

While several retrospective studies have demonstrated that inappropriate therapy of bacteremic septic shock yields increased mortality,[4,10,44–47] none have suggested that early narrowing of therapy is detrimental if the organism is identified or if the patient is responding well clinically. This approach maximizes appropriate antibiotic coverage of inciting pathogens in septic shock while minimizing selection pressure toward resistant organisms. Although it is tempting to continue a broad-spectrum regimen in the one third of patients who are culture-negative for a potential pathogen even as they clinically improve, intensivists must recognize that a strategy of broad-spectrum initial antimicrobial therapy will only be sustainable if overuse of these agents can be avoided.

Where Possible, Early Source Control Should be Implemented in Patients with Severe Sepsis, Septic Shock, and Other Life-threatening Infections

Source control is a critical issue in the management of infection associated with severe sepsis. Infections found in intensive care unit patients frequently require source control for optimal management. The need for such source control may initially be overlooked in many infections commonly found in the intensive care unit (eg, pneumonia-associated bacterial empyema, decubitus ulcers, *C difficile* colitis). Causes of septic shock where source control may be required are noted in **Box 1**.

Source control may include removal of implanted or tunneled devices, open surgical/ percutaneous drainage of infected fluids or abscesses, and surgical resection of infected tissues. In a broader sense, source control includes elimination of inciting chemotherapies (eg, antibiotics driving *C difficile* colitis or chemotherapy

Box 1
Common sources of severe sepsis/septic shock requiring urgent source control
Toxic megacolon or *C difficile* colitis with shock
Ischemic bowel
Perforated viscus
Intra-abdominal abscess
Ascending cholangitis
Gangrenous cholecystitis
Necrotizing pancreatitis with infection
Bacterial empyema
Mediastinitis
Purulent tunnel infections
Purulent foreign body infections
Obstructive uropathy
Complicated pyelonephritis/perinephric abscess
Necrotizing soft tissue infections (necrotizing fasciitis)
Clostridial myonecrosis

causing gut injury). Efforts to identify infections requiring invasive forms of source control frequently require rapid (<2 hour) radiographic imaging (often computerized axial tomography [CT] scan) or, if clinical status and findings are supportive, direct and immediate surgical intervention without an imaging effort. With rare exceptions, surgical source control should follow aggressive resuscitative efforts to minimize intraoperative morbidity and mortality. In some cases (eg, rapidly progressive necrotizing soft tissue infections, bowel infarction), optimal management mandates simultaneous aggressive resuscitation and surgical intervention. Subgroup analysis in at least one large prospective severe sepsis study has suggested that failure to implement adequate source control is associated with increased mortality.[93] Earlier surgical intervention has been shown to have a significant impact on outcome in certain rapidly progressive infections, such as necrotizing fasciitis.[94,95] In a large retrospective study, time from hypotension to implementation of source control was found to be highly correlated with outcome.[96]

The necessity for or efficacy of source control efforts should be reassessed within 12 to 36 hours following admission and/or source control efforts based on clinical response.

SUMMARY

Every patient with sepsis and septic shock must be evaluated thoroughly at presentation before the initiation of antibiotic therapy. However, in most situations, an abridged initial assessment focusing on critical diagnostic and management planning elements is sufficient. Intravenous antibiotics should be administered as early as possible, and always within the first hour of recognizing severe sepsis and septic shock. Broad-spectrum antibiotics must be selected with one or more agents active against likely bacterial or fungal pathogens and with good penetration into the presumed source. Antimicrobial therapy should be reevaluated daily to optimize efficacy, prevent resistance, avoid toxicity, and minimize costs. Consider combination therapy in *Pseudomonas* infections, and combination empiric therapy in neutropenic patients. Combination therapy should be continued for no more than 3 to 5 days and de-escalation should occur following availability of susceptibilities. The duration of antibiotic therapy typically is limited to 7 to 10 days; longer duration is considered if response is slow, if there is inadequate surgical source control, or in the case of immunologic deficiencies. Antimicrobial therapy should be stopped if infection is not considered the etiologic factor for a shock state.

REFERENCES

1. Angus DC, Linde-Zwirble WT, Lidicker J, et al. Epidemiology of severe sepsis in the United States: analysis of incidence, outcome, and associated costs of care. Crit Care Med 2001;29:1303–10.
2. Finland M, Jones WF, Barnes MW. Occurrence of serious bacterial infections since the introduction of antibacterial agents. JAMA 1959;84:2188–97.
3. Hemminki E, Paakkulainen A. Effect of antibiotics on mortality from infectious diseases in Sweden and Finland. Am J Public Health 1976;66:1180–4.
4. Kreger BE, Craven DE, McCabe WR. Gram-negative bacteremia. IV. Re-evaluation of clinical features and treatment in 612 patients. Am J Med 1980;68:344–55.
5. Martin GS, Mannino DM, Eaton S, et al. The epidemiology of sepsis in the United States from 1979 through 2000. N Engl J Med 2003;348:1546–54.
6. Minino AM, Heron MP, Murphy SL, et al. Deaths: final results for 2004. National Vital Statistics Report 2007;55:1–120.
7. Friedman G, Silva E, Vincent JL. Has the mortality of septic shock changed with time? Crit Care Med 1998;26:2078–86.
8. Kumar A, Roberts D, Wood KE, et al. Duration of hypotension before initiation of effective antimicrobial therapy is the critical determinant of survival in human septic shock. Crit Care Med 2006;34:1589–96.
9. Meehan TP, Fine MJ, Krumholz HM, et al. Quality of care, process, and outcomes in elderly patients with pneumonia. JAMA 1997;278:2080–4.
10. Ibrahim EH, Sherman G, Ward S, et al. The influence of inadequate antimicrobial treatment of bloodstream infections on patient outcomes in the ICU setting. Chest 2000;118:146–55.
11. Kollef MH, Sherman G, Ward S, et al. Inadequate antimicrobial treatment of infections: a risk factor for hospital mortality among critically ill patients. Chest 1999;115:462–74.
12. Kollef MH. Inadequate antimicrobial treatment: an important determinant of outcome for hospitalized patients. Clin Infect Dis 2000;31(Suppl 4):S131–8.
13. Drusano GL. Antimicrobial pharmacodynamics: critical interactions of 'bug and drug'. Nat Rev Microbiol 2004;2:289–300.
14. Pinder M, Bellomo R, Lipman J, et al. Pharmacological principles of antibiotic prescription in the critically ill. Anaesth Intensive Care 2002;30:134–44.
15. Li RC. New pharmacodynamic parameters for antimicrobial agents. Int J Antimicrob Agents 2000;13:229–35.
16. Solomkin JS, Miyagawa CI. Principles of antibiotic therapy. Surg Clin North Am 1994;74(3):497–517.
17. Craig WA. Pharmacokinetic/pharmacodynamic parameters: rationale for antibacterial dosing of mice and men. Clin Infect Dis 1998;26:1–10.

18. Chelluri L, Jastremski MS. Inadequacy of standard aminoglycoside loading doses in acutely ill patients. Crit Care Med 1987;15:1143–5.
19. Harbarth S, Garbino J, Pugin J, et al. Inappropriate initial antimicrobial therapy and its effect on survival in a clinical trial of immunomodulating therapy for severe sepsis. Am J Med 2003;115:529–35.
20. Bartlett JG. Anti-anaerobic antibacterial agents. Lancet 1982;2(8296): 478–81.
21. Lumish RM, Norden CW. Therapy of neutropenic rats infected with pseudomonas aeruginosa. J Infect Dis 1976;133:538–47.
22. Mylonakis E, Calderwood SB. Infective endocarditis in adults. N Engl J Med 2001; 345(18):1318–30.
23. Geraci JE, Martin WJ. Antibiotic therapy of bacterial endocarditis: VI. Subacute enterococcal endocarditis: clinical, pathologic and therapeutic consideration of 33 cases. Circulation 1954;10:173–94.
24. Moreillon P, Que YA. Infective endocarditis. Lancet 2004;363(9403): 139–49.
25. Klastersky J, Zinner SH. Synergistic combinations of antibiotics in gram-negative bacillary infections. Rev Infect Dis 1982;4:294–301.
26. Paul M, Soares-Weiser K, Leibovici L. Beta-lactam monotherapy versus b-lactam-aminoglycoside combination therapy for fever with neutropenia: systematic review and meta-analysis. Br Med J 2003;326:1111–8.
27. Safdar N, Handelsman J, Maki DG, et al. Does combination antimicrobial therapy reduce mortality in gram-negative bacteraemia? A meta-analysis. Lancet Infect Dis 2004;4:519–27.
28. Drusano GL. Pharmacokinetics and pharmacodynamics of antimicrobials. Clin Infect Dis 2007;45(Suppl 1):S89–95.
29. Roberts JA, Lipman J. Pharmacokinetic issues for antibiotics in the critically ill patient. Crit Care Med 2009;37(3):840–51, quiz 859.
30. Roberts JA, Lipman J, Blot S, et al. Better outcomes through continuous infusion of time-dependent antibiotics to critically ill patients? Curr Opin Crit Care 2008; 14(4):390–6.
31. Falagas ME, Siempos II, Tsakoumis I. Cure of persistent, post-appendectomy Klebsiella pneumoniae septicaemia with continuous intravenous administration of meropenem. Scand J Infect Dis 2006;38:807–10.
32. Craig WA, Ebert SC. Continuous infusion of beta-lactam antibiotics. Antimicrob Agents Chemother 1992;36:2577–83.
33. Bodey GP, Ketchel SJ, Rodriguez V. A randomized study of carbenicillin plus cefamandole or tobramycin in the treatment of febrile episodes in cancer patients. Am J Med 1979;67:608–16.
34. Kollef MH, Fraser VJ. Antibiotic resistance in the intensive care unit. Ann Intern Med 2001;134(4):298–314.
35. Kaye KS, Engemann JJ, Fraimow HS, et al. Pathogens resistant to antimicrobial agents: epidemiology, molecular mechanisms, and clinical management. Infect Dis Clin North Am 2004;18(3):467–511.
36. Dandekar PK, Quintiliani R, Nightingale CH, et al. Extended-spectrum beta-lactamases (ESBL). Conn Med 2002;66:13–5.
37. Sanders CC, Sanders WE Jr. Microbial resistance to newer generation beta-lactam antibiotics: clinical and laboratory implications. J Infect Dis 1985;151(3): 399–406.
38. Schlossberg D. Clinical approach to antibiotic failure. Med Clin North Am 2006; 90(6):1265–77.

39. Lepper MH, Dowling HF. Treatment of pneumoccic meningitis with penicillin compared with penicillin plus aureomycin. Studies including observations on an apparent antagonism between penicillin and aureomycin. Arch Intern Med 1951;88:489–94.
40. Acar JF. Antibiotic synergy and antagonism. Med Clin North Am 2000;84(6): 1391–406.
41. Matthews T. Antibiotic antagonism and synergy. Lancet 1978;2(8085):376–7.
42. Neu HC. Synergy and antagonism of fluoroquinolones with other classes of antimicrobial agents. Drugs 1993;45(Suppl 3):54–8.
43. Kumar A, Ellis P, Arabi Y, et al. Initiation of inappropriate antimicrobial therapy results in a 5-fold reduction of survival in human septic shock. Chest 2009; in press.
44. Young LS, Martin WJ, Meyer RD, et al. Gram-negative rod bacteremia: microbiologic, immunologic, and therapeutic considerations. Ann Intern Med 1977;86: 456–71.
45. Romero-Vivas J, Rubio M, Fernandez C, et al. Mortality associated with nosocomial bacteremia due to methicillin-resistant Staphylococcus aureus. Clin Infect Dis 1995;21:1417–23.
46. Nguyen MH, Peacock JE Jr, Tanner DC, et al. Therapeutic approaches in patients with candidemia. Evaluation in a multicenter, prospective, observational study. Arch Intern Med 1995;155:2429–35.
47. Vergis EN, Hayden MK, Chow JW, et al. Determinants of vancomycin resistance and mortality rates in enterococcal bacteremia. A prospective multicenter study. Ann Intern Med 2001;135:484–92.
48. Parkins MD, Sabuda DM, Elsayed S, et al. Adequacy of empirical antifungal therapy and effect on outcome among patients with invasive Candida species infections. J Antimicrob Chemother 2007;60:613–8.
49. Byl B, Clevenbergh P, Jacobs F, et al. Impact of infectious diseases specialists and microbiological data on the appropriateness of antimicrobial therapy for bacteremia [comment]. Clin Infect Dis 1999;29:60–6.
50. Raineri E, Pan A, Mondello P, et al. Role of the infectious diseases specialist consultant on the appropriateness of antimicrobial therapy prescription in an intensive care unit. Am J Infect Control 2008;36(4):283–90.
51. Aronin SI, Peduzzi P, Quagliarello VJ. Community-acquired bacterial meningitis: risk stratification for adverse clinical outcome and effect of antibiotic timing. Ann Intern Med 1998;129:862–9.
52. Miner JR, Heegaard W, Mapes A, et al. Presentation, time to antibiotics, and mortality of patients with bacterial meningitis at an urban county medical center. J Emerg Med 2001;21:387–92.
53. Proulx N, Frechette D, Toye B, et al. Delays in the administration of antibiotics are associated with mortality from adult acute bacterial meningitis. QJM 2005;98: 291–8.
54. Houck PM, Bratzler DW, Nsa W, et al. Timing of antibiotic administration and outcomes for Medicare patients hospitalized with community-acquired pneumonia. Arch Intern Med 2004;164:637–44.
55. Natsch S, Kullberg BJ, Van der Meer JW, et al. Delay in administering the first dose of antibiotics in patients admitted to hospital with serious infections. Eur J Clin Microbiol Infect Dis 1998;17(10):681–4.
56. Pimentel FL, Abelha F, Trigo MA, et al. Determination of plasma concentrations of amikacin in patients of an intensive care unit. J Chemother 1995;7:45–9.
57. Whipple JK, Ausman RK, Franson T, et al. Effect of individualized pharmacokinetic dosing on patient outcome. Crit Care Med 1991;19:1480–5.

58. Joukhadar C, Frossard M, Mayer BX, et al. Impaired target site penetration of beta-lactams may account for therapeutic failure in patients with septic shock. Crit Care Med 2001;29:385–91.
59. Franson TR, Quebbeman EJ, Whipple J, et al. Prospective comparison of traditional and pharmacokinetic aminoglycoside dosing methods. Crit Care Med 1988;16:840–3.
60. Tegeder I, Schmidtko A, Brautigam L, et al. Tissue distribution of imipenem in critically ill patients. Clin Pharmacol Ther 2002;71:325–33.
61. Moore RD, Smith CR, Lietman PS. The association of aminoglycoside plasma levels with mortality in patients with gram-negative bacteremia. J Infect Dis 1984;149:443–8.
62. Moore RD, Smith CR, Lietman PS. Association of aminoglycoside plasma levels with therapeutic outcome in gram-negative pneumonia. Am J Med 1984;77: 657–62.
63. Forrest A, Nix DE, Ballow CH, et al. Pharmacodynamics of intravenous ciprofloxacin in seriously ill patients. Antimicrob Agents Chemother 1993;37: 1073–81.
64. Preston SL, Drusano GL, Berman AL, et al. Pharmacodynamics of levofloxacin: a new paradigm for early clinical trials. JAMA 1998;279:125–9.
65. Drusano GL, Preston SL, Fowler C, et al. Relationship between fluoroquinolone area under the curve: minimum inhibitory concentration ratio and the probability of eradication of the infecting pathogen, in patients with nosocomial pneumonia. J Infect Dis 2004;189:1590–7.
66. Moore RD, Lietman PS, Smith CR. Clinical response to aminoglycoside therapy: importance of the ratio of peak concentration to minimal inhibitory concentration. J Infect Dis 1987;155:93–9.
67. Kashuba AD, Nafziger AN, Drusano GL, et al. Optimizing aminoglycoside therapy for nosocomial pneumonia caused by gram-negative bacteria. Antimicrobial Agents & Chemotherapy 1999;43:623–9.
68. Schentag JJ, Smith IL, Swanson DJ, et al. Role for dual individualization with cefmenoxime. Am J Med 1984;77:43–50.
69. Craig WA. Once-daily versus multiple-daily dosing of aminoglycosides. J Chemother 1995;7(Suppl 2):47–52.
70. Kashuba AD, Bertino JS Jr, Nafziger AN. Dosing of aminoglycosides to rapidly attain pharmacodynamic goals and hasten therapeutic response by using individualized pharmacokinetic monitoring of patients with pneumonia caused by gram-negative organisms. Antimicrobial Agents & Chemotherapy 1998;42: 1842–4.
71. Daenen S, Vries-Hospers H. Cure of Pseudomonas aeruginosa infection in neutropenic patients by continuous infusion of ceftazidime. Lancet 1988;1: 937.
72. Egerer G, Goldschmidt H, Hensel M, et al. Continuous infusion of ceftazidime for patients with breast cancer and multiple myeloma receiving high-dose chemotherapy and peripheral blood stem cell transplantation. Bone Marrow Transplant 2002;30:427–31.
73. Benko AS, Cappelletty DM, Kruse JA, et al. Continuous infusion versus intermittent administration of ceftazidime in critically ill patients with suspected gram-negative infections. Antimicrobial Agents & Chemotherapy 1996;40:691–5.
74. Thalhammer F, Traunmuller F, El M, et al. Continuous infusion versus intermittent administration of meropenem in critically ill patients. J Antimicrob Chemother 1999;43:523–7.

75. Sfeir T, Saha DC, Astiz M, et al. Role of interleukin-10 in monocyte hyporesponsiveness associated with septic shock. Crit Care Med 2001;29:129–33.
76. Haupt W, Riese J, Mehler C, et al. Monocyte function before and after surgical trauma. Dig Surg 1998;15:102–4.
77. Brandtzaeg P, Osnes L, Ovstebo R, et al. Net inflammatory capacity of human septic shock plasma evaluated by a monocyte-based target cell assay: identification of interleukin-10 as a major functional deactivator of human monocytes. J Exp Med 1996;184:51–60.
78. Williams MA, Withington S, Newland AC, et al. Monocyte anergy in septic shock is associated with a predilection to apoptosis and is reversed by granulocyte-macrophage colony-stimulating factor ex vivo. J Infect Dis 1998;178:1421–33.
79. Tavares-Murta BM, Zaparoli M, Ferreira RB, et al. Failure of neutrophil chemotactic function in septic patients. Crit Care Med 2002;30:1056–61.
80. Holzer K, Konietzny P, Wilhelm K, et al. Phagocytosis by emigrated, intra-abdominal neutrophils is depressed during human secondary peritonitis. Eur Surg Res 2002;34:275–84.
81. Benjamim CF, Ferreira SH, Cunha FQ. Role of nitric oxide in the failure of neutrophil migration in sepsis. J Infect Dis 2000;182:214–23.
82. Barriere SL. Monotherapy versus combination antimicrobial therapy: a review. Pharmacotherapy 1991;11:64S–71S.
83. Hughes WT, Armstrong D, Bodey GP, et al. 2002 guidelines for the use of antimicrobial agents in neutropenic patients with cancer. Clin Infect Dis 2002;34:730–51.
84. Bochud PY, Glauser MP, Calandra T, et al. Antibiotics in sepsis. Intensive Care Med 2001;27(Suppl 1):S33–48.
85. Hilf M, Yu VL, Sharp J, et al. Antibiotic therapy for Pseudomonas aeruginosa bacteremia: outcome correlations in a prospective study of 200 patients. Am J Med 1989;87:540–6.
86. Chow JW, Fine MJ, Shlaes DM, et al. Enterobacter bacteremia: clinical features and emergence of antibiotic resistance during therapy. Ann Intern Med 1991;115:585–90.
87. Korvick JA, Bryan CS, Farber B, et al. Prospective observational study of Klebsiella bacteremia in 230 patients: outcome for antibiotic combinations versus monotherapy. Antimicrobial Agents & Chemotherapy 1992;36:2639–44.
88. Anderson ET, Young LS, Hewitt WL. Antimicrobial synergism in the therapy of gram-negative rod bacteremia. Chemotherapy 1978;24:45–54.
89. Baddour LM, Yu VL, Klugman KP, et al. Combination antibiotic therapy lowers mortality among severely ill patients with pneumococcal bacteremia. Am J Respir Crit Care Med 2004;170(4):440–4.
90. Waterer GW, Somes GW, Wunderink RG. Monotherapy may be suboptimal for severe bacteremic pneumococcal pneumonia. Arch Intern Med 2001;161:1837–42.
91. Martinez JA, Horcajada JP, Almela M, et al. Addition of a macrolide to a beta-lactam-based empirical antibiotic regimen is associated with lower in-hospital mortality for patients with bacteremic pneumococcal pneumonia. Clin Infect Dis 2003;36:389–95.
92. Rodriguez A, Mendia A, Sirvent JM, et al. Combination antibiotic therapy improves survival in patients with community-acquired pneumonia and shock. Crit Care Med 2007;35:1493–8.
93. Sprung CL, Finch RG, Thijs LG, et al. International sepsis trial (INTERSEPT): role and impact of a clinical evaluation committee. Crit Care Med 1996;24:1441–7.

94. Sudarsky LA, Laschinger JC, Coppa GF, et al. Improved results from a standardized approach in treating patients with necrotizing fasciitis. Ann Surg 1987;206: 661–5.
95. Moss RL, Musemeche CA, Kosloske AM. Necrotizing fasciitis in children: prompt recognition and aggressive therapy improve survival. J Pediatr Surg 1996;31: 1142–6.
96. Kumar A, Wood K, Gurka D, et al. Outcome of septic shock correlates with duration of hypotension prior to source control implementation. ICAAC Proceedings 2004;350:K-1222.

Principles of Source Control in the Management of Sepsis

John C. Marshall, MD, FRCSC[a,b,c,*], Abdullah al Naqbi, MD[b]

KEYWORDS

• Source control • Sepsis • Abscess • Surgery
• Percutaneous drainage • Debridement • Foreign body

The term "source control" encompasses a spectrum of interventions whose objective is the physical control of foci of infection and the restoration of optimal function and quality of life. Adequate source control – in conjunction with antibiotics, resuscitation and support of vital organ function – is a cornerstone of the successful management of the septic patient. It is also the oldest mode of infection control: the Edwin Smith papyrus from the seventeenth century BCE describes the role of spontaneous drainage in the treatment of an abscess of the chest wall.

The spectrum of source-control options is large, and their utility in an individual patient is heavily dependent not only on the site and nature of the inciting infection but also on the premorbid state of the patient, and the local availability of human and technological resources.[1] Optimal decision-making requires the application of core principles in the biology of the host inflammatory response; these principles are the focus of this article.

BIOLOGIC CONSIDERATIONS

Infection and other stimuli evoke a response that has evolved to contain the insult, to limit damage, and to activate the necessary processes that will lead to tissue repair and sustain survival. In aggregate, these processes, which include inflammation, coagulation, and tissue repair, constitute the innate immune response.

Local tissue invasion by microorganisms results in an acute inflammatory response, characterized by the classic manifestations of *rubor* (redness), *calor* (warmth), *dolor*

[a] Department of Surgery, Li Ka Shing Knowledge Institute, St Michael's Hospital, University of Toronto, 30 Bond Street, Toronto, Ontario, M5B 1W8, Canada
[b] Department of Critical Care Medicine, Li Ka Shing Knowledge Institute, St Michael's Hospital, University of Toronto, 30 Bond Street, Toronto, Ontario, M5B 1W8, Canada
[c] The Keenan Research Centre, Li Ka Shing Knowledge Institute, St Michael's Hospital, University of Toronto, 30 Bond Street, Toronto, Ontario, M5B 1W8, Canada
* Corresponding author. St Michael's Hospital, 4th Floor Bond Wing, Room 4-007, 30 Bond Street, Toronto, Ontario, M5B 1W8, Canada.
E-mail address: marshallj@smh.toronto.on.ca (J.C. Marshall).

Crit Care Clin 25 (2009) 753–768
doi:10.1016/j.ccc.2009.08.001
criticalcare.theclinics.com
0749-0704/09/$ – see front matter

(pain), *tumor* (swelling), and *functio laesa* (loss of function). The consequence is an increase in local blood flow, and the influx of polymorphonuclear neutrophils, recruited though the release of chemokines such as interleukin-8, and retained following the reciprocal upregulation of adhesion molecules on the local vascular endothelium and on the infiltrating neutrophil.[2] Coincident with this, tissue factor is expressed on the activated endothelial cells, and initiates local activation of the coagulation cascade.[3] These processes can lead to the elimination of the invading pathogen, or to a biologic standoff, in which the organism is not eliminated, but is contained within an abscess cavity. The structure of the abscess reflects these preceding processes (**Fig. 1**). Activation of coagulation leads to the deposition of fibrin, which forms the wall of the abscess and contains its contents (a mixture of bacteria, infiltrating neutrophils, serum, and tissue debris). The process serves to limit bacterial spread and to isolate the abscess contents from systemic host defenses.

Drainage

The contents of an abscess are typically liquid, and the formation of an abscess allows the successful use of drainage, one of the 3 core elements of source control (**Table 1**). Succssful drainage converts a closed-space abscess into a controlled sinus (a cavity that communicates with an epithelially lined surface) or fistula (an abnormal communication between 2 epithelially lined surfaces). A fistula will persist if any of several conditions is present: distal obstruction, epithelialization of the tract, a foreign body, uncontrolled infection or inflammation, malignancy, or radiation injury. In the absence of these factors, the fistulous tract will close. Thus following successful drainage of an abscess, and its conversion into a controlled fistula, the fistula is maintained open by the presence of the drainage tube, and when the tube is removed, provided that none of the other factors is present, the fistula should close (**Fig. 2**). The principles underlying the development and persistence or resolution of a fistula are some of the most fundamental upon which the craft of surgery is based. In addition to their use

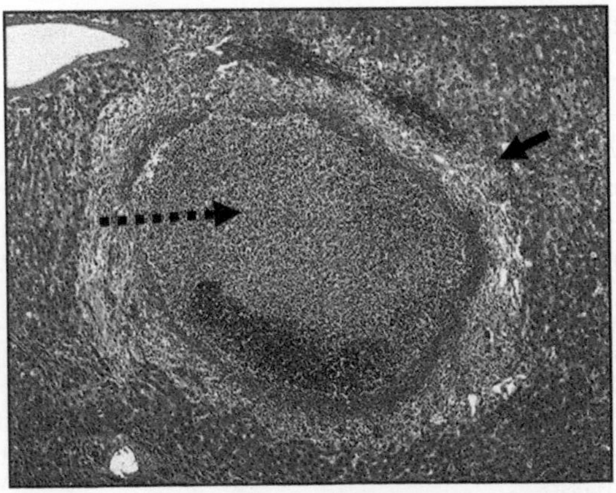

Fig. 1. A photomicrograph of a liver abscess illustrates the key structural features of an abscess. The abscess contents (*dotted arrow*) are a mixture of neutrophils, bacteria, tissue debris, and tissue fluid, colloquially called pus. Local activation of inflammation induces activation of the coagulation cascade resulting in fibrin deposition at the periphery of this process, and creating the characteristic fibrin capsule that walls off an abscess (*solid arrow*). *From* the CDC Public Health Image Library, image credit CDC/Rodney M. Donlan, PhD; Janice Carr (PHIL #7488), 2005.

Table 1 Core elements of source control	
Drainage	The evacuation of infected fluid through the opening of an abscess, by incision or by the insertion of a drain. Drainage converts a closed abscess into a controlled sinus or fistula
Examples	Incision and drainage of an ischiorectal abscess Percutaneous drainage of a diverticular abscess Open surgical drainage of a subphrenic abscess
Debridement	The removal of devitalized or infected solid tissue
Examples	Wet-to-dry dressings of an infected surgical wound Surgical excision of infected pancreatic necrosis Excision of gangrenous soft tissue or intestine
Device removal	The removal of a prosthetic device that has become colonized by microorganisms living in a biofilms
Examples	Removal of an infected central venous or urinary catheter Excision of an infected vascular graft Replacement of an endotracheal tube by a tracheostomy tube
Definitive measures	Other interventions performed to remove a focus of infection and to restore optimal function and quality of life
Examples	Excision of diverticular disease and restoration of intestinal continuity Decortication following drainage of an empyema Repair of an abdominal wall hernia following treatment of peritonitis

in the source-control management of an abscess, they represent the biologic basis for the success of intestinal anastomoses or stomas (epithelialization of a fistulous tract maintains its patency) or for procedures such as tracheostomy or gastrostomy, in which a foreign body enables a fistulous tract to persist.

Debridement

Small amounts of necrotic tissue are degraded by enzymes from phagocytic cells, and comprise one of the components of an abscess. Larger volumes of necrotic

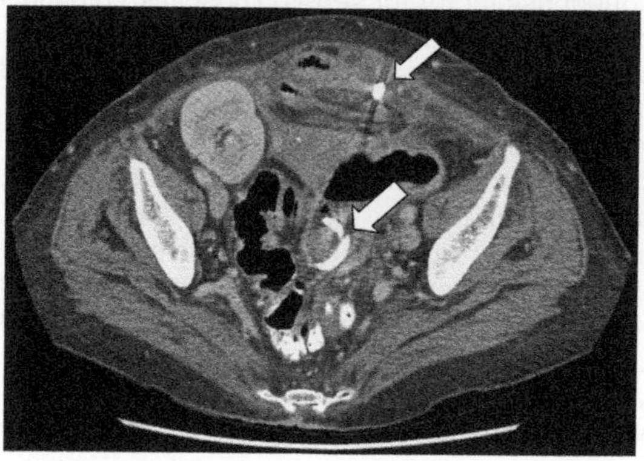

Fig. 2. Percutaneous drainage of a diverticular abscess in a patient with diverticulitis has created a colocutaneous fistula. The fistula remains open, because of the presence of a foreign body (the drain, *arrows*). In the absence of distal obstruction in the sigmoid colon or rectum, epithelialization of the tract, malignancy, or uncontrolled inflammation, the tract should close following drain removal, permitting an elective sigmoid resection at a later date to remove the diseased colon and prevent recurrent diverticulitis.

tissue, however, overwhelm the capacity of the host innate immune system, and so must be removed surgically. Although microbial products, interacting with pattern recognition receptors on host innate immune cells, are the best-known triggers of the inflammatory response resulting in sepsis, necrotic tissue can evoke a similar response by inducing the release of interleukin-1α (IL-1α).[4] The mechanisms promoting the activation of an inflammatory response by noninfectious stimuli are poorly understood, and challenging to elucidate. It is known that host-derived substances such as uric acid,[5] heat shock proteins,[6] and oxidized phospholipids[7] induce an inflammatory response through the activation of toll-like receptor signaling pathways. A potent systemic inflammatory response with massive neutrophil accumulation in the lung is the result of ischemia-reperfusion injury of the intestine[8] or extremity.[9] It is unclear whether that response results from the release of endogenous substances from the ischemic tissue, or from the secondary effects of the injury on the gastrointestinal tract, leading to the translocation of endotoxin or bacteria from the gut lumen.

It is apparent, however, that removal of necrotic tissue, and particularly infected necrotic tissue, plays an important role in eliminating the trigger of an ongoing inflammatory response. In some cases, notably gangrene of the distal extremities in patients with peripheral vascular disease, the ischemic tissue is isolated from the systemic circulation by virtue of the occlusion of the arteries and veins of the region; under these circumstances, the systemic response is minimal, and urgent intervention is not needed. In other circumstances, for example necrotizing soft tissue infections or intestinal infarction, the systemic response to the necrotic infected tissue is dramatic and life threatening, and emergent intervention is required. Yet in other infections such as infected retroperitoneal necrosis following severe acute pancreatitis, debridement of infected necrotic tissue may be necessary for the resolution of the infection, but may be safely deferred until it can be performed with minimal morbidity.[10]

Device Removal

Although device-related infections causing sepsis in ambulatory individuals are uncommon, they are the most common cause of nosocomial infection in the critically ill patient, and a frequent risk factor for sepsis in hospitalized patients. Removal of the infected device is desirable, because the device typically harbours microorganisms in a biofilm, and so serves as a source of continuous bacterial shedding, and because the presence of a foreign body impairs local host defenses.

Many microorganisms are capable of living independently (in a planktonic state) or within an exopolymeric matrix known as a biofilm (in a sessile state). The transition between the 2 states is regulated by environmental factors such as nutrient availability, through microbial quorum-sensing mechanisms that provide the organism with information about the external milieu.[11] The formation of a biofilm enables a colony of microorganisms to establish residence on an indwelling foreign body, and biofilms have been implicated in the pathogenesis and persistence of device-related infections, including those involving prosthetic joints,[12] prosthetic heart valves,[13] central venous catheters,[14] urinary catheters,[15] and endotracheal tubes (**Fig. 3**).[16]

Microorganisms present within a biofilm are less sensitive to antibiotics than those in the planktonic or free state.[17] This reduced susceptibility results not only from the physical barrier created by the biofilm but also from secondary effects of the biofilm on the local oxygen availability. The presence of a foreign body impairs neutrophil oxidative killing capacity, and so impedes innate antimicrobial host defenses.[18]

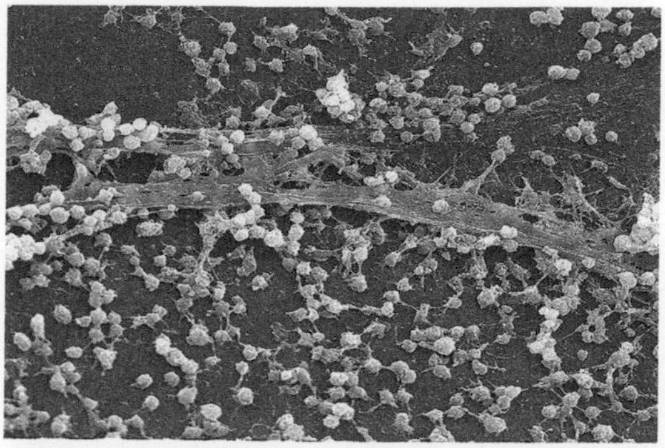

Fig. 3. *Staphylococcus aureus* growing within a biofilm on a vascular catheter. (*From* the CDC Public Health Image Library, image credit CDC/Rodney M. Donlan, PhD; Janice Carr (PHIL #7488), 2005).

PRINCIPLES OF CLINICAL MANAGEMENT

Diagnosis

Effective source control presumes an ability to diagnose a local focus of infection that is amenable to source-control measures. The history and physical examination remain the most important initial diagnostic maneuvers. New onset of pain may aid in localizing the site of infection in a patient with systemic manifestations of sepsis. A history of a recent surgical procedure suggests an infectious complication at the surgical site, or in the surgical wound. A history of peripheral vascular disease, or recent myocardial infarction, atrial fibrillation, or invasive arteriographic procedure raises the possibility of arterial thrombosis or embolus respectively. A careful history from the patient, family, or caregivers will often enable a presumptive diagnosis to be established.

Tenderness or other local signs of inflammation are characteristic manifestations of an infectious process that may benefit from source-control measures. Invasive devices raise the possibility of a device-related infection such as catheter-related bacteremia, endocarditis, or sinusitis secondary to a nasogastric tube. Crepitus in the tissues suggests the possibility of a gas-forming necrotizing soft tissue infection.

However, physical examination alone is rarely sufficient to diagnose an infectious focus and to plan its optimal treatment. Contrast-enhanced computed tomography (CT) has emerged as the single most useful diagnostic modality, because it not only identifies a pathologic process resulting in infection but also provides information on the nature of the local infectious process: is there a discrete, walled-off abscess or diffuse nonlocalized infected fluid?; is there tissue necrosis with evidence of nonperfused tissue? CT scanning provides a means of accessing an infectious focus using percutaneous techniques.

Other radiologic techniques provide useful information in selected circumstances. A plain film of the chest or abdomen may show free intraperitoneal air, and so establish a diagnosis of a perforated viscus (typically a duodenal ulcer or sigmoid diverticulitis) (**Fig. 4**). Ultrasonography is particularly useful in evaluating the biliary tree.

Drainage

Drainage techniques are useful when there is a well-localized collection of infected fluid, for example, an intra-abdominal abscess, a liquid empyema, or an infected joint. The optimal approach to drainage is one that creates a controlled sinus or fistula with the least trauma to the patient. Image-guided percutaneous drainage is generally the

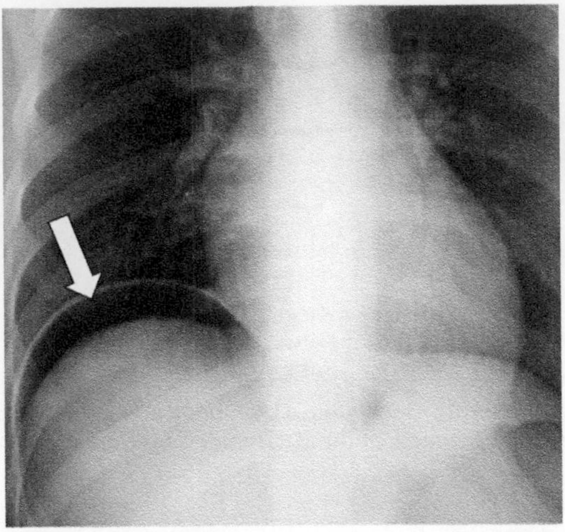

Fig. 4. Upright chest X-ray demonstrating free air under the right hemidiaphragm of a patient with a perforated duodenal ulcer.

approach of choice; however, operating may be preferred if the collection is inaccessible to radiologic drainage, if there are multiple loculated or diffuse poorly localized collections, if percutaneous techniques have failed, if there is a significant component of infected solid tissue, or if operating can safely expedite the definitive management of the source of infection.

Percutaneous drainage is accomplished under local anesthesia using CT or ultrasound imaging.[19] The collection is visualized, and an access route selected that avoids passing the drain through the bowel or other structures. After the abscess cavity has been entered using a finder needle, the tract is dilated using a Seldinger technique, and a flexible pigtail catheter inserted. The technique causes minimal injury to surrounding tissues; however, the small lumen of the catheter makes it susceptible to occlusion by local fibrin plugs. For the patient with multiple abscesses or a single complex multiloculated collection, several drains may be needed to accomplish adequate drainage.

The optimal surgical approach depends on the clinical context. For the patient presenting with a complex intra-abdominal process, a midline laparotomy provides optimal exposure and access, and so facilitates management. Laparoscopic approaches are an alternative to open exploration in centers where the expertise is available, and are particularly useful in the management of perforated ulcers.[20] However, the need for pneumoperitoneum, with its adverse effects on venous return, limits the role of laparoscopy in a hemodynamically unstable patient. Anastomotic leaks or postoperative collections are usually approached through the original surgical incision, provided that exposure is adequate; a new midline incision is a useful alternative if access through the original incision is restricted. Percutaneous techniques have largely eliminated the extraperitoneal approaches classically employed for the management of subphrenic abscesses.[21]

Open-abdomen approaches have fallen out of favor in the management of intra-abdominal infection.[22] They have not been shown to improve outcome, and are associated with an increased risk of fistulas, and an increased nursing workload. Most surgeons leave the abdomen open only when closure is not technically possible or would result in abdominal compartment syndrome.

Debridement

Only liquids can pass through a drainage tube; infected or necrotic solid tissue must be physically excised, a process known as debridement. This goal can be accomplished through the use of wet-to-dry dressings or chemical debriding agents, but surgery is the mainstay of therapy.

When an infectious process is of sufficient severity to result in life-threatening sepsis, surgical excision is invariably needed, although the timing of intervention may vary with the anatomic site of origin. Certain infections (notably necrotizing soft tissue infections or intestinal necrosis) follow a rapid course to a fatal outcome in the absence of intervention; emergent surgical intervention is life saving. Debridement of a necrotizing soft tissue infection requires the resources of an operating room and general anesthesia. The involved area is incised, and necrotic tissue excised back to viable tissues, identified by bleeding from the wound edges.[23,24] It is often difficult to assess the extent of necrosis at the initial procedure, and so the patient should be returned to the operating room in 24 hours and on a daily basis for further debridement, until the tissue necrosis is fully controlled, and granulation tissue is forming at the wound margins.[25] Subsequent wound management is aided by the use of a negative pressure wound vacuum device.[26] The need for amputation in necrotizing soft tissue infections of the extremity is dictated by the amount of muscle excised, and the prospects for functional recovery; amputation can be avoided in the majority of cases.

Intestinal infarction requires the excision of the necrotic bowel, and should be performed as rapidly as possible. The demarcation between viable and nonviable bowel is usually clear if the cause of the infarction is a closed-loop obstruction or arterial embolism, but may be more difficult to determine in cases of arterial or venous thrombosis, or in infarction associated with a low-flow state. If the extent of ischemia cannot be reliably assessed at the time of the initial operation, the patient should be taken back to the operating room in 24 to 48 hours for a second-look laparotomy or laparoscopy.[27,28] In an unstable patient, it is often safest to resect bowel that is visibly necrotic, leaving the ends stapled off in the peritoneal cavity, and closing the abdomen with a temporary abdominal-closure device. Further resection and anastomosis with formal abdominal closure can then be accomplished at the time of second-look laparotomy.

Device Removal

Although removal of a colonized device provides optimal source control in device-related infections, it is apparent that the morbidity of removal of a urinary or vascular catheter is significantly less than that of an infected vascular graft or heart valve (**Fig. 5**). In many patients, vascular access is challenging to obtain because of venous thrombosis and prior catheter use, and it may be preferable to leave the device in situ, and treat instead with a prolonged course of antibiotics.

SOURCE CONTROL IN INFECTIONS THAT ARE COMMON CAUSES OF SEPSIS

INTRA-ABDOMINAL INFECTION

Source-control decisions are often defined by multiple factors, and guided by the application of principles rather than normative data from large clinical trials. Some of those principles are discussed earlier in this article, but a few scenarios that are relatively common in patients with sever sepsis merit further comment. Decisions regarding optimal source control should be made by an experienced surgeon who can assess the relative merits of operative versus nonoperative management in an individual patient.

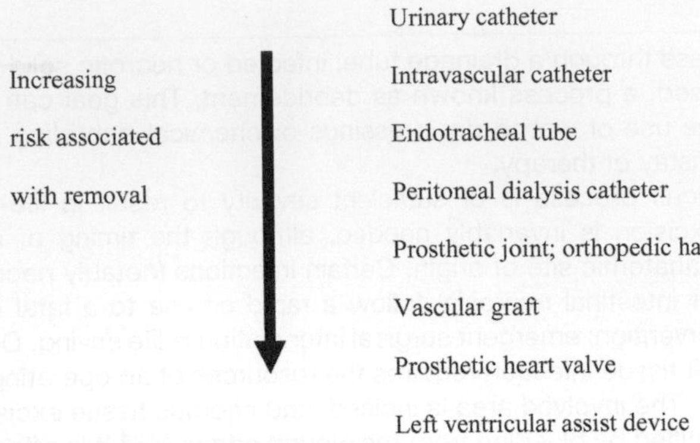

Fig. 5. Ease of removal of colonized devices.

Gastrointestinal Perforation

Perforation of the stomach or duodenum secondary to ulcer disease, or of the sigmoid colon secondary to diverticulitis, is a common community-acquired cause of intra-abdominal infection leading to sepsis. Although it is the most common cause of the acute abdomen, appendicitis typically runs a more benign clinical course, and is rarely the cause of severe sepsis or significant clinical morbidity.[29]

The diagnosis of a perforation of the gastrointestinal tract is typically presumptive, based on evidence of free intraperitoneal air or radiographic contrast material (**Fig. 6**). The need for surgery is dictated by the extent to which the procedure is localized, and the urgency of intervention by the clinical state of the patient. Thus a walled-off collection can usually be managed by percutaneous drainage, whereas evidence of diffuse peritoneal contamination identifies a situation that requires surgical intervention. The clinical state of the patient (not the findings of radiographic investigations) is the prime factor in deciding about the timing of intervention. A hemodynamically unstable patient with rapidly evolving organ dysfunction should have immediate intervention, whereas a patient who is clinically stable can be dealt with after deliberation.

In the stable patient, a walled-off perforation of a duodenal ulcer can be managed nonoperatively,[30] because normal peritoneal defenses have accomplished the objective of creating a controlled sinus. Poor localization, suggested by diffuse pain on abdominal examination or physiologic instability, suggests that operative intervention is needed. Current approaches are to patch a duodenal ulcer defect with omentum, or excise a perforated gastric ulcer; open and laparoscopic approaches are employed.[31]

Spontaneous colonic perforations most commonly arise in an area of diverticular disease, and originate within the sigmoid colon; resection of the sigmoid removes the focus of ongoing contamination and prevents future episodes. Nonetheless, if the perforation is localized, initial management by percutaneous drainage is the preferred approach (see **Fig. 2**), with definitive resection deferred to a later date.[32] When percutaneous techniques are not possible, there are several options. Historically, a 3-stage approach was preferred, consisting of an initial laparotomy to drain the abscess and a proximal colostomy to defunction the sigmoid colon, a second procedure to resect the sigmoid and anastomose the descending colon to the rectum, and finally a third stage, the closure of the colostomy. This 3-stage approach has given way to a 2- stage approach comprising an initial laparotomy with resection of the diseased sigmoid colon and drainage of the abscess, closure of the rectal stump, and creation of an end colostomy from the end of the descending colon (the so-called

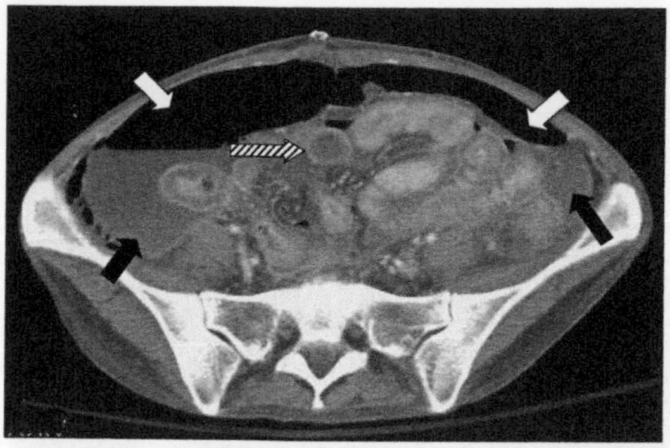

Fig. 6. CT scan demonstrating sequelae of an anastomotic leak following an ileocecal resection for Crohn disease, and demonstrating extensive free intraperitoneal air (*white arrows*) and fluid (*black arrows*); dotted arrow demonstrates enhancement of the small bowel serosa secondary to the local inflammatory process. Lack of localization of the infective process precluded percutaneous drainage, and so the patient was managed by laparotomy, peritoneal irrigation, and conversion of the leaking anastomosis to an ileostomy (a controlled enterocutaneous fistula).

Hartmann procedure). A small randomized trial[33] and a synthesis of data from a series of comparative studies[34] suggest that the 2-stage procedure results in lower rates of morbidity and mortality, particularly when the morbidity and mortality of the subsequent procedures necessary to restore intestinal continuity are considered. More recent case series suggest that resection and primary anastomosis is at least as good, if not better, than a 2-stage approach.[35–37] Another alternative in an unstable patient is a damage-control approach, consisting of sigmoid resection alone, leaving the stapled-off ends of the colon within the abdomen. The abdomen is closed with a temporary closure device, and the patient taken back to the operating room 24 to 48 hours later to complete the anastomosis and close the abdominal wall.[38]

Gastrointestinal Ischemia

Gut ischemia is a common and potentially lethal cause of an acute abdomen. Bacteria and their products can escape from the ischemic gut, and are absorbed through regional lymphatics and the peritoneal cavity. Gut ischemia can arise from arterial occlusion by embolism or thrombus, venous occlusion, or globally reduced splanchnic perfusion.[39] The responsible mechanism dictates the optimal management approach, and can often be inferred from the clinical presentation.

Acute arterial occlusion can result from embolus or thrombosis, from vasculitis, or from compression of the arterial inflow by adhesive bands or an intestinal volvulus, leading to a closed loop obstruction (**Fig. 7**).[40,41] Because of its gentle takeoff from the aorta, and lack of reliable collateral flow, the superior mesenteric artery is the most commonly affected vessel, with the result that ischemia involves the small bowel and the colon to the level of the distal transverse colon. The diagnosis is suggested by the appropriate clinical setting, reflecting risk factors such as atrial fibrillation, recent myocardial infarction, or antecedent invasive aortic angiographic procedure in the case of embolism, or severe preexisting occlusive vascular disease in the case of thrombosis, and the development of severe midgut abdominal pain, localized to the periumbilical region. Clinical features such as profound leukocytosis or acidosis are suggestive of, but neither sensitive nor specific for, the diagnosis of intestinal

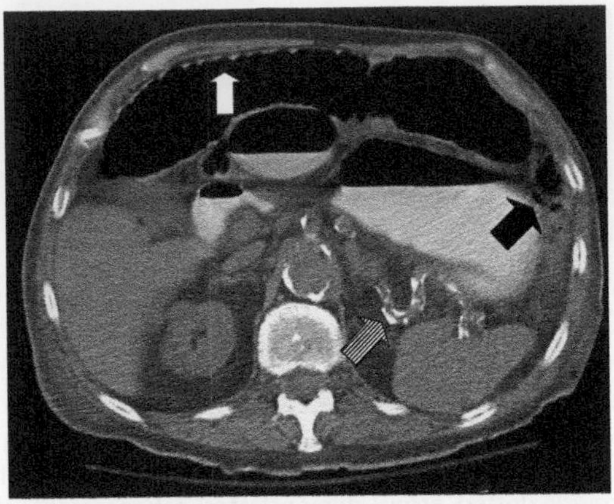

Fig. 7. Nonocclusive mesenteric ischemia secondary to splanchnic hypoperfusion. Note the irregular features of the mucosa of the transverse colon (*white arrow*), evidence of pneumatosis at the splenic flexure (*black arrow*), and the evidence of peripheral vascular disease reflected in calcification of the splenic artery (*hatched arrow*).

ischemia. Thrombosis typically involves the orifice of the takeoff of the superior mesenteric artery, and results in ischemia or infarction that involves the small bowel from the ligament of Treitz through to the midtransverse colon. Emboli characteristically lodge distal to the first jejunal branch of the superior mesenteric artery, and thus approximately 20 to 30 cm of jejunum is spared. Venous infarction arises in patients with preexisting prothrombotic disorders, and is associated with engorgement of the affected gut that can often be identified on ultrasonography. Nonocclusive mesenteric ischemia occurs in patients with hypotension, and more commonly involves the colon.

The diagnosis is suggested by the clinical setting and is most commonly confirmed by CT scan. Clinical judgment is paramount, for radiologic investigations are not completely sensitive,[41] and conversely, intuitively ominous findings such as portal venous gas do not necessarily imply gut ischemia.[42] The key to successful source-control management of gut ischemia is emergent intervention to restore vascular flow or resect gangrenous intestine. The appropriate clinical setting and a high index of clinical suspicion are key to initiating the investigations and surgical interventions that can accomplish this objective.

Infected Pancreatic Necrosis

Secondary infection of necrotic pancreatic and peripancreatic tissue is a common complication of necrotizing pancreatitis of sufficient severity to warrant admission to the intensive care unit. Infection is a late complication, typically arising several weeks after the onset of illness,[43] and involving enteric organisms that have translocated from the adjacent gastrointestinal tract.[44]

Contemporary management of the patient with suspected infected necrosis has changed dramatically in recent decades.[45] The diagnosis is suspected on the basis of CT findings of necrosis and gas, and confirmed by fine-needle aspiration of the involved area.[46] Case series[47,48] and a single randomized controlled trial[49] support contemporary approaches to surgical management based on delaying intervention until the area of necrosis has become well walled-off from surrounding tissues, a process that typically is not evident for 3 or 4 weeks or longer after the onset of the disease. Percutaneous drainage of the liquid component of a complex pancreatic infection can temporize (**Fig. 8**), and may in some circumstances suffice to effect resolution of, the illness.[50]

Other Intra-Abdominal Infections

Cholangitis secondary to occlusion of the common bile duct by a gallstone produces a characteristic clinical syndrome of jaundice, fever, and right upper quadrant pain, and, in severe cases, hypotension and changes in mental status. Relief of the obstruction, usually by endoscopic retrograde pancreatography with papillotomy and stone extraction, results in rapid correction of the physiologic derangements.[51] Acute cholecystitis or liver abscess is an uncommon cause of severe sepsis and septic shock; percutaneous drainage is effective initial management for both.[52]

The management of postoperative peritonitis poses unique challenges arising from the nature of the antecedent procedure that led to the infection, the timing of diagnosis, the stability of the patient, and the skills and experience of the surgeon. Treatment must be individualized based on core principles articulated earlier in this article: the establishment of a controlled sinus or fistula by the simplest approach possible, and the removal of necrotic infected tissue.

The patient with suspected intra-abdominal infection but a nondiagnostic or negative abdominal CT scan is a common clinical scenario, and a particular source of friction between intensivists and surgeons. As a general principle, an intra-abdominal complication of sufficient severity to produce a clinical picture of severe sepsis or septic shock reflects a significant anatomic derangement that will be evident using modern CT scan techniques, and there is no credible evidence that nondirected or "blind" laparotomy is beneficial.[53] On the other hand, when imaging resources are not available, or in the rare situation where the clinical picture suggests a specific cause, laparotomy may be diagnostic and therapeutic. The decision is difficult, because a nontherapeutic laparotomy carries risk, and so the active involvement of an experienced surgeon is critical.

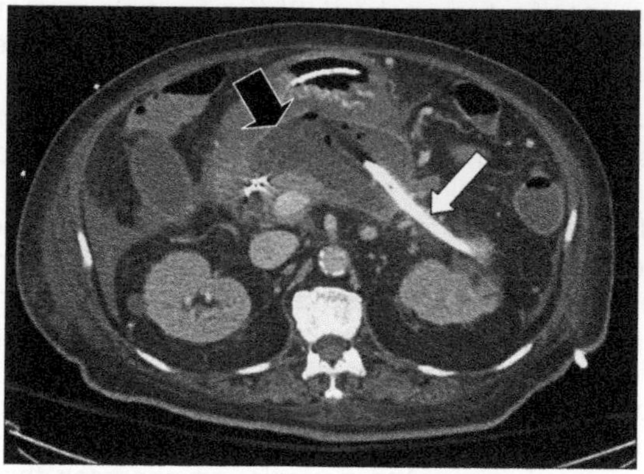

Fig. 8. Percutaneous drainage of a pancreatic abscess. The use of a percutaneous drain permits decompression of a complex pancreatic composed of infected pancreatic fluid and necrotic peripancreatic fact, allowing definitive surgical management to be delayed until the abscess cavity has become well demarcated from surrounding viable tissue. (*Black arrow* identifies the abscess cavity, and the *white arrow*, the percutaneous drain).

THORACIC INFECTIONS

The role of source control in patients with pneumonia is limited. Physiotherapy may be considered a form of source control directed at mobilizing pulmonary secretions, but it has not been shown to improve prognosis or hasten the resolution of community-acquired pneumonia.[54,55] Similarly, tracheal suctioning does not seem to alter the outcome in cases of established pneumonia, although it has been shown to reduce rates of development of ventilator-associated pneumonia in several clinical trials.[56,57] Since ventilator-associated pneumonia is a device-related infection, minimizing the duration of intubation and mechanical ventilation, or changing a colonized endotracheal tube, are logical management strategies, although they are difficult to evaluate, and so primarily of theoretical interest.

Source-control measures are important in the management of pleural or mediastinal infections. During the early course of an empyema, the infected pleural fluid is readily controlled by percutaneous drainage using a chest tube or an image-guided catheter. With time, activation of coagulation within the cavity results in the deposition of fibrin, which can entrap the lung and prevent its full reexpansion. In the early phases of fibrinopurulent empyema, video-assisted drainage is often successful, but with further organization, formal surgical decortication becomes necessary.[58]

Mediastinitis most commonly arises following open cardiac surgery. Although a bacteriologic diagnosis can usually be established by percutaneous sampling, adequate source control generally necessitates open surgical drainage.[59] Mediastinitis can also be a consequence of inferior extension of infection arising in the head and neck; successful management of these infections with percutaneous catheter drainage has been reported.[60]

NECROTIZING SOFT TISSUE INFECTIONS

Necrotizing soft tissue infections include a variety of clinical syndromes that have in common the development of necrosis of the skin, subcutaneous fat, fascia, and, in some cases, underlying muscle. The terminology applied to such infections is confusing, and includes descriptions based on the infecting organism (for example, gas gangrene caused by *Clostridia*), the anatomic site involved (for example, Fournier gangrene), and the specific tissues involved (for example, necrotizing fasciitis). In reality these are overlapping syndromes, for which the key issue with respect to source control is the presence of necrosis, rather than simply inflammation. Infections with *Clostridia* or group A streptococci are particularly virulent and evolve rapidly; emergent diagnosis and management are essential to minimize morbidity and mortality.

The presence of underlying necrosis may be suggested by bullae, ecchymosis, or discoloration of the overlying skin, or by crepitus on physical examination; however, these findings are not particularly sensitive. Radiographic examination may reveal air in the tissues, but this finding too lacks sensitivity and specificity for the diagnosis.[61] Fascial thickening and edema on CT scan suggest the diagnosis,[62] and biopsy or aspiration of the suspected area may establish a bacteriologic diagnosis. Nonetheless, it is not uncommon that the diagnosis is established through surgical exploration of the area of suspected necrosis, an approach that is sensitive and specific, and curative when positive, with only minimal additional morbidity when it is not.

The treatment of a necrotizing soft tissue infection entails wide debridement of all necrotic tissue.[63] Because the extent of tissue necrosis may not be apparent at the initial operation, initial debridement back to bleeding tissue should be followed by reexploration in 24 hours with further debridement as indicated. Reexploration is repeated as long as significant amounts of newly necrotic tissue are encountered.

URINARY TRACT INFECTIONS

Urinary tract infections typically carry a better prognosis than other infections that produce the clinical syndromes of severe sepsis and septic shock. Source-control measures are indicated in the event of abscess or obstruction, and in cystitis arising in association with a colonized urinary catheter.

The diagnosis of urinary tract infection is established based on clinical features, supplemented by urinalysis and culture, and appropriate imaging studies. Ultrasonography and CT scanning have emerged as the preferred diagnostic modalities for infections involving the kidney and upper urinary tract.[64]

Most infections of the upper urinary tract can be managed adequately by a combination of systemic antibiotics and percutaneous drainage of an obstructed ureter or renal abscess.[65] The need for nephrectomy is uncommon. Cystitis is readily managed by catheter change.

SUMMARY

This brief overview of the role of source control in sepsis emphasizes the underlying principles rather than the empiric evidence from well-performed clinical studies. The reasons for this are several. First there is a paucity of high-level published evidence, with few rigorous large clinical series, and even fewer clinical trials. Second, the decision-making process in the individual patient is complex, and often not amenable to study using the design of a randomized controlled trial, for decisions involve consideration not only of the underlying disease but of the stability of the patient, the presence of comorbidities, and the prior surgical history, all factors that can heavily influence the decision to choose one therapeutic option rather than another. The scope of the topic is large, and the space limited. Interested readers are referred to more detailed discussions such as that found in the background to the recommendations on source control in the guidelines of the Surviving Sepsis Campaign.[1]

Source control is a core treatment modality in the management of the patient with severe sepsis or septic shock. Its optimal use assumes a comprehensive knowledge of biologic principles, the complexities of the septic response, and the range of surgical and nonsurgical options, and a combination of therapeutic aggressiveness and judicious caution in the clinician charged with making the decision. As every intensivist learns, appropriate source-control intervention can rapidly alter the course of sepsis to a more favorable direction, and suboptimal decision-making can change a difficult clinical challenge into a nightmare.

REFERENCES

1. Marshall JC, Maier RV, Jimenez M, et al. Source control in the management of severe sepsis and septic shock: an evidence-based review. Crit Care Med 2004;32(Suppl 11):S513–26.
2. Marshall JC. Neutrophils in the pathogenesis of sepsis. Crit Care Med 2005; 33(Suppl 12):S502–5.
3. Schouten M, Wiersinga WJ, Levi M, et al. Inflammation, endothelium, and coagulation in sepsis. J Leukoc Biol 2008;83(3):536–45.

4. Chen CJ, Kono H, Golenbock D, et al. Identification of a key pathway required for the sterile inflammatory response triggered by dying cells. Nat Med 2007;13(7): 851–6.
5. Martinon F, Pétrilli V, Mayor A, et al. Gout-associated uric acid crystals activate the NALP3 inflammasome. Nature 2006;440(7081):237–41.
6. Chase MA, Wheeler DS, Lierl KM, et al. Hsp72 induces inflammation and regulates cytokine production in airway epithelium through a TLR4- and NF-kappaB-dependent mechanism. J Immunol 2007;179(9):6318–24.
7. Imai Y, Kuba K, Neely GG, et al. Identification of oxidative stress and Toll-like receptor 4 signaling as a key pathway of acute lung injury. Cell 2008;133(2): 235–49.
8. Sookhai S, Wang JJ, McCourt M, et al. A novel therapeutic strategy for attenuating neutrophil-mediated lung injury in vivo. Ann Surg 2002;235(2):285–91.
9. Vega VL, Mardones L, Maldonaldo M, et al. Xanthine oxidase released from reperfused hind limbs mediate kupffer cell activation, neutrophil sequestration, and hepatic oxidative stress in rats subjected to tourniquet shock. Shock 2000; 14(5):565–71.
10. Adler DG, Chari ST, Dahl TJ, et al. Conservative management of infected necrosis complicating severe acute pancreatitis. Am J Gastroenterol 2003;98(1):98–103.
11. Lynch AS, Rbertson GT. Bacterial and fungal biofilm infections. Annu Rev Med 2008;59:415–28.
12. Gristina AG, Costerton JW. Bacterial adherence to biomaterials and tissue. The significance of its role in clinical sepsis. J Bone Joint Surg Am 1985;67(2): 264-73.
13. Litzler PY, Benard L, Barbier-Frebourg N, et al. Biofilm formation on pyrolytic carbon heart valves: influence of surface free energy, roughness, and bacterial species. J Thorac Cardiovasc Surg 2007;134(4):1025–32.
14. Donlam RM. Biofilms on central venous catheters: is eradication possible? Curr Top Microbiol Immunol 2008;322:133–61.
15. Hatt JK, Rather PN. Role of bacterial biofilms in urinary tract infections. Curr Top Microbiol Immunol 2008;322:163–92.
16. Feldman C, Kassel M, Cantrell J, et al. The presence and sequence of endotracheal tube colonization in patients undergoing mechanical ventilation. Eur Respir J 1999;13(3):546–51.
17. Stewart PS, Costerton JW. Antibiotic resistance of bacteria in biofilms. Lancet 2001;358(9276):135–8.
18. Zimmerli W, Lew PD, Waldvogel FA. Pathogenesis of foreign body infection. Evidence for a local granulocyte defect. J Clin Invest 1984;73(4):1191–200.
19. vanSonnenberg E, Wittich GR, Goodacre BW, et al. Percutaneous abscess drainage: update. World J Surg 2001;25(3):362–72.
20. Sanabria AE, Morales CH, Villegas MI. Laparoscopic repair for perforated peptic ulcer disease. Cochrane Database Syst Rev 2005;(4):CD004778.
21. Spain DA, Martin RC, Carrillo EH, et al. Twelfth rib resection. Preferred therapy for subphrenic abscess in selected surgical patients. Arch Surg 1997;132(11): 1203–6.
22. Adkins AL, Robbins J, Villalba M, et al. Open abdomen management of intra-abdominal sepsis. Am Surg 2004;70(2):137–40.
23. Elliott DC, Kufera JA, Myers RAM. Necrotizing soft tissue infections. Risk factors for mortality and strategies for management. Ann Surg 1996;224(5):672–83.
24. Cainzos M, Gonzalez-Rodriguez FJ. Necrotizing soft tissue infections. Curr Opin Crit Care 2007;13(4):433–9.

25. Bilton BD, Zibari GB, McMillan RW, et al. Aggressive surgical management of necrotizing fasciitis serves to decrease mortality: a retrospective study. Am Surg 1998;64:397–400.
26. Gregor S, Maegaele M, Sauerland S, et al. Negative pressure wound therapy: a vacuum of evidence? Arch Surg 2008;143(2):189–96.
27. Ward D, Vernava AM, Kamisnki DL, et al. Improved outcome by identification of high-risk nonocclusive mesenteric ischemia, aggressive reexploration, and delayed anastomosis. Am J Surg 1995;170(6):577–80.
28. Yanar H, Taviloglu K, Ertekin C, et al. Planned second-look laparoscopy in the management of acute mesenteric ischemia. World J Gastroenterol 2007;13(24): 3350–3.
29. Davies GM, Dasbach EJ, Teutsch S. The burden of appendicitis-related hospitalizations in the United States in 1997. Surg Infect (Larchmt) 2004;5(2):160–5.
30. Crofts TJ, Park KG, Steele RJ, et al. A randomized trial of nonoperative treatment for perforated peptic ulcer. N Engl J Med 1989;321(15):970–3.
31. Lunevicius R, Morkevicius M. Systematic review comparing laparoscopic and open repair for perforated peptic ulcer. Br J Surg 2005;92(10):1195–207.
32. Singh B, May K, Coltart I, et al. The long-term results of percutaneous drainage of diverticular abscess. Ann R Coll Surg Engl 2008;90(4):297–301.
33. Kronborg O. Treatment of perforated sigmoid diverticulitis: a prospective randomized trial. Br J Surg 1993;80(4):505–7.
34. Jimenez MF, Marshall JC. Source control in the management of sepsis. Intensive Care Med 2001;27:S49–62.
35. Biondo S, Jaurrieta E, Marti Rague J, et al. Role of resection and primary anastomosis of the left colon in the presence of peritonitis. Br J Surg 2000;87(11): 1580–4.
36. Schilling MK, Maurer CA, Kollmar O, et al. Primary vs. secondary anastomosis after sigmoid colon resection for perforated diverticulitis (Hinchey Stage III and IV): a prospective outcome and cost analysis. Dis Colon Rectum 2001;44(5): 699–703.
37. Gooszen AW, Tollenaar RA, Geelkerken RH, et al. Prospective study of primary anastomosis following sigmoid resection for suspected acute complicated diverticular disease. Br J Surg 2001;88(5):693–7.
38. van Goor H. Interventional management of abdominal sepsis: when and how. Langenbecks Arch Surg 2002;387(5-6):191–200.
39. Menon MJ, Amin AM, Mohammed A, et al. Acute mesenteric ischaemia. Acta Chir Belg 2005;105(4):344–54.
40. Herbert GS, Steele SR. Acute and chronic mesenteric ischemia. Surg Clin North Am 2007;87(5):1115–34.
41. Oldenburg WA, Lau LL, Rodenberg TJ, et al. Acute mesenteric ischemia: a clinical review. Arch Intern Med 2004;164(10):1054–62.
42. Nelson AL, Millington TM, Sahani D, et al. Hepatic portal venous gas: the ABCs of management. Arch Surg 2009;144(6):575–81.
43. Beger HG, Bittner R, Block S, et al. Bacterial contamination of pancreatic necrosis. A prospective clinical study. Gastroenterology 1986;91(2):433–8.
44. Ammori BJ. Role of the gut in the course of severe acute pancreatitis. Pancreas 2003;26(2):122–9.
45. Dugernier T, Dewaele J, Laterre PF. Current surgical management of acute pancreatitis. Acta Chir Belg 2006;106(2):165–71.
46. Uhl W, Warshaw A, Imrie C, et al. IAP guidelines for the surgical management of acute pancreatitis. Pancreatology 2002;2(6):565–73.

47. Hungness ES, Robb BW, Seeskin C, et al. Early debridement for necrotizing pancreatitis: is it worthwhile? J Am Coll Surg 2002;194(6):740–4.
48. Ashley SW, Perez A, Pierce EA, et al. Necrotizing pancreatitis: contemporary analysis of 99 consecutive cases. Ann Surg 2001;234(4):572–80.
49. Mier J, Leon EL, Castillo A, et al. Early versus late necrosectomy in severe necrotizing pancreatitis. Am J Surg 1997;173(2):71–5.
50. Loveday BP, Mittal A, Phillips A, et al. Minimally invasive management of pancreatic abscess, pseudocyst, and necrosis: a systematic review of current guidelines. World J Surg 2008;32(11):2383–94.
51. Lai EC, Mok FP, Tan ES, et al. Endoscopic biliary drainage for severe acute cholangitis. N Engl J Med 1992;326(24):1582–6.
52. Yusoff IF, Barkun JS, Barkun AN. Diagnosis and management of cholecystitis and cholangitis. Gastroenterol Clin North Am 2003;32(4):1145–68.
53. Bunt TJ. Non-directed relaparotomy for intraabdominal sepsis: a futile procedure. Am Surg 1986;52(6):294–8.
54. Britton S, Bejstedt M, Vedin L. Chest physiotherapy in primary pneumonia. Br Med J 1985;290(6483):1703–4.
55. Siempos II, Vardakas KZ, Kopterides P, et al. Adjunctive therapies for community-acquired pneumonia: a systematic review. J Antimicrob Chemother 2008;62(4):661–8.
56. Caruso P, Denari S, Ruiz SA, et al. Saline instillation before tracheal suctioning decreases the incidence of ventilator-associated pneumonia. Crit Care Med 2009;37(1):32–8.
57. Smulders K, van der Hoeven H, Weers-Pothoff I, et al. A randomized clinical trial of intermittent subglottic secretion drainage in patients receiving mechanical ventilation. Chest 2002;121(3):858–62.
58. Molnar TF. Current surgical treatment of thoracic empyema in adults. Eur J Cardiothorac Surg 2007;32(3):422–30.
59. Luskraz H, Murphy F, Bryant S, et al. Vacuum-assisted closure as a treatment modality for infections after cardiac surgery. J Thorac Cardiovasc Surg 2003;125(2):301–5.
60. Sumi Y, Ogura H, Nakamori Y, et al. Nonoperative catheter management for cervical necrotizing fasciitis with and without descending necrotizing mediastinitis. Arch Otolaryngol Head Neck Surg 2008;134(7):750–6.
61. Lille ST, Sato TT, Engrav LH, et al. Necrotizing soft tissue infections: obstacles in diagnosis. J Am Coll Surg 1996;182(1):7–11.
62. Beauchamp NJ Jr, Scott WW Jr, Gottlieb LM, et al. CT evaluation of soft tissue and muscle infection and inflammation: a systematic compartmental approach. Skeletal Radiol 1995;24:317–24.
63. Sarani B, Strong M, Pascual J, et al. Necrotizing fasciitis: current concepts and review of the literature. J Am Coll Surg 2009;208(2):279–88.
64. Browne RF, Zwirewich C, Torreggiani WC. Imaging of urinary tract infection in the adult. Eur Radiol 2004;14(Suppl 3):E168–83.
65. Somani BK, Nabi G, Thorpe P, et al. Is percutaneous drainage the new gold standard in the management of emphysematous pyelonephritis? Evidence from a systematic review. J Urol 2008;179(5):1844–9.

Sepsis-Induced Tissue Hypoperfusion

Alan E. Jones, MD*, Michael A. Puskarich, MD

KEYWORDS

• Sepsis • Septic shock • Resuscitation • Lactate
• Hypoperfusion • Infection • Emergency

It is been estimated that severe sepsis occurs at an incidence of 3.0 cases per 1000 persons per year, resulting in approximately 750,000 affected persons annually in the United States. Of those affected, 500,000 (67%) require intensive or intermediate care unit (ICU) services.[1] Recent estimates indicate that the rate of severe sepsis hospitalizations doubled during the last decade and that age-adjusted population-based mortality is increasing.[2] Sepsis affects the cardiovascular system through multiple mechanisms, and often these derangements result in tissue hypoperfusion. Tissue hypoperfusion is often present in the setting of overt shock, but it can also be present in patients without obvious shock physiology. If left untreated, tissue hypoperfusion contributes to the development of multiple organ dysfunction and ultimately, death. This article provides an overview of the pathophysiology, recognition, and treatment of sepsis-induced hypoperfusion.

PATHOPHYSIOLOGY

The clinician identifies tissue hypoperfusion by synthesizing the clinical impression with quantitative data, such as vital signs, urine output, and direct measurements of oxygenation. When the clinical impression and quantitative data suggest widespread organ hypoperfusion, emergent resuscitation must restore normal tissue oxygenation, and substrate delivery must occur to prevent further deterioration.[3] At the cellular level, hypoperfusion first affects the mitochondria.[4] The vast majority of aerobic chemical energy comes from mitochondrial combustion of fuel substrates (fats, carbohydrates, ketones) plus oxygen into carbon dioxide, and water. Mitochondria are affected first in conditions of inadequate tissue perfusion, and when they are provided inadequate oxygen, the cell catabolizes fuels to lactate, which accumulates and diffuses into the blood.[3,4]

One of the key components in identifying and treating tissue hypoperfusion in sepsis is understanding the cardiovascular derangements encountered during sepsis.

Department of Emergency Medicine, Carolinas Medical Center, 1000 Blythe Boulevard, MEB 304e, Charlotte, NC 28203, USA
* Corresponding author.
E-mail address: alan.jones@carolinas.org (A.E. Jones).

Crit Care Clin 25 (2009) 769–779
doi:10.1016/j.ccc.2009.06.003
criticalcare.theclinics.com

Although the understanding of sepsis pathophysiology has evolved dramatically over the past several decades,[5,6] the understanding of sepsis-induced cardiovascular derangements and how they develop continues to be incomplete. Understanding these cardiovascular manifestations is important in as much as they are the targets of therapeutic intervention in patients with tissue hypoperfusion.

Sepsis causes 2 major hemodynamic effects that must be considered: relative hypovolemia and cardiovascular depression. Sepsis produces relative hypovolemia from venous and arterial dilatation, which reduces right ventricular filling. Additionally, there is often absolute hypovolemia from insensible losses and sepsis-induced capillary leak, which leads to relative loss of intravascular volume into third spaces.[3] If volume resuscitation is initiated, it will lead to low systemic vascular resistance, normal or increased cardiac output, and elevated mixed venous oxygenation—a constellation known as hyperdynamic shock syndrome—in most patients. These hemodynamic abnormalities are collectively referred to as distributive shock because of the presumed hypoperfusion to various tissues due to maldistribution of flow.[5,7]

Evidence has shown that septic shock causes myocardial dysfunction simultaneously with vasodepression and capillary leak. Through direct measurements of cardiac contractility, investigators have shown reduced left ventricular ejection fraction, increased end-diastolic and end-systolic volumes (increased compliance) and normal or decreased stroke volume, reduced systemic vascular resistance, and compensatory tachycardia as the characteristic pattern of sepsis-induced heart dysfunction.[5,8,9] Fluid therapy will usually modify this pattern by increasing stroke volume; however, in normotensive and hypotensive subjects, impaired ejection fraction and ventricular dilation remain present, and their presence peaks in the first few days and reverses within the first week of sepsis onset in survivors.[10,11]

Tissue hypoperfusion can be present even in the presence of normal blood pressure and adequate cardiac output, a state sometimes referred to as cryptic shock.[12–15] This hypoperfusion may be related to preferential maldistribution of blood flow at the regional or microvascular level.[13] It also may be related to mitochondrial dysfunction in the presence of adequate substrate delivery.[16] Derangements of small vessel perfusion are largely a function of intrinsic events in the microcirculation. The causes of microcirculatory flow alterations in sepsis are multifactorial and include endothelial cell dysfunction, increased leukocyte and platelet adhesion, fibrin deposition, erythrocyte stiffness, altered local perfusion pressures due to regional redistribution of blood flow, and functional shunting.[17–20] Although research on septic shock is classically focused on macrocirculatory hemodynamics that reflect the distribution of blood flow globally throughout the body, a functioning microcirculation is another critical component of the cardiovascular system that is necessary for effective oxygen delivery to tissues. Regardless of the cause, it seems as if early and aggressive hemodynamic intervention can impart the best opportunity to limit the damage caused by tissue hypoperfusion, including attenuating the inflammatory response and endothelial injury.[21,22]

CLINICAL FEATURES

If effective tissue perfusion is not restored in a timely manner, the incipient cellular dysfunction and organ failure may become irreversible. Therefore, rapid recognition of tissue hypoperfusion requires the integration of information from bedside assessment synthesized with quantitative data. Heart rate can be normal or low in states of hypoperfusion, especially in cases complicated by prescribed drugs that depress heart rate. Arterial blood pressure can be normal or even high when significant tissue hypoperfusion is present, probably due to adrenergic reflexes. Although arterial blood pressure as a sole indicator of hypoperfusion is an unreliable marker, its presence can be an important indicator of tissue hypoperfusion. A recent study found that nonsustained hypotension in the emergency department confers a significantly increased risk of death during hospitalization in patients admitted with sepsis. This should impart reluctance to dismiss nonsustained hypotension, including a single measurement, as not clinically significant or meaningful.[23] The heart rate to systolic blood pressure ratio (shock index) may provide greater evidence of hypoperfusion, especially in the setting of normotension, than either measurement alone; a normal ratio is less than 0.8. Urine output provides an excellent indicator of regional (organ) tissue perfusion and is readily available in most patients.[3] A scoring system for the detection of tissue hypoperfusion in sepsis was proposed by Spronk and colleagues,[17] and it includes hemodynamic variables, peripheral circulation, microcirculatory variables, systemic markers of tissue oxygenation, and organ dysfunction. Although the bedside calculation of a score for tissue hypoperfusion is not likely to be necessary, the incorporation of an indicator of tissue hypoperfusion into the clinical assessment may improve identification of hypoperfusion, particularly in subtle cases. **Table 1** provides a list of variables that can assist with detecting tissue hypoperfusion. Regional tissue hypoperfusion can be, and often is, present in the absence of evidence of global hypoperfusion. Several of these common variables will be covered with more depth.

Lactate

Lactate is a commonly used indicator of tissue hypoperfusion, particularly in sepsis. Lack of oxygen delivery to the cell prompts a stall in transfer of electrons to the mitochondrial electron transport chain, subsequently decreasing acetyl coenzyme A entry into the tricarboxylic acid cycle.[4] As mitochondrial oxidative phosphorylation fails and energy metabolism becomes dependent on anaerobic glycolysis, the production of cellular lactate increases sharply, resulting in eventual diffusion into the blood during prolonged cell ischemia. Elevated circulating lactate concentration thus indicates

Table 1
Variables that can assist with detecting tissue hypoperfusion

Global	Organ or Regional
Hypotension	Low urine output
Tachycardia	Elevated levels of bilirubin or liver transaminases
Low cardiac output	Elevated levels of cardiac enzymes
Mottled skin	Impaired microcirculatory flow (sidestream dark-field video microscopy)
Delayed capillary refill	Increased tonometric CO_2 gap (gastric tonometry)
Altered mental state	Increased sublingual CO_2 gap (sublingual capnometry)
Hyperlactemia	Decreased tissue oxygenation or delayed occlusion test slope (near infrared spectroscopy)
Low mixed venous oxygen saturation	—
Low central venous oxygen saturation	—

42. Nguyen HB, Rivers EP, Knoblich BP, et al. Early lactate clearance is associated with improved outcome in severe sepsis and septic shock. Crit Care Med 2004;32:1637–42.
43. Arnold RC, Shapiro NI, Jones AE, et al. Multi-center study of early lactate clearance as a determinant of survival in patients with presumed sepsis. Shock 2009;34:36–40.
44. Jones A, Shapiro N, Trzeciak S, et al. Multi-center randomized controlled trial of lactate clearance versus central venous oxygen saturation as the endpoint of early sepsis resuscitation. Acad Emerg Med 2009;16(4 Suppl 1):S143.
45. Gattinoni L, Brazzi L, Pelosi P, et al. A trial of goal-oriented hemodynamic therapy in critically ill patients. SvO2 Collaborative Group. N Engl J Med 1995;333:1025–32.
46. Rhodes A, Cusack RJ, Newman PJ, et al. A randomized, controlled trial of the pulmonary artery catheter in critically ill patients [see comment]. Intensive Care Med 2002;28:256–64.
47. Richard C, Warszawski J, Anguel N, et al. Early use of the pulmonary artery catheter and outcomes in patients with shock and acute respiratory distress syndrome: a randomized controlled trial. JAMA 2003;290:2713–20.
48. Harvey S, Harrison DA, Singer M, et al. Assessment of the clinical effectiveness of pulmonary artery catheters in management of patients in intensive care (PAC-Man): a randomized controlled trial. Lancet 2005;366:472–7.
49. Binanay C, Califf RM, Hasselblad V, et al. Evaluation study of congestive heart failure and pulmonary artery catheterization effectiveness: the ESCAPE trial. JAMA 2005;294:1625–33.
50. Ardsnet, Wheeler AP, Bernard GR, et al. Pulmonary-artery versus central venous catheter to guide treatment of acute lung injury. N Engl J Med 2006;354:2213–24.
51. Rivers EP, Ander DS, Powell D. Central venous oxygen saturation monitoring in the critically ill patient. Curr Opin Crit Care 2001;7:204–11.
52. Scheinman MM, Brown MA, Rapaport E. Critical assessment of use of central venous oxygen saturation as a mirror of mixed venous oxygen in severely ill cardiac patients. Circulation 1969;40:165–72.
53. Dueck MH, Klimek M, Appenrodt S, et al. Trends but not individual values of central venous oxygen saturation agree with mixed venous oxygen saturation during varying hemodynamic conditions. Anesthesiology 2005;103:249–57.
54. Bellomo R, Reade MC, Warrillow SJ. The pursuit of a high central venous oxygen saturation in sepsis: growing concerns. Crit Care 2008;12:130.
55. Creteur J, Carollo T, Soldati G, et al. The prognostic value of muscle StO2 in septic patients. Intensive Care Med 2007;33:1549–56.
56. Doerschug KC, Delsing AS, Schmidt GA, et al. Impairments in microvascular reactivity are related to organ failure in human sepsis. Am J Physiol Heart Circ Physiol 2007;293:H1065–71.
57. Skarda DE, Mulier KE, Myers DE, et al. Dynamic near-infrared spectroscopy measurements in patients with severe sepsis. Shock 2007;27:348–53.
58. Marik PE. Sublingual capnography: a clinical validation study. Chest 2001;120: 923–7.
59. Creteur J, De BD, Sakr Y, et al. Sublingual capnometry tracks microcirculatory changes in septic patients. Intensive Care Med 2006;32:516–23.
60. Marik PE, Bankov A. Sublingual capnometry versus traditional markers of tissue oxygenation in critically ill patients. Crit Care Med 2003;31:818–22.
61. Groner W, Winkelman JW, Harris AG, et al. Orthogonal polarization spectral imaging: a new method for study of the microcirculation. Nat Med 1999;5: 1209–12.

62. Harris AG, Sinitsina I, Messmer K. The Cytoscan Model E-II, a new reflectance microscope for intravital microscopy: comparison with the standard fluorescence method. J Vasc Res 2000;37:469–76.
63. Mathura KR, Vollebregt KC, Boer K, et al. Comparison of OPS imaging and conventional capillary microscopy to study the human microcirculation. J Appl Phys 2001;91:74–8.
64. Lehmann KG, Gelman JA, Weber MA, et al. Comparative accuracy of three automated techniques in the noninvasive estimation of central blood pressure in men. Am J Cardiol 1998;81:1004–12.
65. Hayes MA, Timmins AC, Yau EH, et al. Elevation of systemic oxygen delivery in the treatment of critically ill patients. N Engl J Med 1994;330:1717–22.
66. Jones AE, Brown MD, Trzeciak S, et al. The effect of a quantitative resuscitation strategy on mortality in patients with sepsis: a meta-analysis. Crit Care Med 2008;36:2734–9.
67. Sevransky JE, Nour S, Susia GM, et al. Hemodynamic goals in randomized clinical trials in patients with sepsis: a systematic review of the literature. Crit Care 2007;11:R67.
68. Dellinger RP, Levy MM, Carlet JM, et al. Surviving sepsis campaign: International guidelines for management of severe sepsis and septic shock: 2008. Crit Care Med 2008;36:296–327.

GENERAL APPROACH

Septic shock requires early, vigorous resuscitation. An integrated approach directed at rapidly restoring systemic oxygen delivery and improving tissue oxygenation has been shown to improve survival significantly in septic shock.[4] Although the specific approach that is used may vary, certain critical elements should be incorporated in any resuscitative effort. Therapy should be guided by parameters that reflect the adequacy of tissue and organ perfusion. Fluid infusion should be vigorous and titrated to clinical end points of volume repletion. Systemic oxygen delivery should be supported by ensuring arterial oxygen saturation, maintaining adequate levels of hemoglobin, and by using vasoactive agents directed to physiologic and clinical end points.

In shock states, estimation of blood pressure using a cuff may be inaccurate; use of an arterial cannula provides a more appropriate and reproducible measurement of arterial pressure.[5–7] Arterial catheters also allow beat-to-beat analysis so that decisions regarding therapy can be based on immediate and reproducible blood pressure information, facilitating the administration of large quantities of fluids and potent vasopressor and inotropic agents to critically ill patients.[1]

Although patients with shock and mild hypovolemia may be treated successfully with rapid fluid replacement alone, hemodynamic monitoring may be useful to provide a diagnostic hemodynamic assessment in patients with moderate or severe shock. In addition, because hemodynamics can change rapidly in sepsis, and because noninvasive evaluation is frequently incorrect in estimating filling pressures and cardiac output, hemodynamic monitoring is often useful for monitoring the response to therapy.

Changes in systolic arterial pressure or pulse arterial pressure caused by positive pressure ventilation can predict which patients respond to fluid loading (increased preload) with an increase in their cardiac output.[8] Echocardiography can also provide information on left ventricular size and systolic performance, right ventricular size and function, and valvular and pericardial abnormalities; and echo Doppler allows for estimation of stroke volume, pulmonary systolic pressure, the severity of valvular stenosis or regurgitation, and diastolic function. This information can be useful to assess myocardial function, cardiac output, and fluid status in patients with septic shock, and is complementary to hemodynamic assessment.

Goals and Monitoring of Vasopressor Therapy

When fluid administration fails to restore an adequate arterial pressure and organ perfusion, therapy with vasopressor agents should be initiated.[6] The ultimate goals of hemodynamic therapy in shock are to restore effective tissue perfusion and to normalize cellular metabolism. In septic shock, tissue hypoperfusion may result not only from decreased perfusion pressure attributable to hypotension but also from abnormal shunting of a normal or increased cardiac output.[1] Cellular alterations may also occur. Hemodynamic support of sepsis requires consideration of both global and regional perfusion.

Arterial pressure is the end point of vasopressor therapy, and the restoration of adequate pressure is the criterion of effectiveness. Blood pressure, however, does not always equate to blood flow, and the precise level of mean arterial pressure to aim for is not necessarily the same in all patients. Animal studies suggest that below a mean arterial pressure of 60 mm Hg, autoregulation in the coronary, renal, and central nervous system vascular beds is compromised, and flow may become linearly dependent on pressure.[9,10] Loss of autoregulation can occur at different levels in different organs, however, and the degree to which septic patients retain intact autoregulation is uncertain. Some patients (especially those with pre-existing hypertension) may require higher blood pressures to maintain adequate perfusion.

The precise blood pressure goal to target in septic shock remains uncertain. Most experts agree, largely on the basis of the animal studies cited previously and on physiologic reasoning, that in septic patients with evidence of hypoperfusion, mean arterial pressure should be maintained above 60[6] or 65 mm Hg.[11] There are no data from randomized clinical trials that demonstrate that failure to maintain blood pressure at this level worsens outcome, but it seems unlikely that such a clinical trial will be conducted soon. It should be recognized that individual patients may have blood pressures somewhat lower than these thresholds without hypoperfusion; it is clinical shock in the presence of hypotension that merits vasopressor support.

Higher blood pressure targets may be warranted in some patients. The renal circulation may be especially sensitive to perfusion pressure, and vasopressor therapy to augment renal perfusion pressure has been shown to increase urine output or creatinine clearance in a number of open-label clinical series; the targeted mean blood pressure varied, but was as high as 75 mm Hg.[12–19] Improvements in renal function with increased perfusion pressure, however, have not been demonstrated in prospective, randomized studies. Randomized trials comparing norepinephrine titrated to either 65 or 85 mm Hg in patients with septic shock have found no significant differences in metabolic variables or renal function.[20,21]

It is important to supplement end points, such as blood pressure, with assessment of regional and global perfusion. Bedside clinical assessment provides a good indication of global perfusion. Indications of decreased perfusion include oliguria, clouded sensorium, delayed capillary refill, and cool skin. Some caution is necessary in interpreting these signs in septic patients, however, because organ dysfunction can occur in the absence of global hypoperfusion. Clinical assessments can be supplemented by other measures, such as serum lactate levels and mixed venous oxygen saturation. Elevated lactate in sepsis may result from global hypoperfusion or from cellular metabolic alterations that may or may not represent tissue hypoxia,[22] but its prognostic value, particularly of the trend of lactate concentrations, has been well established in septic shock patients.[23–25] Mixed venous oxyhemoglobin saturation (SvO_2) reflects the balance between oxygen delivery and consumption, and can be elevated in septic patients because of maldistribution of blood flow, so values must be interpreted in the context of the wider hemodynamic picture. Low values, however, suggest increased oxygen extraction and potentially incomplete resuscitation. A recent study showed that monitoring of central venous oxygen saturation ($ScvO_2$) can be a valuable guide to early resuscitation.[4] The correlation between $ScvO_2$ and SvO_2 is reasonable,[26] but may not always be reliable.[27]

Adequacy of regional perfusion is usually assessed clinically.[1] Methods of measuring regional perfusion more directly have been under investigation, with a focus on the splanchnic circulation, which is especially susceptible to ischemia and may drive organ failure.[28] Measurements of oxygen saturation in the hepatic vein have revealed oxygen desaturation in a subset of septic patients, suggesting that hepatosplanchnic oxygen supply may be inadequate in some patients, even when more global parameters seem adequate.[29] Direct visualization of the sublingual circulation[30] or sublingual capnometry[31] may be useful to monitor the restoration of microvascular perfusion in patients with sepsis.

ADRENERGIC AGENTS

There has been longstanding debate about whether one catecholamine vasopressor agent is superior to another. These discussions may be enlightening in that they tend to highlight differences in pharmacology among the agents, but sometimes the arguments tend to focus on the agents themselves when the therapeutic strategy is actually what differs. Different catecholamine agents have different effects on α- and β-adrenergic receptors, as shown in **Fig. 1**. The hemodynamic actions of these receptors are well known, with α-adrenergic receptors promoting vasoconstriction, β_1-adrenergic receptors increasing heart rate and myocardial contractility, and β_2-adrenergic receptors causing peripheral vasodilation.

The result of these differential effects on adrenergic receptors is that the different agents have different effects on pressure and flow, as shown in **Fig. 2**. Conceived in these terms, the argument about which catecholamine is best in a given situation is transformed into a discussion about which agent is best suited to implement the therapeutic strategy chosen. This may or may not make the choice easier, but it does emphasize the need to define the goals and end points of therapy and to identify how those end points will be monitored.

INDIVIDUAL VASOPRESSOR AGENTS

Dopamine

Dopamine, the natural precursor of norepinephrine and epinephrine, has distinct dose-dependent pharmacologic effects. At doses less than 5 μg/kg/min, dopaminergic receptors are activated, leading to vasodilation in the renal and mesenteric beds.[32] At doses of 5 to 10 μg/kg/min, β_1-adrenergic effects predominate, increasing cardiac contractility and heart rate. At doses above 10 μg/kg/min, α_1-adrenergic effects predominate, leading to arterial vasoconstriction and an increase in blood pressure. There is a great deal of overlap in these effects, particularly in critically ill patients.

Dopamine increases mean arterial pressure and cardiac output, primarily by an increase in stroke volume, and to a lesser extent by an increase in heart rate.[33–43] In open-label trials, dopamine (median dose, 15 μg/kg/min) increased mean arterial pressure by 24% in septic patients who remained hypotensive after optimal fluid resuscitation.[33–43] Dopamine has been shown to increase oxygen delivery, but its effects on calculated or measured oxygen consumption have been mixed, suggesting that tissue oxygenation may not always be improved, perhaps because of failure to

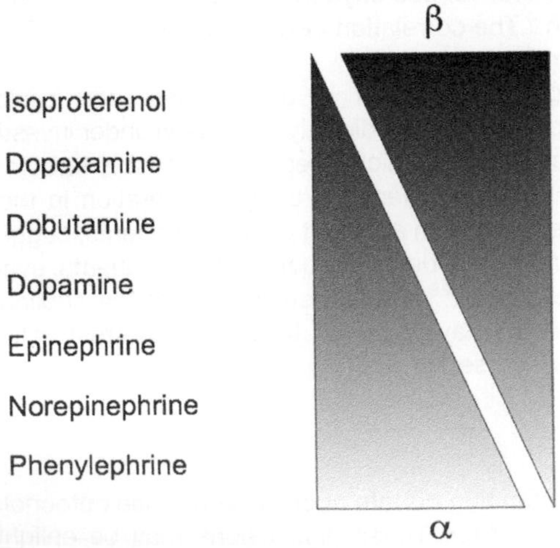

Fig. 1. α- and β-adrenergic effects of vasoactive catecholamines.

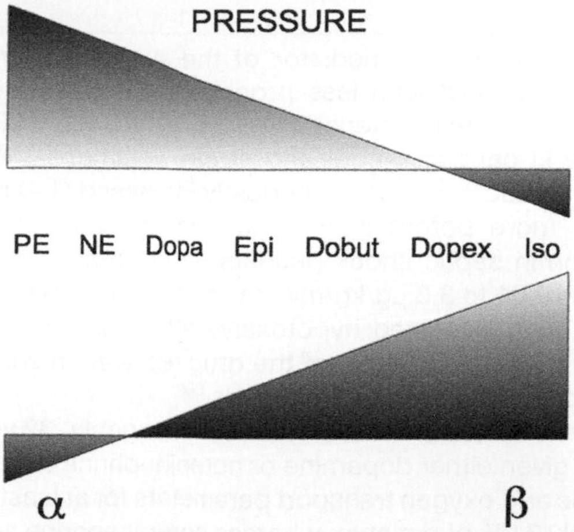

Fig. 2. Effects of vasoactive catecholamines on pressure and blood flow.

improve microcirculatory flow.[34,35,44,45] The effect of dopamine on splanchnic perfusion has also been mixed. Increases in splanchnic blood flow have been reported, but have not always been associated with increases in splanchnic oxygen consumption, beneficial effects on gastric intramucosal pH, or improvement in hepatosplanchnic energy balance.[33,34,36,46–48]

Low doses of dopamine increase renal blood flow and glomerular filtration rate in laboratory animals and healthy volunteers, supporting the idea that dopamine can reduce the risk of renal failure in critically ill patients by increasing renal blood flow. This notion has now been put to rest by a definitive clinical trial that randomized 328 critically ill patients with early renal dysfunction to low ("renal") dose dopamine (2 μg/kg/min) or placebo.[49] No difference was found in either the primary outcome (peak serum creatinine); other renal outcomes (increase in creatinine, need for renal replacement, urine output); or secondary outcomes (survival to either ICU or hospital discharge, ICU or hospital stay, arrhythmias).[49]

Dopamine effectively increases mean arterial pressure in patients who remain hypotensive after optimal volume expansion, largely as a result of increasing cardiac index, so it may be chosen in patients with compromised cardiac function or cardiac reserve. Its major side effects are tachycardia and arrhythmogenesis, both of which are more prominent than with other vasopressor agents. Safety concerns have also been raised concerning extracardiac side effects. Dopamine has the potential to decrease prolactin release, favoring lymphocyte apoptosis with consequent immunosuppression.[50,51]

Dopamine use was associated with increased mortality in patients with shock in an observational cohort study of 198 European ICUs, and remained a significant predictor after multivariate analysis.[52] Another, similarly sized observational cohort of 17 Portuguese ICUs showed decreased mortality in septic shock patients treated with dopamine compared with norepinephrine, however, a finding that also persisted after multivariate analysis.[53] These observational studies have known limitations. A large prospective randomized clinical trial comparing dopamine with norepinephrine in 1603 pressor-dependent patients with septic shock has recently been completed, and presented but not yet published.[54] No significant difference in mortality between use of dopamine and norepinephrine was observed, although there were more arrhythmias in the dopamine group.[54]

Norepinephrine

Norepinephrine, the endogenous mediator of the sympathetic nervous system, is a potent α-adrenergic agonist with less pronounced β-adrenergic agonist effects. Norepinephrine increases mean arterial pressure by vasoconstriction, with a small (10%–15%) increase in cardiac output and stroke volume.[12–14,18,55,56] Filling pressures are either unchanged[12–14,18,57] or modestly increased (1–3 mm Hg).[17,19,34,36,38]

Norepinephrine is more potent than dopamine and may be more effective at reversing hypotension in septic shock patients. In open-label trials, norepinephrine at doses ranging from 0.01 to 3.3 μg/kg/min has been shown to increase mean arterial pressure in patients who remained hypotensive after fluid resuscitation and dopamine.[13,14,18,19,36,56–59] The large doses of the drug required in some patients may be caused by α-receptor down-regulation in sepsis.[60]

In the only randomized trial comparing vasopressor agents, 32 volume-resuscitated septic patients were given either dopamine or norepinephrine to achieve and maintain normal hemodynamic and oxygen transport parameters for at least 6 hours. Dopamine was successful in only 31% of patients, whereas norepinephrine administration (1.5 ± 1.2 mg/kg/min) was successful in 93% (P<.001). Of the 11 patients who did not respond to dopamine, 10 responded when norepinephrine was added. Serum lactate levels were also decreased, suggesting that norepinephrine improved tissue oxygenation.[38]

The vasoconstrictive effects of norepinephrine can have detrimental effects on renal hemodynamics in patients with hypotension and hypovolemia, with the potential for renal ischemia.[61–63] The situation may differ in adequately resuscitated, hyperdynamic septic shock.[17] Norepinephrine has a greater effect on efferent than afferent renal arteriolar resistance and increases the filtration fraction. Several studies have shown increases in urine output and renal function in patients with septic shock treated with norepinephrine alone or norepinephrine added to dobutamine.[12,15,17,19,34,38,39,57,64]

Results of studies of the effects of norepinephrine on splanchnic blood flow in patients with septic shock have been mixed. Effects of norepinephrine on both splanchnic blood flow and oxygen consumption have been unpredictable both among patients and within groups.[33,36] Comparisons between norepinephrine and other vasoactive agents have also been variable. One pilot study found that gastric mucosal pHi was significantly increased during a 3-hour treatment with norepinephrine but significantly decreased during treatment with dopamine.[34] A more recent study compared the effects of norepinephrine, epinephrine, and dopamine in 20 patients with septic shock.[65] In the 10 patients with moderate shock, no differences in splanchnic blood flow or gastric-arterial P_{CO_2} difference were observed. In the 10 with severe shock, the effects of norepinephrine and dopamine were similar: epinephrine increased cardiac index more than norepinephrine but splanchnic blood flow was lower despite this higher cardiac index.[65]

Norepinephrine can increase blood pressure in patients with septic shock without causing deterioration in cardiac index and organ function. Although the effect of the drug on oxygen transport variables and splanchnic parameters has varied in different studies, other clinical parameters of peripheral perfusion, such as urine flow and lactate concentration, are significantly improved in most studies. In a recent multivariate analysis including 97 septic shock patients, mortality was favorably influenced by the use of norepinephrine; use of high-dose dopamine, epinephrine, or dobutamine had no significant effect.[66]

Controlled data comparing norepinephrine with other catecholaminergic agents were limited to one small randomized study[38] until completion of the large randomized trial comparing dopamine with norepinephrine.[54] This trial showed no difference in mortality, but fewer arrhythmias with norepinephrine.[54] Because randomized data do not suggest large differences in overall outcomes across broad populations, individualization of vasopressor agents based on clinical and hemodynamic factors still seems warranted.

Phenylephrine

Phenylephrine, a selective α_1-adrenergic agonist, increases blood pressure by vasoconstriction. Its rapid onset, short duration, and primary vascular effects make it an attractive agent in the management of hypotension associated with sepsis, but there are concerns about its potential to reduce cardiac output in these patients.

Data concerning the use of phenylephrine in hyperdynamic sepsis are sparse. Phenylephrine has been shown to increase blood pressure when given to normotensive hyperdynamic septic patients at doses of 0.5 to 8 μg/kg/min, with little change in cardiac output or stroke volume.[67,68] A small 13-patient study in hypotensive septic patients showed that phenylephrine added to either low-dose dopamine or dobutamine increased mean arterial pressure and cardiac index without a change in heart rate.[69] Recently, a crossover pilot study compared systemic hemodynamics, gastric tonometry, and renal function in 15 patients with septic shock changed from norepinephrine to phenylephrine titrated to maintain a similar blood pressure, and then back again.[70] Systemic hemodynamics were similar (although heart rate, as expected, was slightly lower), but indices of hepatosplanchnic perfusion and function were decreased with phenylephrine, as was renal function.[70] A 32-patient randomized control trial comparing phenylephrine with norepinephrine for initial support of patients with septic shock by the same group, however, showed no significant difference in global or regional hemodynamics, or in renal function, which might suggest potential differences between delayed and early administration.[71]

The limited information available with phenylephrine suggests that this drug can increase blood pressure modestly in fluid-resuscitated septic shock patients, and may be a good option when tachyarrhythmias limit therapy with other vasopressors.[6]

Epinephrine

Epinephrine, which is synthesized, stored, and released from the chromaffin cells of the adrenal medulla, is a potent α- and β-adrenergic agent that increases mean arterial pressure by increasing both cardiac index and peripheral vascular tone.[16,72–74] Epinephrine increases oxygen delivery, but oxygen consumption also may be increased.[72–76] Lactate levels can be increased after use of epinephrine in sepsis, although whether this results from excess vasoconstriction and compromised perfusion or increased lactate production remains uncertain.[58,72,76]

The main concern with the use of epinephrine in sepsis is the potential to decrease regional blood flow, particularly in the splanchnic circulation.[58,77–79] In a recent study of patients with severe septic shock, epinephrine increased global oxygen delivery and consumption but caused a lower absolute and fractional splanchnic blood flow and lower indocyanine green clearance, validating the adverse effects of epinephrine alone on the splanchnic circulation.[65] Another group has reported improved gastric mucosal perfusion with epinephrine compared with norepinephrine-dobutamine combination,[80] but the same group subsequently reported superiority of a norepinephrine-dopexamine combination over epinephrine.[81]

A randomized clinical trial comparing epinephrine with norepinephrine in 280 critically ill patients with shock found no difference in time to achieve arterial pressure goals, 28-day mortality, or 90-day mortality, although 13% of the patients in the epinephrine group were withdrawn from the study because of lactic acidosis or tachycardia.[82] When a prespecified analysis of the 158 patients with septic shock was performed, results were similar, with no differences in hemodynamics or mortality.[82]

Another fairly large (N = 330) randomized clinical trial compared epinephrine with norepinephrine with or without dobutamine, with drugs titrated to maintain a mean arterial pressure above 70 and a cardiac index above 2.5 L/min, in patients with septic shock.[83] Metabolic abnormalities were transient in this trial, and no patients were withdrawn for this reason. There was no significant difference in time to hemodynamic success, vasopressor withdrawal, or mortality at 28 days in the ICU or in the hospital between epinephrine and norepinephrine with dobutamine.[83]

Epinephrine can increase blood pressure in patients unresponsive to traditional agents. It increases heart rate and has the potential to induce tachyarrhythmias, ischemia, and hypoglycemia. Because of its effects on gastric blood flow and its propensity to increase lactate concentrations, epinephrine has been considered a second-line agent whose use should be considered in patients failing to respond to traditional therapies.[6] Recent clinical trials, however, have cast some doubt on whether epinephrine is inferior to other agents.

Vasopressin

Vasopressin is a peptide hormone synthesized in the hypothalamus and then transported to and stored in the pituitary gland. Released in response to decreases in blood volume, decreased intravascular volume, and increased plasma osmolality, vasopressin constricts vascular smooth muscle directly by V1 receptors and also increases responsiveness of the vasculature to catecholamines.[84,85] Vasopressin may also increase blood pressure by inhibition of vascular smooth muscle nitric oxide production[86] and K^+-ATP channels.[85,87]

Normal levels of vasopressin have little effect on blood pressure in physiologic conditions[84] but vasopressin helps maintain blood pressure during hypovolemia,[88] and seems to restore impaired hemodynamic mechanisms and also inhibit pathologic vascular responses in shock.[85] Increased levels of vasopressin have been documented in hemorrhagic shock,[89] but a growing body of evidence indicates that this response is abnormal or blunted in septic shock. One study found markedly increased levels of circulating vasopressin in 12 patients with cardiogenic shock, but much lower levels in 19 patients with septic shock, levels that were hypothesized to be inappropriately low.[90] One potential mechanism for this relative vasopressin deficiency is depletion of pituitary stores, possibly in conjunction with impaired synthesis. Depletion of vasopressin stores in the neurohypophysis evaluated by MRI has been described in a small group of septic shock patients.[91] A recent prospective cohort study of patients with septic shock found that vasopressin levels were almost always elevated in the initial hours of septic shock and decreased afterward; one third of patients developed relative vasopressin deficiency as defined by the investigators.[92]

Given this theoretical rationale, observational studies demonstrated that the addition of a low dose of vasopressin (0.01–0.04 U/min) to catecholamines can raise blood pressure in patients with pressor-refractory septic shock.[93–95] Several small randomized studies comparing vasopressin with norepinephrine have demonstrated that initiation of vasopressin decreases catecholamine requirements,[96,97] and one showed improved renal function.[96] Similar data are available for terlipressin, a synthetic vasopressin analog.[98] There is concern, however, that vasopressin infusion in septic patients may either decrease splanchnic perfusion or redistribute blood flow away from the splanchnic mucosa.[99,100] Vasopressin should be thought of as replacement therapy for relative deficiency rather than as a vasopressor agent to be titrated to effect.

A large randomized clinical trial (VASST) has now been completed comparing vasopressin with norepinephrine in 776 patients with pressor-dependent septic shock.[101] Patients were randomized to vasopressin (0.03 U/min) or 15 μg/min norepinephrine in addition to their original vasopressor infusion; the primary end point was 28-day mortality; a prespecified subgroup analysis was done on patients with less severe (NE 5–14 μg/min) and more severe (NE >15 μg/min) septic shock. For the group as a whole, there was no difference in mortality, but vasopressin seemed to be better in the less severe subgroup.[101]

Vasopressin (0.03 U/min) added to norepinephrine seems to be as safe and effective as norepinephrine in fluid-resuscitated patients with septic shock. Vasopressin may be more effective in patients on lower doses of norepinephrine than when started as rescue therapy, although what to do in patients with high vasopressor requirements despite vasopressin infusion remains uncertain.

INOTROPIC THERAPY

Background

The broad outlines of myocardial dysfunction in patients with septic shock have been well defined. Despite the fact that cardiac output is usually normal or high, there is evidence that myocardial contractility may be impaired in a subgroup of septic patients. In the initial report, performed with serial radionuclide scans, left ventricular ejection fraction was decreased, and the left ventricle was dilated, so stroke volume was preserved.[102] Subsequent reports using echocardiography found a similarly decreased ejection fraction in a subset of septic patients, but less prominent ventricular dilation, and some of these patients were reported to have low stroke volumes.[103,104] In reports from both groups, myocardial depression developed 24 to 48 hours after the onset of septic shock and was reversible in survivors. In addition to depressed left ventricular ejection fraction, some studies in septic patients have suggested abnormalities in ventricular responses to fluid loading, with lower increases in left ventricular performance (measured by left ventricular stroke work index) increased less in septic shock patients than in controls.[105]

The reversibility of myocardial dysfunction in sepsis suggests the involvement of circulating mediators, but the precise mechanisms of myocardial dysfunction remain unclear. A role for inflammatory cytokines has been suggested by studies showing that tumor necrosis factor,[106] interleukin-1,[107] and other inflammatory cytokines, either alone or in combination,[108] depress contractility of isolated cardiac myocytes. The time course of myocardial depression in large animal models and in patients with sepsis, with onset between 24 and 48 hours, along with evidence for its induction by cytokines, suggests the possibility of cytokine-inducible nitric oxide synthase as a mediator.[108] Studies have implicated both nitric oxide production and reactive oxygen species in cytokine-induced myocardial depression, and have further suggested a role for peroxynitrite.[109] Other studies have implicated decreased myocyte myofilament calcium responsiveness, possibly mediated by abnormal protein kinase A phosphorylation.[110] Regardless of the mechanism, the reversibility of myocardial depression in septic patients suggests the feasibility of a strategy of inotropic support while awaiting recovery.

The challenge in interpreting myocardial dysfunction in sepsis is that the most important physiologic parameter is cardiac output, not ejection fraction. Some patients, especially those with pre-existing cardiac dysfunction, may have decreased cardiac output, and those patients are clearly candidates for inotropic therapy to improve cardiac performance. For other patients, the clinical issue is not so much

Phosphodiesterase Inhibitors

Phosphodiesterase inhibitors increase intracellular cyclic AMP and have inotropic effects independent of β-adrenergic receptors. In view of recent data suggesting the potential for decreased myocardial adrenergic responsiveness in septic shock,[122] their use might be considered in some settings. Most of the available case series are confounded by concomitant use of adrenergic agents, but one small randomized trial of 12 pediatric patients was able to demonstrate increased cardiac output with milrinone in sepsis.[123] Phosphodiesterase inhibitors have vasodilatory effects that might exacerbate hypotension in sepsis, mandating caution in their use, especially given their relatively long half-lives. The decision to use this drug in septic shock patients to increase cardiac output is expected to increase vasopressor requirements.

Levosimendan

Levosimendan is a novel agent that increases cardiac myocyte calcium responsiveness and also opens ATP-dependent potassium channels, giving the drug both inotropic and vasodilatory properties. Levosimendan has been most extensively studied in acute heart failure, but given the potential role for abnormal calcium handling in sepsis-induced myocardial depression, its use also has been proposed in sepsis. Studies in animal models of endotoxin infusion have suggested that levosimendan can improve myocardial performance with relatively modest decreases in arterial pressure.[124] One clinical trial randomized 30 patients with septic shock and ejection fraction less than 45% to dobutamine or levosimendan, with norepinephrine used to maintain blood pressure.[125] Levosimendan improved ejection fraction, stroke volume, and cardiac index and also improved urine output and gastric mucosal PO_2 compared with dobutamine.[125] Another trial by the same group randomized 35 patients with septic shock and acute respiratory distress syndrome to levosimendan or placebo.[126] Levosimendan improved right ventricular performance, and mixed venous oxygen saturation also was improved, suggesting that its effects on cardiac function translated into a systemic effect.[126]

Levosimendan is not currently approved for use in the United States. Despite a reasonable rationale for its use, and some experimental data suggesting some beneficial effects, larger randomized trials with patient-centered end points, such as survival and length of stay, are needed before it can be considered for widespread use as an inotropic agent in sepsis.

COMPLICATIONS OF VASOPRESSOR THERAPY

All of the catecholamine agents can cause significant tachycardia, especially in patients who are inadequately volume resuscitated. In patients with significant coronary atherosclerosis, catecholamine-induced coronary artery constriction may precipitate myocardial ischemia and infarction; this is of particular concern in patients treated with vasopressin. In the presence of myocardial dysfunction, excessive vasoconstriction can decrease stroke volume, cardiac output, and oxygen delivery. Should this occur, the dose should be lowered, or the addition of an inotropic agent should be considered.[56] Excessive doses of vasopressors can also cause limb ischemia and necrosis.

Administration of vasopressor agents may potentially impair blood flow to the splanchnic system, and this can be manifested by stress ulceration, ileus, malabsorption, and even bowel infarction.[58,76] Gut mucosal integrity occupies a key position in the pathogenesis of multiple organ failure, and countercurrent flow in splanchnic microcirculation gives the gut a higher critical threshold for oxygen delivery than other organs. It makes sense to avoid episodes of intramucosal acidosis, which might be detected either by a fall in gastric mucosal pHi or an increase in gastric mucosal P_{CO_2}. Whether to monitor these parameters routinely is less certain, because pHi or gastric P_{CO_2}-directed care has not been shown to reduce mortality in patients with septic shock in prospective randomized controlled trials.

At inotropic doses, catecholamines can trigger tachyarrythmias, including supraventricular tachycardias, atrial fibrillation, and ventricular tachycardia. The phosphodiesterase inhibitors and levosimendan also have the potential to produce hypotension, especially in patients with inadequate fluid resuscitation. As such, monitoring stroke volume and cardiac output with these agents, so as to obtain the desired therapeutic effect at the minimal dosage, is advisable. Patients in septic shock may manifest severe clinical manifestations of disseminated intravascular coagulation including loss of digits and extremities. These patients may also be on significant doses of vasopressors, leading to a false conclusion that the limb loss is caused by the vasopressors.

CONSENSUS RECOMMENDATIONS

Consensus recommendations regarding vasopressor support in patients with septic shock have been put forth by the American College of Critical Care Medicine[6] and the Surviving Sepsis campaign[11]; these recommendations differ more in wording than in substance, and are compiled in **Table 1**. The Surviving Sepsis campaign will likely amend the vasopressin section to take the VASST trial results under consideration.

SUMMARY

The ultimate goals of hemodynamic therapy in shock are to restore effective tissue perfusion and to normalize cellular metabolism. In sepsis, both global and regional perfusion must be considered. In addition, mediators of sepsis can perturb cellular metabolism, leading to inadequate use of oxygen and other nutrients despite adequate perfusion; one would not expect organ dysfunction mediated by such abnormalities to be corrected by hemodynamic therapy.

Despite the complex pathophysiology of sepsis, an underlying approach to its hemodynamic support can be formulated that is particularly pertinent with respect to vasoactive agents. Both arterial pressure and tissue perfusion must be taken into account when choosing therapeutic interventions and the efficacy of hemodynamic therapy should be assessed by monitoring a combination of clinical and hemodynamic parameters. It is relatively easy to raise blood pressure, but somewhat harder to raise cardiac output in septic patients. How to optimize regional blood and microcirculatory blood flow remains uncertain. Specific end points for therapy are debatable and are likely to evolve. Nonetheless, the idea that clinicians should define specific goals and end points, titrate therapies to those end points, and evaluate the results of their interventions on an ongoing basis remains a fundamental principle. The practice parameters were intended to emphasize the importance of such an approach so as to provide a foundation for the rational choice of vasoactive agents in the context of evolving monitoring techniques and therapeutic approaches.

REFERENCES

1. Hollenberg SM, Parrillo JE. Shock. In: Fauci AS, Braunwald E, Isselbacher KJ, et al, editors. Harrison's principles of internal medicine. 14th edition. New York: McGraw-Hill; 1997. p. 214–22.

43. Wilson RF, Sibbald WJ, Jaanimagi JL. Hemodynamic effects of dopamine in critically ill septic patients. J Surg Res 1976;20:163–72.
44. Meier-Hellmann A, Reinhart K. Effects of catecholamines on regional perfusion and oxygenation in critically ill patients. Acta Anaesthesiol Scand Suppl 1995; 107:239–48.
45. Hiltebrand LB, Krejci V, Sigurdsson GH. Effects of dopamine, dobutamine, and dopexamine on microcirculatory blood flow in the gastrointestinal tract during sepsis and anesthesia. Anesthesiology 2004;100:1188–97.
46. Maynard ND, Bihari DJ, Dalton RN, et al. Increasing splanchnic blood flow in the critically ill. Chest 1995;108:1648–54.
47. Neviere R, Chagnon JL, Vallet B, et al. Dobutamine improves gastrointestinal mucosal blood flow in a porcine model of endotoxic shock. Crit Care Med 1997;25:1371–7.
48. Guerin JP, Levraut J, Samat-Long C, et al. Effects of dopamine and norepinephrine on systemic and hepatosplanchnic hemodynamics, oxygen exchange, and energy balance in vasoplegic septic patients. Shock 2005;23:18–24.
49. Bellomo R, Chapman M, Finfer S, et al. Care Society (ANZICS) Clinical Trials Group. Low-dose dopamine in patients with early renal dysfunction: a placebo-controlled randomised trial. Lancet 2000;356:2139–43.
50. Van den Berghe G, de Zegher F. Anterior pituitary function during critical illness and dopamine treatment. Crit Care Med 1996;24:1580–90.
51. Oberbeck R, Schmitz D, Wilsenack K, et al. Dopamine affects cellular immune functions during polymicrobial sepsis. Intensive Care Med 2006;32:731–9.
52. Sakr Y, Reinhart K, Vincent JL, et al. Does dopamine administration in shock influence outcome? Results of the Sepsis Occurrence in Acutely Ill Patients (SOAP) Study. Crit Care Med 2006;34:589–97.
53. Povoa PR, Carneiro AH, Ribeiro OS, et al. Influence of vasopressor agent in septic shock mortality: results from the Portuguese Community-Acquired Sepsis Study (SACiUCI study). Crit Care Med 2009;37:410–6.
54. DeBacker D. Comparison of dopamine and norepinephrine as the first vasopressor agent in the management of shock. Presented, European Society of Intensive Care Medicine 2008.
55. Martin C, Perrin G, Saux P, et al. Effects of norepinephrine on right ventricular function in septic shock patients. Intensive Care Med 1994;20:444–7.
56. Martin C, Saux P, Eon B, et al. Septic shock: a goal-directed therapy using volume loading, dobutamine and/or norepinephrine. Acta Anaesthesiol Scand 1990;34:413–7.
57. Schreuder WO, Schneider AJ, Groeneveld ABJ, et al. Effect of dopamine vs norepinephrine on hemodynamics in septic shock. Chest 1989;95:1282–8.
58. Levy B, Bollaert PE, Charpentier C, et al. Comparison of norepinephrine and dobutamine to epinephrine for hemodynamics, lactate metabolism, and gastric tonometric variables in septic shock: a prospective, randomized study. Intensive Care Med 1997;23:282–7.
59. Martin C, Viviand X, Arnaud S, et al. Effects of norepinephrine plus dobutamine or norepinephrine alone on left ventricular performance of septic shock patients. Crit Care Med 1999;27:1708–13.
60. Chernow B, Roth BL. Pharmacologic manipulation of the peripheral vasculature in shock: clinical and experimental approaches. Circ Shock 1986;18: 141–55.
61. Murakawa K, Kobayashi A. Effects of vasopressors on renal tissue gas tensions during hemorrhagic shock in dogs. Crit Care Med 1988;16:789–92.

62. Conger JD, Robinette JB, Guggenheim SJ. Effect of acetylcholine on the early phase of reversible norepinephrine-induced acute renal failure. Kidney Int 1981;19:399–409.
63. Schaer GL, Fink MP, Parrillo JE. Norepinephrine alone versus norepinephrine plus low-dose dopamine: enhanced renal blood flow with combination pressor therapy. Crit Care Med 1985;13:492–6.
64. Albanese J, Leone M, Garnier F, et al. Renal effects of norepinephrine in septic and nonseptic patients. Chest 2004;126:534–9.
65. De Backer D, Creteur J, Silva E, et al. Effects of dopamine, norepinephrine, and epinephrine on the splanchnic circulation in septic shock: which is best? Crit Care Med 2003;31:1659–67.
66. Martin C, Viviand X, Leone M, et al. Effect of norepinephrine on the outcome of septic shock. Crit Care Med 2000;28:2758–65.
67. Yamazaki T, Shimada Y, Taenaka N, et al. Circulatory responses to afterloading with phenylephrine in hyperdynamic sepsis. Crit Care Med 1982;10:432–5.
68. Flancbaum L, Dick M, Dasta J, et al. A dose-response study of phenylephrine in critically ill, septic surgical patients. Eur J Clin Pharmacol 1997;51:461–5.
69. Gregory JS, Bonfiglio MF, Dasta JF, et al. Experience with phenylephrine as a component of the pharmacologic support of septic shock. Crit Care Med 1991;19:1395–400.
70. Morelli A, Lange M, Ertmer C, et al. Short-term effects of phenylephrine on systemic and regional hemodynamics in patients with septic shock: a crossover pilot study. Shock 2008;29:446–51.
71. Morelli A, Ertmer C, Rehberg S, et al. Phenylephrine versus norepinephrine for initial hemodynamic support of patients with septic shock: a randomized, controlled trial. Crit Care 2008;12:R143.
72. Wilson W, Lipman J, Scribante J, et al. Septic shock: does adrenaline have a role as a first-line inotropic agent? Anesth Intens Care 1992;20:470–4.
73. Moran JL, O'Fathartaigh MS, Peisach AR, et al. Epinephrine as an inotropic agent in septic shock: a dose-profile analysis. Crit Care Med 1993;21:70–7.
74. Mackenzie SJ, Kapadia F, Nimmo GR, et al. Adrenaline in treatment of septic shock: effects on haemodynamics and oxygen transport. Intensive Care Med 1991;17:36–9.
75. Le Tulzo Y, Seguin P, Gacouin A, et al. Effects of epinephrine on right ventricular function in patients with severe septic shock and right ventricular failure: a preliminary study. Intensive Care Med 1997;23:664–70.
76. Day NP, Phu NH, Bethell DP, et al. The effects of dopamine and adrenaline infusions on acid-base balance and systemic haemodynamics in severe infection. Lancet 1996;348:219–23.
77. Meier-Hellmann A, Reinhart K, Bredle DL, et al. Epinephrine impairs splanchnic perfusion in septic shock. Crit Care Med 1997;25:399–404.
78. Zhou SX, Qiu HB, Huang YZ, et al. Effects of norepinephrine, epinephrine, and norepinephrine-dobutamine on systemic and gastric mucosal oxygenation in septic shock. Acta Pharmacol Sin 2002;23:654–8.
79. Martikainen TJ, Tenhunen JJ, Giovannini I, et al. Epinephrine induces tissue perfusion deficit in porcine endotoxin shock: evaluation by regional CO(2) content gradients and lactate-to-pyruvate ratios. Am J Physiol Gastrointest Liver Physiol 2005;288:G586–92.
80. Seguin P, Bellissant E, Le Tulzo Y, et al. Effects of epinephrine compared with the combination of dobutamine and norepinephrine on gastric perfusion in septic shock. Clin Pharmacol Ther 2002;71:381–8.

81. Seguin P, Laviolle B, Guinet P, et al. Dopexamine and norepinephrine versus epinephrine on gastric perfusion in patients with septic shock: a randomized study [NCT00134212]. Crit Care 2006;10:R32.
82. Myburgh JA, Higgins A, Jovanovska A, et al. A comparison of epinephrine and norepinephrine in critically ill patients. Intensive Care Med 2008;34:2226–34.
83. Annane D, Vignon P, Renault A, et al. Norepinephrine plus dobutamine versus epinephrine alone for management of septic shock: a randomised trial. Lancet 2007;370:676–84.
84. Holmes CL, Patel BM, Russell JA, et al. Physiology of vasopressin relevant to management of septic shock. Chest 2001;120:989–1002.
85. Barrett BJ, Parfrey PS. Clinical practice: preventing nephropathy induced by contrast medium. N Engl J Med 2006;354:379–86.
86. Kusano E, Tian S, Umino T, et al. Arginine vasopressin inhibits interleukin-1 beta-stimulated nitric oxide and cyclic guanosine monophosphate production via the V1 receptor in cultured rat vascular smooth muscle cells. J Hypertens 1997;15:627–32.
87. Wakatsuki T, Nakaya Y, Inoue I. Vasopressin modulates K(+)-channel activities of cultured smooth muscle cells from porcine coronary artery. Am J Physiol 1992;263:H491–6.
88. Abboud FM, Floras JS, Aylward PE, et al. Role of vasopressin in cardiovascular and blood pressure regulation. Blood Vessels 1990;27:106–15.
89. Wang BC, Flora-Ginter G, Leadley RJ Jr, et al. Ventricular receptors stimulate vasopressin release during hemorrhage. Am J Physiol 1988;254:R204–11.
90. Landry DW, Levin HR, Gallant EM, et al. Vasopressin deficiency contributes to the vasodilation of septic shock. Circulation 1997;95:1122–5.
91. Sharshar T, Carlier R, Blanchard A, et al. Depletion of neurohypophyseal content of vasopressin in septic shock. Crit Care Med 2002;30:497–500.
92. Sharshar T, Blanchard A, Paillard M, et al. Circulating vasopressin levels in septic shock. Crit Care Med 2003;31:1752–8.
93. Landry DW, Levin HR, Gallant EM, et al. Vasopressin pressor hypersensitivity in vasodilatory septic shock. Crit Care Med 1997;25:1279–82.
94. Tsuneyoshi I, Yamada H, Kakihana Y, et al. Hemodynamic and metabolic effects of low-dose vasopressin infusions in vasodilatory septic shock. Crit Care Med 2001;29:487–93.
95. Holmes CL, Walley KR, Chittock DR, et al. The effects of vasopressin on hemodynamics and renal function in severe septic shock: a case series. Intensive Care Med 2001;27:1416–21.
96. Patel BM, Chittock DR, Russell JA, et al. Beneficial effects of short-term vasopressin infusion during severe septic shock. Anesthesiology 2002;96:576–82.
97. Dunser MW, Mayr AJ, Ulmer H, et al. Arginine vasopressin in advanced vasodilatory shock: a prospective, randomized, controlled study. Circulation 2003;107:2313–9.
98. Albanese J, Leone M, Delmas A, et al. Terlipressin or norepinephrine in hyperdynamic septic shock: a prospective, randomized study. Crit Care Med 2005;33:1897–902.
99. van Haren FM, Rozendaal FW, van der Hoeven JG. The effect of vasopressin on gastric perfusion in catecholamine-dependent patients in septic shock. Chest 2003;124:2256–60.
100. Klinzing S, Simon M, Reinhart K, et al. High-dose vasopressin is not superior to norepinephrine in septic shock. Crit Care Med 2003;31:2646–50.
101. Russell JA, Walley KR, Singer J, et al. Vasopressin versus norepinephrine infusion in patients with septic shock. N Engl J Med 2008;358:877–87.

102. Parker MM, Shelhamer JH, Bacharach SL, et al. Profound but reversible myocardial depression in patients with septic shock. Ann Intern Med 1984;100:483–90.
103. Jardin F, Fourme T, Page B, et al. Persistent preload defect in severe sepsis despite fluid loading: a longitudinal echocardiographic study in patients with septic shock. Chest 1999;116:1354–9.
104. Vieillard-Baron A, Caille V, Charron C, et al. Actual incidence of global left ventricular hypokinesia in adult septic shock. Crit Care Med 2008;36:1701–6.
105. Ognibene FP, Parker MM, Natanson C, et al. Depressed left ventricular performance. Response to volume infusion in patients with sepsis and septic shock. Chest 1988;93:903–10.
106. Hollenberg SM, Cunnion RE, Lawrence M, et al. Tumor necrosis factor depresses myocardial cell function: results using an in vitro assay of myocyte performance [abstract]. Clin Res 1989;37:528A.
107. Kumar A, Thota V, Dee L, et al. Tumor necrosis factor-a and interleukin-1b are responsible for in vitro myocardial cell depression induced by human septic shock serum. J Exp Med 1996;183:949–58.
108. Balligand J-L, Ungureanu-Longrois D, Simmons WW, et al. Cytokine-inducible nitric oxide synthase (iNOS) expression in cardiac myocytes. J Biol Chem 1994;269:27580–8.
109. Ferdinandy P, Danial H, Ambrus I, et al. Peroxynitrite is a major contributor to cytokine-induced myocardial contractile failure. Circ Res 2000;87:241–7.
110. Layland J, Cave AC, Warren C, et al. Protection against endotoxemia-induced contractile dysfunction in mice with cardiac-specific expression of slow skeletal troponin I. FASEB J 2005;19:1137–9.
111. Astiz M, Rackow EC, Weil MH, et al. Early impairment of oxidative metabolism and energy production in severe sepsis. Circ Shock 1988;26:311–20.
112. Tuchschmidt J, Fried J, Astiz M, et al. Elevation of cardiac output and oxygen delivery improves outcome in septic shock. Chest 1992;102:216–20.
113. Gattinoni L, Brazzi L, Pelosi P, et al. A trial of goal-oriented hemodynamic therapy in critically ill patients. N Engl J Med 1995;333:1025–32.
114. Hayes MA, Timmins AC, Yau EHS, et al. Elevation of systemic oxygen delivery in the treatment of critically ill patients. N Engl J Med 1994;330:1717–22.
115. Dellinger RP, Levy MM, Carlet JM, et al. Surviving Sepsis Campaign: international guidelines for management of severe sepsis and septic shock: 2008. Crit Care Med 2008;36:296–327.
116. Bakker J, Coffemils M, Leon M, et al. Blood lactates are superior to oxygen-derived variables in predicting outcome in human septic shock. Chest 1992; 99:956–62.
117. Jardin F, Sportiche M, Bazin M, et al. Dobutamine: a hemodynamic evaluation in human septic shock. Crit Care Med 1981;9:329–32.
118. Vincent JL, Roman A, Kahn RJ. Dobutamine administration in septic shock: addition to a standard protocol. Crit Care Med 1990;18:689–93.
119. De Backer D, Berre J, Zhang H, et al. Relationship between oxygen uptake and oxygen delivery in septic patients: effects of prostacyclin versus dobutamine. Crit Care Med 1993;21:1658–64.
120. Vallet B, Chopin C, Curtis SE, et al. Prognostic value of the dobutamine test in patients with sepsis syndrome and normal lactate values: a prospective, multicenter study. Crit Care Med 1993;21:1868–75.
121. Gutierrez G, Clark C, Brown SD, et al. Effect of dobutamine on oxygen consumption and gastric mucosal pH in septic patients. Am J Respir Crit Care Med 1994;150:324–9.

122. Cariou A, Pinsky MR, Monchi M, et al. Is myocardial adrenergic responsiveness depressed in human septic shock? Intensive Care Med 2008;34:917–22.
123. Barton P, Garcia J, Kouatli A, et al. Hemodynamic effects of I.V. milrinone lactate in pediatric patients with septic shock: a prospective, double-blinded, randomized, placebo- controlled, interventional study. Chest 1996;109:1302–12.
124. Pinto BB, Rehberg S, Ertmer C, et al. Role of levosimendan in sepsis and septic shock. Curr Opin Anaesthesiol 2008;21:168–77.
125. Morelli A, De Castro S, Teboul JL, et al. Effects of levosimendan on systemic and regional hemodynamics in septic myocardial depression. Intensive Care Med 2005;31:638–44.
126. Morelli A, Teboul JL, Maggiore SM, et al. Effects of levosimendan on right ventricular afterload in patients with acute respiratory distress syndrome: a pilot study. Crit Care Med 2006;34:2287–93.

Hemodynamic Monitoring in Sepsis

Brian Casserly, MD[a], Richard Read, MD[b], Mitchell M. Levy, MD[b,*]

KEYWORDS

• Hemodynamic • Monitoring • Sepsis • Goal-directed
• Intensive care • Physiologic

The hemodynamics of sepsis (ie, blood flow and tissue perfusion) is complicated because of the phasic nature of sepsis. Cardiovascular derangements lead to development of tissue hypoperfusion.[1] Tissue hypoperfusion is an important factor in the development of multiple organ failure. Therefore, recognition of sepsis-induced tissue hypoperfusion and timely clinical intervention to prevent and correct this are fundamental aspects of managing patients with sepsis and septic shock. Hemodynamic monitoring plays a key role in the management of the critically ill and is used to identify hemodynamic instability and its cause and to monitor the response to therapy. However, the utility of many forms of hemodynamic monitoring that are commonly used in management of sepsis and septic shock remain controversial and unproven.[2]

RATIONALE FOR HEMODYNAMIC MONITORING

There are an increasing number of different technological advances available that allow monitoring and assessment of a wide range physiologic variables[3]; however, most intensive care (ICU) monitors display only blood pressure (BP), heart rate (HR), and oxygen saturation by pulse oximetry (SpO2). These monitors serve to alert the patient's caregivers to vital signs that require further attention but are not sufficiently sensitive to drive treatment protocols. For example, blood pressure alone is not sufficient in identifying the presence or absence of tissue hypoperfusion in patients with sepsis; patients with sepsis-induced hypoperfusion can present with normal blood pressures.[4,5] It is therefore important to monitor other signs that are indicative of tissue hypoperfusion and hemodynamic instability.[6] Because the primary goal of the cardiovascular system is to supply adequate amounts of oxygen to meet the metabolic demands of the body, calculation of systemic oxygen delivery (DO2) and oxygen consumption (VO2), identifying tissue ischemia (usually monitored by mixed venous

[a] Division of Pulmonary and Critical Care Medicine, The Memorial Hospital of Rhode Island, Pawtucket, RI, USA
[b] Division of Pulmonary and Critical Care Medicine, Rhode Island Hospital, Providence, RI, USA
* Corresponding author.
E-mail address: mitchell_levy@brown.edu (M.M. Levy).

Crit Care Clin 25 (2009) 803–823
doi:10.1016/j.ccc.2009.08.006
criticalcare.theclinics.com

dysfunction and "cell stunning," with a subsequent reduction in oxygen consumption at the cellular levels.[43] This phenomenon is likely unresponsive to alterations in the macrocirculation[44]; however, patients with sepsis may also present with a low or normal SvO2. Following SvO2 in patients with sepsis is useful because a low SvO2 is often associated with inadequate CO and should trigger aggressive interventions to increase oxygen delivery to the tissues and minimize sepsis-induced tissue hypoperfusion. However, measurement of SvO2 involves placement of a pulmonary artery catheter with a risk/benefit relationship that is still a matter of controversy.[45–47] In comparison, measuring central venous oxygen saturation (ScvO2) requires a central venous catheter, which is routinely inserted in critically ill patients for monitoring of central venous pressure and administration of inotropes/vasopressors and parenteral nutrition. In principle, measuring ScvO2 reflects the degree of oxygen extraction from the brain and the upper part of the body. In healthy humans, the oxygen saturation in the inferior vena cava (IVC) is higher than in the superior vena cava owing to the increased metabolic demand of the brain. Because the pulmonary artery contains a mixture of blood from both the superior as well as the IVC, SvO2 is greater than the oxygen saturation in the superior vena cava. The reversal of the physiologic difference between ScvO2 and SvO2 can be observed in septic shock. During hemodynamic deterioration, mesenteric blood flow decreases followed by an increase of O2 extraction in these organs.[48,49] Naturally, this goes along with venous desaturation in the lower body. On the other hand, cerebral blood flow is maintained over some period in shock causing a delayed drop of ScvO2 in comparison with SvO2. This effect can be demonstrated in several types of shock.[50]

However, more important than the precise prediction of SvO2 is the question of whether changes in SvO2 indicating a hemodynamic derangement or a treatment effect are mirrored by changes in the ScvO2. In a dog model, various clinical conditions such as hypoxia and hemorrhagic shock were investigated regarding their effects on these parameters.[51] This study confirmed that ScvO2 differed from SvO2 but changes in SvO2 were accompanied by parallel changes in ScvO2. This has also been demonstrated in the clinical setting where 32 critically ill surgical patients were monitored for a total of 1097 hours. A good agreement between SvO2 and ScvO2 was shown.[50] Therefore, measurement of ScvO2 seems to be an attractive alternative to monitoring of SvO2 because it can be performed more easily and is less risky. Thus, the guidelines of the Surviving Sepsis Campaign[32] stated that the use of SvO2 and ScvO2 is equivalent in the management of patients with severe sepsis and septic shock. Monitoring of ScvO2 has been successfully used as a hemodynamic goal in the management of early sepsis.[12]

In the trial by Rivers and colleagues[12] the use of an ScvO2 above 70% was the only difference in hemodynamic monitoring parameters used in the treatment arm compared with the control group, which resulted in an absolute reduction of mortality by 15%.

Pulmonary Artery Catheter

A debate continues over the utility of pulmonary artery catheters (PACs) in the management of critically ill patients. In large part, this controversy surrounding PAC use has been driven by several prospective, randomized clinical trials,[2,45,52,53] indicating that using a PAC does not influence outcomes, ie, it is neither inherently dangerous nor beneficial. The interpretation of these studies is made difficult by their design. As investigators may still prefer to insert a PAC when they are convinced it may help, only those patients for whom there is equipoise, ie, when the clinician feels uncertain about the beneficial aspects, can be randomized. Thus, in these studies,[2,52–54] only a fraction of patients considered were actually enrolled and randomized, creating a significant treatment bias. These trials demonstrate risks of PAC insertion are similar to those for central venous catheter insertion with the exception of increased incidence of transient cardiac arrythmias that appear to have minimal clinical consequences.[55] There is no evidence that catheter-associated infections are greater with the PAC than with central venous catheterization. The other specific PAC complications like pulmonary artery rupture with balloon inflation and catheter knotting occur very infrequently.[55] If we consider that the evidence supports a lack of benefit associated with the use of the PAC, how likely is it that less invasive monitoring systems will result in better outcomes?[56]

There is clearly no justification for invasive monitoring if there is little likelihood of deriving benefit from the information obtained; however, a critical point when reviewing these studies is that the insertion of a PAC and simply monitoring hemodynamic indices does not improve outcomes.[3,16,57] In addition, it may be insufficient to specify end points as goals to be met and not specify the most effective treatment regimen to reach these end points.[58] Hemodynamic indices (to include perfusion indices) should be used as a part of an evidence-based treatment plan aimed at optimizing tissue perfusion before organ dysfunction occurs, as exemplified by the improved outcomes associated with goal-directed therapy for patients with septic shock,[12] high-risk surgical patients,[59–61] and postcardiac surgery patients.[42,62] Unfortunately, designing global protocols to guide therapy for every patient that also accounts for the limitations of the information obtained from a PAC is a difficult task.

Despite the ongoing debate surrounding use of the PAC, it is still used and when used appropriately, can provide important information to assist in choosing hemodynamic interventions in patients with sepsis. The hemodynamic variables measured by a PAC include SvO2, CO, right ventricular ejection fraction (with some catheters), and intrapulmonary vascular pressures. Modern catheters are fitted with a heating filament that intermittently heats and measures the thermodilution curve providing serial CO measurement, but these are displayed after a delay of 2 to 3 minutes. Integration of the hemodynamic data from the PAC can be useful in diagnosing different causes of shock as well as monitoring disease progression and response to therapeutic interventions.[63]

However, there is one important area that limits the utility of PA pressure monitoring. Critical care clinicians (nurses and physicians) may incorrectly gather and interpret the data.[64–68] This opinion is supported by studies that documented better outcome in the centers that had the largest experience with the PAC.[53,58] Correct measurement: zeroing, calibration, elimination of artifacts and proper reading of the values are crucial in the effective utility of a PAC. Regrettably, these errors in data collection,[69,70] degrade the usefulness of subsequent clinical decision making. It is important to recognize the effects of respiratory variation, positive end-expiratory pressure, increased pleural pressure, and the position of the catheter in different lung zones on the hemodynamic information. Correct interpretation of these pressures requires integration of the three PAC elements (pressures, CO, and SvO2). Unfortunately, many clinicians still only monitor single data elements or misinterpret their meaning.

It is probably premature to conclude that PACs have no future role in the management of sepsis and septic shock despite the advent of new noninvasive techniques that measure CO. These techniques, which will be discussed in the forthcoming paragraphs, still do not provide any assessment of cardiac filling pressures or adequacy of perfusion.

Fluid Responsiveness

Before beginning a description of any further hemodynamic monitoring techniques it is important to familiarize ourselves with the concept of fluid responsiveness. This has become very popular over the past few years, likely because this is a very pragmatic approach to fluid therapy. Restoration and maintenance of adequate circulating blood volume are essential goals in the proper management of the septic patient[20,71]; however, it is difficult to determine which level of preload is optimal in an "abnormal" situation like sepsis. The key is to detect patients who will turn fluid loading into a significant increase in stroke volume and CO. If not, fluid administration is useless or even potentially harmful (worsening in pulmonary edema). Therefore, fluid infusion has to significantly increase cardiac preload and the increase in cardiac preload has to induce a significant increase in stroke volume. Volumetric markers of cardiac preload are therefore useful for checking whether cardiac preload effectively increases during fluid infusion. Whether this translates into a predictor of fluid responsiveness remains uncertain.[72] As a consequence, functional measurements like monitoring pulse pressure have been developed to better predict the response to fluid resuscitation.

The traditional approach of assessing preload responsiveness is the intravascular fluid challenge, wherein a bolus of fluid is rapidly infused and the subsequent changes in specific flow-dependent variables (CO, MAP, HR, SvO2, CVP, pulmonary artery occlusion pressure) are measured. Reversible fluid challenges including the use of positive pressure to cyclically alter venous return and passive leg raising are being increasing investigated. These are being coupled to less invasive measures of stroke volume responsiveness (a marker of preload responsiveness) to predict patients who would benefit from further fluid resuscitation.[73,74] Stroke volume variation (SVV) during positive pressure ventilation occurs as a consequence of tidal volume–induced changes in venous return.[75] Positive pressure ventilation when applied to a patient at rest and with no spontaneous respiratory effort is associated with a cyclic decrease in right ventricle (RV) filling and subsequently left ventricle (LV) filling. Several studies have documented that SVV is highly predictive of preload responsiveness.[76–80] However SVV can only be assessed directly by either esophageal Doppler echocardiography[79] or echocardiographic measures of aortic velocity[77] or complex analysis of the arterial waveform analysis these will be discussed in more detail later in this article.

Because the primary determinant of arterial pulse pressure is stroke volume, pulse pressure variation (PPV) can be used as accurate measure of stroke volume variation. A 13% PPV predicts a 15% increase in CO for a 500-mL volume bolus in septic patients with circulatory shock[81] and it requires only the insertion of an arterial catheter and monitoring pulse pressure measurements over time.[82–85] There are, however, a few important caveats. Because respiratory changes in preload are induced by changes in pleural pressure, in patients ventilated with a low tidal volume (6 mL/kg, for example), the respiratory changes in pleural pressure may not be sufficient to induce significant changes in preload.[86] These parameters will lose their predictive value under conditions of varying R-R intervals (atrial fibrillation), and they may also lose accuracy if tidal volume varies from breath to breath as may occur with assisted and spontaneous ventilation.[87,88] These represent significant limitations for broad applicability in critically ill patients.

A simplified approach is to use passive leg raising (PLR) as a transient and reversible increase in venous return.[89] PLR causes an approximate 300-mL blood bolus in a 70-kg man that persists for about 2 to 3 minutes before resulting in intravascular volume redistribution. The immediate hemodynamic response from before to during the PLR is taken to reflect preload response.[90] To minimize the need for a constant HR and tidal volume, measures of mean aortic flow averaged over 20 to 30 seconds can be measured by esophageal Doppler and is clearly superior in predicting fluid responsiveness compared with SVV and PPV measures in subjects breathing spontaneously.[88] One of the major limitations of this technique is that in severely hypovolemic patients, the blood volume mobilized by leg raising, which is dependent on total blood volume. could be small, which, in turn, can show minimal to no increase in CO and blood pressure, even in responders.[91] It is clear that all these techniques require clinical validation but less invasive functional hemodynamic monitoring likely represents the future of goal-directed therapy in sepsis.

VOLUMETRIC MEASURES OF PRELOAD

There has been recent interest in less invasive alternatives— catheter-related, bedside-device volume estimates, using thermodilution to assess cardiac preload in septic shock.[73,92] The original transpulmonary indicator dilution (TPID) technique introduced is the double indicator dilution approach, which is based on two indicators injected simultaneously: a plasma-bound indicator (indocyanine green dye) and a freely diffusible indicator.[93,94] The determination of flow and volume by this method is based on the simultaneous application of the two indicators: one that is diffusible into the extravascular pulmonary tissue compartments (temperature) and the other that is not diffusible (dye). The volume of distribution of thermal indicator will include not only the intravascular but also the extravascular lung water (EVLW) space (without any distinction between interstitial and alveolar water), as water is a very good thermal conductor. Injecting simultaneously through a central venous catheter a thermal and a strictly intravascular indicator (for instance, indocyanine green dye), detecting the respective dilution curves in the femoral artery, and comparing the volume of distribution of these two indicators gives an estimate of the EVLW content (**Fig. 1**).[95]

Several studies have demonstrated that these volumetric parameters can be useful for predicting fluid responsiveness—but only when they are very low or very high.[73,96,97] For example, it has been shown that the rate of positive response to a fluid challenge is high when the right ventricular end-diastolic volume (RVEDV) index is below 90 mL/m^2, but low when the RVEDV index is greater than 140 mL/m^2.[96,97] Similar findings have been recently reported with the global end-diastolic volume (GEDV) index, which reflects the volume of blood contained in the four heart chambers during diastole. When the GEDV index is below 600 mL/m^2, a positive response to a fluid challenge is very likely; in contrast, when the GEDV index is greater than 800 mL/m^2, a positive response is very unlikely.[73] However, in all these studies, intermediate values are not very predictive. The recent multicenter randomized National Institutes of Health trial[98] conducted in patients with acute lung injury demonstrated that fluid restriction and diuresis improve lung function and shorten the duration of mechanical ventilation and intensive care, emphasizing the potential value of EVLW measurement as a tool to guide such a therapeutic strategy.[99,100] The development of a single indicator dilution technique extensively used in pulse power and pulse contour estimates of stroke volume will be discussed later.

MEASURES OF CARDIAC OUTPUT

An accurate and noninvasive measurement of CO has become the primary focus of the most of the emerging techniques of hemodynamic assessment. Invasive methods are available, but as mentioned earlier there is little clinical evidence that these methods are effective in guiding therapy.[2,45,52,53,101] As a result, there are a number of new techniques, now commercially available, that are less invasive than direct intracardiac catheterization (**Table 1**). Ideally, these techniques would allow continuous

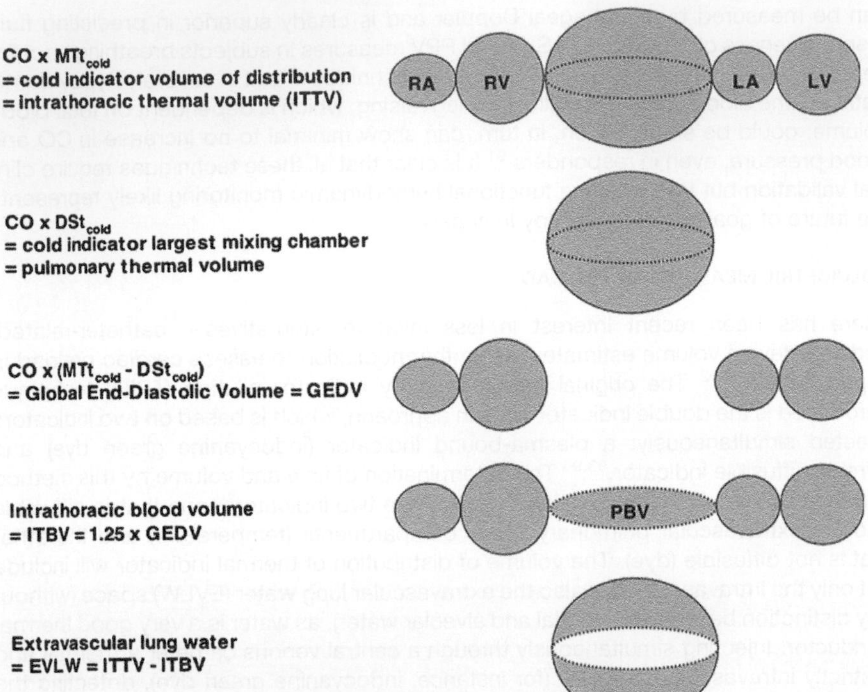

Fig. 1. Principles of extravascular lung water (EVLW) estimation by the single-indicator dilution method. The intrathoracic blood volume (ITBV) is derived from the measurement of the global end-diastolic volume (GEDV) with the equation ITBV = 1.25 × GEDV. The difference between the volume of distribution of the thermal indicator and ITBV yields EVLW. CO, cardiac output; MTt, mean transit time; Dst, down slope time; RA, right atrium; RV, right ventricle; PBV, pulmonary blood volume; LA, left atrium; LV, left ventricle. (*From* Michard F. Bedside assessment of extravascular lung water by dilution methods: temptations and pitfalls. Crit Care Med 2007;35(4):1186–92; with permission.)

monitoring of central circulation, and because of their less invasive nature, allow earlier assessment of patients at risk for hemodynamic instability. It should be acknowledged that large outcome studies using less invasive CO monitoring devices for hemodynamic optimization are still lacking. However, the concept of a "goal-directed hemodynamic therapy," applied to selected patient groups at risk of inadequate tissue perfusion, is promising.[60–62] Comprehensive evaluation of these new methods requires an insight into their unique strengths and weaknesses. They have been shown to be able to adequately replace the PAC under certain clinical circumstances. Unfortunately, relative comparisons are limited by the absence of a widely accepted "gold standard" measurement. The Fick principle involves calculating the oxygen (VO2) consumed over a given period of time from measurement of the oxygen content of the venous blood (Cv) and the arterial blood (Ca), CO can be derived from the following equation:

$$CO = (VO_2/[C_A - C_V]) * 100$$

While considered to be the most accurate method for CO measurement, Fick is invasive, requires time for the sample analysis, and accurate oxygen consumption

Table 1
Summary of advantages and disadvantages of the techniques used to measure cardiac output in sepsis

Name of Technique	Advantage	Disadvantage
Thermodilution	The validity of the thermodilution cardiac output technique for cardiac output measurement is based on a high correlation (r = 0.91 to 0.98) with the direct Fick method.	In conditions of low cardiac output states and in patients with valvular heart diseases and intracardiac shunts, the values may be erroneous about 20% of time.
Esophageal Doppler	Less invasive measure of cardiac output. Validation studies confirm the reliability of this cardiac output measurement in clinical practice.	Only measures the descending thoracic aortic flow and not true cardiac and is therefore influenced by nonlinear changes in cardiac output and systemic vascular resistance. Steep learning curves for probe positioning have been reported. Complete validation of these emerging techniques will require the comparison with "true gold standards" like a calibrated electromagnetic aortic flow probe (an invasive cardiac flowmeter).
Transesophageal echocardiography	Echocardiographic measurement of flow volume is clinically well established and of proven accuracy.	Requires training and is time consuming to perform effectively. The 2D measurement of the aortic valve diameter is challenging and associated with significant error.
Pulse pressure (PP) methods	Less invasive approach compared with thermodilution. Provides continuous cardiac output monitoring.	PP methods measure the combined performance of the heart and the vessels, thus limiting the application of PP methods for measurement of cardiac output. Cannot be used in patients who have poorly defined arterial waveform or presenting arrhythmia because pulse contour methods cannot provide reliable results in such conditions.
Specific pulse pressure (PP) methods Transpulmonary thermodilution and arterial waveform analysis	Gives measurements of cardiac filling volumes (GEDV), intrathoracic blood volume, and extravascular lung water.	Recalibration is recommended after changes in patient position, therapy, or condition.
Specific pulse pressure (PP) methods Transpulmonary lithium indicator dilution and arterial waveform analysis	Lithium dilution uses a peripheral vein to a peripheral arterial line.	Calibration measurements cannot be performed too frequently, and can be subject to error in the presence of certain muscle relaxants. It cannot be used in patients taking lithium.

samples are difficult to acquire. In fact most of the newer techniques have been validated against thermodilution techniques. The validity of the thermodilution CO technique for CO measurement is based on a high correlation ($r = 0.91$ to 0.98) with the direct Fick method.[102] However, the thermodilution CO is actually an average of three values obtained over 3 to 5 minutes. In conditions of low CO states, the values may be erroneous about 20% of times[103,104] and it is during periods of low CO states that accurate measurement is most desirable. Furthermore, in patients with valvular heart diseases and intracardiac shunts, the value of CO measured may, at best, be an approximation of the true CO. Cardiac output can also be affected by the phase of respiration with intrathoracic pressure changes influencing diastolic filling and therefore CO. Other issues that can affect validity of the measurements include the position of the pulmonary artery catheter, the rate of injection of the indicator solution, the volume and temperature of the injectate, the timing of the injection of indicator solution during the respiratory cycle, the position of the subject, and the presence of concomitant infusions.[66,68]

Esophageal Doppler

Esophageal Doppler consists of a sensor on the end of a probe, which can be introduced via the mouth or nose and positioned in the esophagus so the Doppler beam aligns with the descending thoracic aorta at a known angle. The blood velocity through the heart causes a "Doppler shift" in the frequency of the returning ultrasound waves. This Doppler shift can then be used to calculate flow velocity. Because the transducer is close to the blood flow, the signal is clear, however the alignment, and thus reliable signal, can often be difficult to maintain during respiration and patient movement. The estimation of stroke volume using esophageal Doppler relies on the measurement of stroke distance in the descending aorta (= velocity – time integral), which is then converted into systemic stroke volume (**Fig. 2**). It relies on the use of nomograms to determine aortic cross-sectional area. Newer devices have been developed to eliminate this problem by echocardiographic aortic diameter measurement,[105] but optimal adjustment of both the Doppler and the ultrasound can be challenging.[106] This method has good validation, particularly for measuring changes in blood flow, but is limited in that it only measures the descending thoracic aortic flow and not true CO and is therefore influenced by nonlinear changes in CO and SVR. Because coronary and brachiocephalic flows are not measured, CO is calculated assuming a constant partition between caudal and cephalic blood supply areas. The probes are smaller than conventional transesophageal echocardiography (TEE) probes and steep learning curves for probe positioning have been reported.[107] As a consequence, clinical trials in the past few years have shown inconsistent results.[54,108–111] However, a recent meta-analysis by Dark and Singer,[112] who reviewed all the validation studies for esophageal Doppler, confirms the reliability of this CO measurement in clinical practice. Recent studies have demonstrated improved patient outcomes using an esophageal Doppler to guide goal-directed perioperative intravascular resuscitation in high-risk surgical patients.[59,113,114] Esophageal Doppler has also recently been advocated as a tool to manage hemodynamically unstable organ donor patients[115] and to guide early goal-directed therapy in sepsis and trauma patients.[116]

Transesophageal Echocardiography

Echocardiography typically uses a conventional ultrasound machine and a combined two-dimensional (2D) and Doppler approach to measure CO. 2D measurement of the diameter (d) of the aortic annulus allows calculation of the flow CSA (cross-sectional

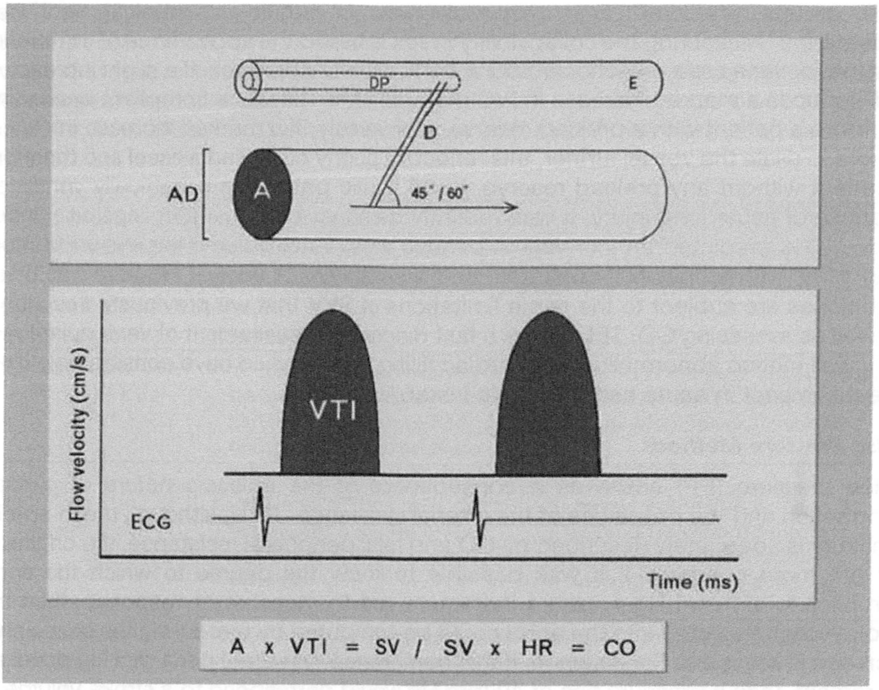

Fig. 2. The Doppler transducer is located at the tip of the probe and the beam is directed at the descending thoracic aorta (angle between Doppler beam and blood flow typically 658 or 458). Cardiac output is determined by Doppler flow measurements and the aortic area calculated from the diameter of the descending aorta either obtained from nomograms or assessed by M-mode echocardiography. A, aortic area (aortic diameter_p/4); AD, aortic diameter; CO, cardiac output; D, Doppler beam; DP, Doppler probe; E, esophagus; ECG, electrocardiogram; HR, heart rate; SV, stroke volume; VTI, velocity time integral. (*From* Hofer CK, Ganter MT, Zollinger A. What technique should I use to measure cardiac output? Curr Opin Crit Care 13:308–17; with permission.)

area), which is then multiplied by the volume time integral of the Doppler flow profile across the aortic valve to determine the flow volume or SV. Multiplying SV by HR produces CO. Prerequisites for optimal measurements are a Doppler beam orientation strictly parallel to the blood flow and an unchanged cross-sectional area over time. This is achieved best at the left ventricular outflow tract or the aortic valve in the transgastric probe position. CO is derived from left ventricular volumes estimated on the basis of a cone-shaped geometric model. Echocardiographic measurement of flow volume is clinically well established[117] and of proven accuracy but requires training and skill, and may be time consuming to perform effectively. The 2D measurement of the aortic valve diameter is challenging and associated with significant error,[118,119] whereas measurement of the pulmonary valve to calculate right-sided CO is even more difficult.

However, echocardiographic parameters of fluid responsiveness have been developed.[120] Because the cross-sectional area of the aortic annulus remains constant during the respiratory cycle, changes in velocity time interval (VTI) directly reflect changes in LV stroke volume. In two clinical trials using Doppler TEE to study changes in left ventricular stroke volume induced by the cyclic positive pressure breathing by measuring the respiratory variation in maximal aortic blood flow velocity,

continuous CO as described by Wesseling and colleagues.[122] This algorithm accounts for the nonlinear shape of the aortic compliance curve that becomes more pronounced in the elderly, in males, and in the presence of arteriosclerosis and increased distending pressures. This technique performed equivalently to thermodilution in a simulated model of septic shock despite concerns about variable vasomotor tone.[123] Several studies support these findings.[124–127] However, recalibration is recommended after changes in patient position, therapy, or condition. Furthermore, this cannot be used in patients who have poorly defined arterial waveform or presenting arrhythmia because pulse contour methods cannot provide reliable results in such conditions.

In the case of transpulmonary lithium indicator dilution and arterial waveform analysis (LiDCO), the independent calibration technique is lithium dilution, again using the Stewart-Hamilton principle. Lithium dilution uses a peripheral vein to a peripheral arterial line; however, it does not provide information on cardiac filling volumes and extravascular lung water. The PulseCO algorithm used by LiDCO is based on pulse power derivation and is not dependent on waveform morphology. Instead it calculates nominal stroke volume from a pressure-volume transform of the entire waveform. The nominal stroke volume is converted to actual stroke volume by calibration of the algorithm with LiDCO trademark. Initial studies indicate good fidelity.[128,129] However, potential drawbacks include that calibration measurements cannot be performed too frequently, and can be subject to error in the presence of certain muscle relaxants. It cannot be used in patients taking lithium because increased lithium background lithium activity causes an overestimation of CO. In both cases, an independent technique is required to provide calibration of the continuous cardiac analysis, as arterial PP analysis cannot account for unmeasured variables such as the changing compliance of the vascular bed. Also, because aortic diameter at maximal pressure as the single parameter that may vary up to ±40% from the population average, the absolute levels of CO cannot be determined with certainty.[130,131]

SUMMARY

Arterial waveform analysis that does not require continuous calibration, impedance cardiography, electrical cardiometry, velocity-encoded phase contrast magnetic resonance imaging (MRI), pulsed dye densitometry, noninvasive pulse pressure analysis using tonometry, suprasternal Doppler, partial CO2 rebreathing techniques, and transcutaneous Doppler are just some of the other emerging technologies not described in this review that may be used routinely in the management of sepsis and septic shock in the very near future. These innovative approaches may further increase our ability to optimize patients' fluid status and hemodynamics. We also have ability to monitor the microcirculation. This increasingly sophisticated approach to the management of sepsis and septic shock will hopefully translate into better patient outcomes. However, optimal use of any hemodynamic monitoring requires an understanding of its physiologic underpinnings. Accurate interpretation of the hemodynamic information coupled with a protocolized management algorithm is the cornerstone of an effective resuscitation effort. Many forms of hemodynamic monitoring have emerged over the past 20 to 30 years with no convincing evidence for the superiority of any single techniques (**Table 2**).

The goal of hemodynamic monitoring and optimization is to combat the systemic imbalance between tissue oxygen supply and demand ranging from global tissue hypoxia to overt shock and multiorgan failure. It remains unproven that hemodynamic monitoring of disease progression can effectively change patient outcome. However, despite our increased understanding of sepsis pathophysiology, mortality and morbidity from the disease remains high. Therefore, the search for the optimal parameters in resuscitation and the best way they can be monitored will continue.

REFERENCES

1. Dellinger RP. Cardiovascular management of septic shock. Crit Care Med 2003; 31(3):946–55.
2. Wheeler AP, Bernard GR, Thompson BT, et al. Pulmonary-artery versus central venous catheter to guide treatment of acute lung injury. N Engl J Med 2006; 354(21):2213–24.
3. Pinsky MR, Payen D. Functional hemodynamic monitoring. Crit Care 2005;9(6): 566–72.
4. Brun-Buisson C, Doyon F, Carlet J, et al. Incidence, risk factors, and outcome of severe sepsis and septic shock in adults. A multicenter prospective study in intensive care units. French ICU Group for Severe Sepsis. J Am Med Assoc 1995;274(12):968–74.
5. Rady MY, Rivers EP, Nowak RM. Resuscitation of the critically ill in the ED: responses of blood pressure, heart rate, shock index, central venous oxygen saturation, and lactate. Am J Emerg Med 1996;14(2):218–25.
6. Trzeciak S, Dellinger RP, Chansky ME, et al. Serum lactate as a predictor of mortality in patients with infection. Intensive Care Med 2007;33(6):970–7.
7. Buwalda M, Ince C. Opening the microcirculation: can vasodilators be useful in sepsis? Intensive Care Med 2002;28(9):1208–17.
8. Lush CW, Kvietys PR. Microvascular dysfunction in sepsis. Microcirculation 2000;7(2):83–101.
9. Rivers EP, Coba V, Visbal A, et al. Management of sepsis: early resuscitation. Clin Chest Med 2008;29(4):689–704, ix–x.
10. Brealey D, Brand M, Hargreaves I, et al. Association between mitochondrial dysfunction and severity and outcome of septic shock. Lancet 2002; 360(9328):219–23.
11. Brealey D, Singer M. Mitochondrial dysfunction in sepsis. Curr Infect Dis Rep 2003;5(5):365–71.
12. Rivers E, Nguyen B, Havstad S, et al. Early goal-directed therapy in the treatment of severe sepsis and septic shock. N Engl J Med 2001;345(19):1368–77.
13. Bland RD, Shoemaker WC, Abraham E, et al. Hemodynamic and oxygen transport patterns in surviving and nonsurviving postoperative patients. Crit Care Med 1985;13(2):85–90.
14. Gattinoni L, Brazzi L, Pelosi P, et al. A trial of goal-oriented hemodynamic therapy in critically ill patients. SvO2 Collaborative Group. N Engl J Med 1995; 333(16):1025–32.
15. Heyland DK, Cook DJ, King D, et al. Maximizing oxygen delivery in critically ill patients: a methodologic appraisal of the evidence. Crit Care Med 1996;24(3): 517–24.
16. Kern JW, Shoemaker WC. Meta-analysis of hemodynamic optimization in high-risk patients. Crit Care Med 2002;30(8):1686–92.
17. Shoemaker WC. A new approach to physiology, monitoring, and therapy of shock states. World J Surg 1987;11(2):133–46.
18. Snell RJ, Parrillo JE. Cardiovascular dysfunction in septic shock. Chest 1991; 99(4):1000–9.

19. Parrillo JE, Parker MM, Natanson C, et al. Septic shock in humans. Advances in the understanding of pathogenesis, cardiovascular dysfunction, and therapy. Ann Intern Med 1990;113(3):227–42.
20. Parrillo JE. Pathogenetic mechanisms of septic shock. N Engl J Med 1993; 328(20):1471–7.
21. Partrick DA, Bensard DD, Janik JS, et al. Is hypotension a reliable indicator of blood loss from traumatic injury in children? Am J Surg 2002;184(6):555–9 [discussion: 559–60].
22. Kumar A, Haery C, Parrillo JE. Myocardial dysfunction in septic shock. Crit Care Clin 2000;16(2):251–87.
23. Carroll GC, Snyder JV. Hyperdynamic severe intravascular sepsis depends on fluid administration in cynomolgus monkey. Am J Phys 1982;243(1): R131–41.
24. Shoemaker WC. Pathophysiology, monitoring, outcome prediction, and therapy of shock states. Crit Care Clin 1987;3(2):307–57.
25. Rivers EP, Coba V, Whitmill M. Early goal-directed therapy in severe sepsis and septic shock: a contemporary review of the literature. Curr Opin Anaesthesiol 2008;21(2):128–40.
26. Pinsky MR. Pathophysiology and therapy of end-organ failure in critical illness. Proc Assoc Am Physicians 1995;107(3):353–60.
27. Shoemaker WC, Appel PL, Kram HB. Tissue oxygen debt as a determinant of lethal and nonlethal postoperative organ failure. Crit Care Med 1988;16(11): 1117–20.
28. Astiz ME, Rackow EC, Kaufman B, et al. Relationship of oxygen delivery and mixed venous oxygenation to lactic acidosis in patients with sepsis and acute myocardial infarction. Crit Care Med 1988;16(7):655–8.
29. Astiz ME, Rackow EC, Weil MH. Oxygen delivery and utilization during rapidly fatal septic shock in rats. Circ Shock 1986;20(4):281–90.
30. Bur A, Hirschl MM, Herkner H, et al. Accuracy of oscillometric blood pressure measurement according to the relation between cuff size and upper-arm circumference in critically ill patients. Crit Care Med 2000;28(2):371–6.
31. Varpula M, Tallgren M, Saukkonen K, et al. Hemodynamic variables related to outcome in septic shock. Intensive Care Med 2005;31(8):1066–71.
32. Dellinger RP, Levy MM, Carlet JM, et al. Surviving Sepsis Campaign: international guidelines for management of severe sepsis and septic shock: 2008. Crit Care Med 2008;36(1):296–327.
33. Kumar A, Anel R, Bunnell E, et al. Pulmonary artery occlusion pressure and central venous pressure fail to predict ventricular filling volume, cardiac performance, or the response to volume infusion in normal subjects. Crit Care Med 2004;32(3):691–9.
34. Vieillard-Baron A, Chergui K, Rabiller A, et al. Superior vena caval collapsibility as a gauge of volume status in ventilated septic patients. Intensive Care Med 2004;30(9):1734–9.
35. Barbier C, Loubières Y, Schmit C, et al. Respiratory changes in inferior vena cava diameter are helpful in predicting fluid responsiveness in ventilated septic patients. Intensive Care Med 2004;30(9):1740–6.
36. Vieillard-Baron A, Augarde R, Prin S, et al. Influence of superior vena caval zone condition on cyclic changes in right ventricular outflow during respiratory support. Anesthesiology 2001;95(5):1083–8.
37. Cortez A, Zito J, Lucas CE, et al. Mechanism of inappropriate polyuria in septic patients. Arch Surg 1977;112(4):471–6.

38. Wo CC, Shoemaker WC, Appel PL, et al. Unreliability of blood pressure and heart rate to evaluate cardiac output in emergency resuscitation and critical illness. Crit Care Med 1993;21(2):218–23.
39. Bauer P, Reinhart K, Bauer M. Significance of venous oximetry in the critically ill. Med Intensiva 2008;32(3):134–42.
40. Creamer JE, Edwards JD, Nightingale P. Hemodynamic and oxygen transport variables in cardiogenic shock secondary to acute myocardial infarction, and response to treatment. Am J Cardiol 1990;65(20):1297–300.
41. Edwards JD. Oxygen transport in cardiogenic and septic shock. Crit Care Med 1991;19(5):658–63.
42. Polonen P, Ruokonen E, Hippeläinen M, et al. A prospective, randomized study of goal-oriented hemodynamic therapy in cardiac surgical patients. Anesth Analg 2000;90(5):1052–9.
43. West MA, Wilson C. Hypoxic alterations in cellular signal transduction in shock and sepsis. New Horiz 1996;4(2):168–78.
44. Marshall JC. Inflammation, coagulopathy, and the pathogenesis of multiple organ dysfunction syndrome. Crit Care Med 2001;29(Suppl 7):S99–106.
45. Harvey S, Harrison DA, Singer M, et al. Assessment of the clinical effectiveness of pulmonary artery catheters in management of patients in intensive care (PAC-Man): a randomised controlled trial. Lancet 2005;366(9484):472–7.
46. Sakr Y, Vincent JL, Reinhart K, et al. Use of the pulmonary artery catheter is not associated with worse outcome in the ICU. Chest 2005;128(4):2722–31.
47. Sandham JD, Hull RD, Brant RF, et al. A randomized, controlled trial of the use of pulmonary-artery catheters in high-risk surgical patients. N Engl J Med 2003; 348(1):5–14.
48. Meier-Hellmann A, Reinhart K, Bredle DL, et al. Epinephrine impairs splanchnic perfusion in septic shock. Crit Care Med 1997;25(3):399–404.
49. Meier-Hellmann A, Specht M, Hannemann L, et al. Splanchnic blood flow is greater in septic shock treated with norepinephrine than in severe sepsis. Intensive Care Med 1996;22(12):1354–9.
50. Reinhart K, Kuhn HJ, Hartog C, et al. Continuous central venous and pulmonary artery oxygen saturation monitoring in the critically ill. Intensive Care Med 2004; 30(8):1572–8.
51. Reinhart K, Rudolph T, Bredle DL, et al. Comparison of central-venous to mixed-venous oxygen saturation during changes in oxygen supply/demand. Chest 1989;95(6):1216–21.
52. Rhodes A, Cusack RJ, Newman PJ, et al. A randomised, controlled trial of the pulmonary artery catheter in critically ill patients. Intensive Care Med 2002; 28(3):256–64.
53. Richard C, Warszawski J, Anguel N, et al. Early use of the pulmonary artery catheter and outcomes in patients with shock and acute respiratory distress syndrome: a randomized controlled trial. J Am Med Assoc 2003;290(20):2713–20.
54. Hullett B, Gibbs N, Weightman W, et al. A comparison of CardioQ and thermodilution cardiac output during off-pump coronary artery surgery. J Cardiothorac Vasc Anesth 2003;17(6):728–32.
55. Elliott CG, Zimmerman GA, Clemmer TP. Complications of pulmonary artery catheterization in the care of critically ill patients. A prospective study. Chest 1979;76(6):647–52.
56. Ospina-Tascon GA, Cordioli RL, Vincent JL. What type of monitoring has been shown to improve outcomes in acutely ill patients? Intensive Care Med 2008; 34(5):800–20.

57. Hall JB. Searching for evidence to support pulmonary artery catheter use in critically ill patients. J Am Med Assoc 2005;294(13):1693–4.
58. Binanay C, Califf RM, Hasselblad V, et al. Evaluation study of congestive heart failure and pulmonary artery catheterization effectiveness: the ESCAPE trial. J Am Med Assoc 2005;294(13):1625–33.
59. Gan TJ, Soppit A, Maroof M, et al. Goal-directed intraoperative fluid administration reduces length of hospital stay after major surgery. Anesthesiology 2002; 97(4):820–6.
60. Pearse R, Dawson D, Fawcett J, et al. Early goal-directed therapy after major surgery reduces complications and duration of hospital stay. A randomised, controlled trial [ISRCTN38797445]. Crit Care 2005;9(6):R687–93.
61. Wakeling HG, McFall MR, Jenkins CS, et al. Intraoperative oesophageal Doppler guided fluid management shortens postoperative hospital stay after major bowel surgery. Br J Anaesth 2005;95(5):634–42.
62. McKendry M, McGloin H, Saberi D, et al. Randomised controlled trial assessing the impact of a nurse delivered, flow monitored protocol for optimisation of circulatory status after cardiac surgery. BMJ 2004;329(7460):258.
63. Shoemaker WC. Monitoring and management of acute circulatory problems: the expanded role of the physiologically oriented critical care nurse. Am J Crit Care 1992;1(1):38–53.
64. Burns D, Shively M. Critical care nurses' knowledge of pulmonary artery catheters. Am J Crit Care 1996;5(1):49–54.
65. Gnaegi A, Feihl F, Perret C. Intensive care physicians' insufficient knowledge of right-heart catheterization at the bedside: time to act? Crit Care Med 1997;25(2): 213–20.
66. Iberti TJ, Daily EK, Leibowitz AB, et al. Assessment of critical care nurses' knowledge of the pulmonary artery catheter. The Pulmonary Artery Catheter Study Group. Crit Care Med 1994;22(10):1674–8.
67. Jain M, Canham M, Upadhyay D, et al. Variability in interventions with pulmonary artery catheter data. Intensive Care Med 2003;29(11):2059–62.
68. Johnston IG, Jane R, Fraser JF, et al. Survey of intensive care nurses' knowledge relating to the pulmonary artery catheter. Anaesth Intensive Care 2004;32(4): 564–8.
69. Morris AH, Chapman RH, Gardner RM. Frequency of wedge pressure errors in the ICU. Crit Care Med 1985;13(9):705–8.
70. Krishnagopalan S, Kumar A, Parrillo JE. Myocardial dysfunction in the patient with sepsis. Curr Opin Crit Care 2002;8(5):376–88.
71. Parrillo JE. Management of septic shock: present and future. Ann Intern Med 1991;115(6):491–3.
72. Reuse C, Vincent JL, Pinsky MR. Measurements of right ventricular volumes during fluid challenge. Chest 1990;98(6):1450–4.
73. Michard F, Alaya S, Zarka V, et al. Global end-diastolic volume as an indicator of cardiac preload in patients with septic shock. Chest 2003;124(5):1900–8.
74. Michard F, Teboul JL, Richard C, et al. Arterial pressure monitoring in septic shock. Intensive Care Med 2003;29(4):659.
75. van den Berg PC, Jansen JR, Pinsky MR. Effect of positive pressure on venous return in volume-loaded cardiac surgical patients. J Appl Phys 2002;92(3): 1223–31.
76. Berkenstadt H, Margalit N, Hadani M, et al. Stroke volume variation as a predictor of fluid responsiveness in patients undergoing brain surgery. Anesth Analg 2001;92(4):984–9.

77. Feissel M, Michard F, Mangin I, et al. Respiratory changes in aortic blood velocity as an indicator of fluid responsiveness in ventilated patients with septic shock. Chest 2001;119(3):867–73.
78. Monnet X, Rienzo M, Osman D, et al. Esophageal Doppler monitoring predicts fluid responsiveness in critically ill ventilated patients. Intensive Care Med 2005;31(9):1195–201.
79. Slama M, Masson H, Teboul JL, et al. Monitoring of respiratory variations of aortic blood flow velocity using esophageal Doppler. Intensive Care Med 2004;30(6):1182–7.
80. Vieillard-Baron A, Chergui K, Augarde R, et al. Cyclic changes in arterial pulse during respiratory support revisited by Doppler echocardiography. Am J Respir Crit Care Med 2003;168(6):671–6.
81. Michard F, Boussat S, Chemla D, et al. Relation between respiratory changes in arterial pulse pressure and fluid responsiveness in septic patients with acute circulatory failure. Am J Respir Crit Care Med 2000;162(1):134–8.
82. Michard F. Changes in arterial pressure during mechanical ventilation. Anesthesiology 2005;103(2):419–28, quiz 449–5.
83. Michard F, Ruscio L, Teboul JL. Clinical prediction of fluid responsiveness in acute circulatory failure related to sepsis. Intensive Care Med 2001;27(7):1238.
84. Cannesson M, Desebbe O, Rosamel P, et al. Pleth variability index to monitor the respiratory variations in the pulse oximeter plethysmographic waveform amplitude and predict fluid responsiveness in the operating theatre. Br J Anaesth 2008;101(2):200–6.
85. Natalini G, Rosano A, Taranto M, et al. Arterial versus plethysmographic dynamic indices to test responsiveness for testing fluid administration in hypotensive patients: a clinical trial. Anesth Analg 2006;103(6):1478–84.
86. De Backer D, Heenen S, Piagnerelli M, et al. Pulse pressure variations to predict fluid responsiveness: influence of tidal volume. Intensive Care Med 2005;31(4): 517–23.
87. Heenen S, De Backer D, Vincent JL. How can the response to volume expansion in patients with spontaneous respiratory movements be predicted? Crit Care 2006;10(4):R102.
88. Monnet X, Rienzo M, Osman D, et al. Passive leg raising predicts fluid responsiveness in the critically ill. Crit Care Med 2006;34(5):1402–7.
89. Thomas M, Shillingford J. The circulatory response to a standard postural change in ischaemic heart disease. Br Heart J 1965;27:17–27.
90. Boulain T, Achard JM, Teboul JL, et al. Changes in BP induced by passive leg raising predict response to fluid loading in critically ill patients. Chest 2002; 121(4):1245–52.
91. Monnet X, Teboul JL. Passive leg raising. Intensive Care Med 2008;34(4):659–63.
92. Sakka SG, Bredle DL, Reinhart K, et al. Comparison between intrathoracic blood volume and cardiac filling pressures in the early phase of hemodynamic instability of patients with sepsis or septic shock. J Crit Care 1999;14(2):78–83.
93. Lichtwarck-Aschoff M, Beale R, Pfeiffer UJ. Central venous pressure, pulmonary artery occlusion pressure, intrathoracic blood volume, and right ventricular end-diastolic volume as indicators of cardiac preload. J Crit Care 1996;11(4):180–8.
94. Lichtwarck-Aschoff M, Zeravik J, Pfeiffer UJ. Intrathoracic blood volume accurately reflects circulatory volume status in critically ill patients with mechanical ventilation. Intensive Care Med 1992;18(3):142–7.
95. Lewis FR, Elings VB, Hill SL, et al. The measurement of extravascular lung water by thermal-green dye indicator dilution. Ann N Y Acad Sci 1982;384:394–410.

96. Della Rocca G, Costa GM, Coccia C, et al. Preload index: pulmonary artery occlusion pressure versus intrathoracic blood volume monitoring during lung transplantation. Anesth Analg 2002;95(4):835–43, table of contents.
97. Della Rocca G, Costa GM, Coccia C, et al. Preload and haemodynamic assessment during liver transplantation: a comparison between the pulmonary artery catheter and transpulmonary indicator dilution techniques. Eur J Anaesthesiol 2002;19(12):868–75.
98. Wiedemann HP, Wheeler AP, Bernard GR, et al. Comparison of two fluid-management strategies in acute lung injury. N Engl J Med 2006;354(24):2564–75.
99. Sakka SG, Klein M, Reinhart K, et al. Prognostic value of extravascular lung water in critically ill patients. Chest 2002;122(6):2080–6.
100. Sakka SG, Rühl CC, Pfeiffer UJ, et al. Assessment of cardiac preload and extravascular lung water by single transpulmonary thermodilution. Intensive Care Med 2000;26(2):180–7.
101. Shah MR, Hasselblad V, Stevenson LW, et al. Impact of the pulmonary artery catheter in critically ill patients: meta-analysis of randomized clinical trials. J Am Med Assoc 2005;294(13):1664–70.
102. Olsson B, Pool J, Vandermoten P, et al. Validity and reproducibility of determination of cardiac output by thermodilution in man. Cardiology 1970;55(3):136–48.
103. Nishikawa T. Alterations in stroke volume during cardiac output determination by thermodilution. Anesthesiology 1994;81(3):786.
104. Nishikawa T, Dohi S. Errors in the measurement of cardiac output by thermodilution. Can J Anaesth 1993;40(2):142–53.
105. Moxon D, Pinder M, van Heerden PV, et al. Clinical evaluation of the HemoSonic monitor in cardiac surgical patients in the ICU. Anaesth Intensive Care 2003;31(4):408–11.
106. Lefrant JY, Bruelle P, Aya AG, et al. Training is required to improve the reliability of esophageal Doppler to measure cardiac output in critically ill patients. Intensive Care Med 1998;24(4):347–52.
107. Berton C, Cholley B. Equipment review: new techniques for cardiac output measurement–oesophageal Doppler, Fick principle using carbon dioxide, and pulse contour analysis. Crit Care 2002;6(3):216–21.
108. Jaeggi P, Hofer CK, Klaghofer R, et al. Measurement of cardiac output after cardiac surgery by a new transesophageal Doppler device. J Cardiothorac Vasc Anesth 2003;17(2):217–20.
109. Kim K, Kwok I, Chang H, et al. Comparison of cardiac outputs of major burn patients undergoing extensive early escharectomy: esophageal Doppler monitor versus thermodilution pulmonary artery catheter. J Trauma 2004;57(5):1013–7.
110. Leather HA, Wouters PF. Oesophageal Doppler monitoring overestimates cardiac output during lumbar epidural anaesthesia. Br J Anaesth 2001;86(6):794–7.
111. Sharma J, Bhise M, Singh A, et al. Hemodynamic measurements after cardiac surgery: transesophageal Doppler versus pulmonary artery catheter. J Cardiothorac Vasc Anesth 2005;19(6):746–50.
112. Dark PM, Singer M. The validity of trans-esophageal Doppler ultrasonography as a measure of cardiac output in critically ill adults. Intensive Care Med 2004;30(11):2060–6.
113. Conway DH, Mayall R, Abdul-Latif MS, et al. Randomised controlled trial investigating the influence of intravenous fluid titration using oesophageal Doppler monitoring during bowel surgery. Anaesthesia 2002;57(9):845–9.

114. Venn R, Steele A, Richardson P, et al. Randomized controlled trial to investigate influence of the fluid challenge on duration of hospital stay and perioperative morbidity in patients with hip fractures. Br J Anaesth 2002;88(1):65–71.
115. de la Torre AN, Fisher A, Wilson DJ, et al. Minimally invasive optimization of organ donor resuscitation: case reports. Prog Transplant 2005;15(1):27–32.
116. Bilkovski RN, Rivers EP, Horst HM. Targeted resuscitation strategies after injury. Curr Opin Crit Care 2004;10(6):529–38.
117. Cholley BP, Vieillard-Baron A, Mebazaa A. Echocardiography in the ICU: time for widespread use! Intensive Care Med 2006;32(1):9–10.
118. Bettex DA, Hinselmann V, Hellermann JP, et al. Transoesophageal echocardiography is unreliable for cardiac output assessment after cardiac surgery compared with thermodilution. Anaesthesia 2004;59(12):1184–92.
119. Zhao X, Mashikian JS, Panzica P, et al. Comparison of thermodilution bolus cardiac output and Doppler cardiac output in the early post-cardiopulmonary bypass period. J Cardiothorac Vasc Anesth 2003;17(2):193–8.
120. Feissel M, Badie J, Merlani PG, et al. Pre-ejection period variations predict the fluid responsiveness of septic ventilated patients. Crit Care Med 2005;33(11):2534–9.
121. Newman EV, Merrell M, Genecin A, et al. The dye dilution method for describing the central circulation. An analysis of factors shaping the time-concentration curves. Circulation 1951;4(5):735–46.
122. Wesseling KH, Jansen JR, Settels JJ, et al. Computation of aortic flow from pressure in humans using a nonlinear, three-element model. J Appl Phys 1993;74(5):2566–73.
123. Jellema WT, Wesseling KH, Groeneveld AB, et al. Continuous cardiac output in septic shock by simulating a model of the aortic input impedance: a comparison with bolus injection thermodilution. Anesthesiology 1999;90(5):1317–28.
124. Godje O, Höke K, Lamm P, et al. Continuous, less invasive, hemodynamic monitoring in intensive care after cardiac surgery. Thorac Cardiovasc Surg 1998;46(4):242–9.
125. Goedje O, Hoeke K, Lichtwarck-Aschoff M, et al. Continuous cardiac output by femoral arterial thermodilution calibrated pulse contour analysis: comparison with pulmonary arterial thermodilution. Crit Care Med 1999;27(11):2407–12.
126. Hamzaoui O, Monnet X, Richard C, et al. Effects of changes in vascular tone on the agreement between pulse contour and transpulmonary thermodilution cardiac output measurements within an up to 6-hour calibration-free period. Crit Care Med 2008;36(2):434–40.
127. Irlbeck M, Forst H, Briegel J, et al. [Continuous measurement of cardiac output with pulse contour analysis]. Anaesthesist 1995;44(7):493–500.
128. Linton R, Band D, O'Brien T, et al. Lithium dilution cardiac output measurement: a comparison with thermodilution. Crit Care Med 1997;25(11):1796–800.
129. Linton RA, Jonas MM, Tibby SM, et al. Cardiac output measured by lithium dilution and transpulmonary thermodilution in patients in a paediatric intensive care unit. Intensive Care Med 2000;26(10):1507–11.
130. Hirschl MM, Binder M, Gwechenberger M, et al. Noninvasive assessment of cardiac output in critically ill patients by analysis of the finger blood pressure waveform. Crit Care Med 1997;25(11):1909–14.
131. Langewouters GJ, Wesseling KH, Goedhard WJ. The pressure dependent dynamic elasticity of 35 thoracic and 16 abdominal human aortas in vitro described by a five component model. J Biomech 1985;18(8):613–20.

Steroid Therapy of Septic Shock

Charles L. Sprung, MD[a,*], Serge Goodman, MD, PhD[b], Yoram G. Weiss, MD[b,c]

KEY WORDS

• Septic shock • Steroids • Corticosteroids
• Mortality • Shock reversal

The treatment of patients in septic shock with corticosteroids has been a controversial subject for many years.[1] The use of high doses of steroids became standard practice in the 1970s and 1980s.[1–3] Subsequently, in the late 1980s and 1990s, studies did not show an improved survival and some even demonstrated detrimental effects for patients treated with steroids.[4–8] At that time corticosteroids stopped being used for patients with sepsis and septic shock. More recently, the importance of inadequate adrenal corticosteroid production has been recognized with the increasing use of medications affecting adrenal cortex function and the decreased use of steroid treatment for sepsis.[9] In the late 1990s and early 2000s studies with lower doses of corticosteroids for longer periods demonstrated hemodynamic benefits.[10–15] Unfortunately, despite their potential benefits, corticosteroids also have adverse affects and the benefits and risks must be balanced in determining whether they should be used or not. Some of the serious adverse affects noted in patients with critically illness have included superinfections[1] and critical illness polyneuromyopathy.[16,17] This article reviews the subject of steroid treatment of patients with septic shock weighing the advantages and disadvantages of steroid treatment.

In evaluating studies of corticosteroids in patients with septic shock, it is important to separate studies of high- and low-dose steroids.

This article is adapted, in part, from Sprung CL, Goodman S, Weiss YG. Corticosteroid treatment of patients in septic shock. In: Vincent JL, editor. Yearbook of intensive care and emergency medicine. Springer; 2009. p. 753–60; with permission.

[a] General Intensive Care Unit, Department of Anesthesiology and Critical Care Medicine, Hadassah Hebrew University Medical Center, P.O. BOX 12000, Jerusalem 91120, Israel
[b] Department of Anesthesiology and Critical Care Medicine, Hadassah Hebrew University Medical Center, P.O. BOX 12000, Jerusalem 91120, Israel
[c] Department of Anesthesia and Critical Care Medicine, University of Pennsylvania School of Medicine, Dulles 781A/HUP 3400 Spruce Street, Philadelphia, PA 19104–4283, USA
* Corresponding author.
E-mail address: sprung@cc.huji.ac.il (C.L. Sprung).

Crit Care Clin 25 (2009) 825–834
doi:10.1016/j.ccc.2009.07.002
0749-0704/09/$ – see front matter

HIGH-DOSE STEROID STUDIES

Beneficial actions of high-dose steroids were believed to be secondary to their antiinflammatory effects. It was thought that corticosteroids interrupted the inflammatory cascade found in septic patients.[18] From the 1950s until the mid-1980s, pharmacologic doses of steroids (methylprednisolone, 30 mg/kg; or dexamethasone 3–6 mg/kg in 2–4 intravenous doses) were used by doctors to treat septic patients. This practice stemmed primarily by the study performed by Schumer,[2] which demonstrated that steroids significantly decreased mortality (from 38% to 10%). Sprung and colleagues[3] showed that septic shock patients receiving high-dose corticosteroids reversed their shock and had an improved survival for a short time. Overall mortality, however, was not significantly different.[3] They suggested that more prolonged steroid therapy might have been beneficial.[3] Subsequently, two large prospective, randomized trials demonstrated that high-dose steroids did not decrease mortality.[4,5] In 1995, two meta-analyses concluded that high-dose steroid treatment for patients with severe sepsis and septic shock were either not effective[6] or harmful.[7] In the trials with the highest quality, patients receiving corticosteroids had the worst outcomes.[7] High-dose corticosteroids were found to be associated with a greater risk of secondary infections[7] and renal and hepatic dysfunction[8] and mortality.[7] After these reports, doctors ceased using high-dose steroids for patients in septic shock (**Fig. 1**).

LOW-DOSE STEROID STUDIES

In the late 1990s and early 2000s, physicians restarted using steroids albeit at lower doses (usually 200–300 mg of intravenous hydrocortisone 3 times a day) for a new indication—relative adrenal insufficiency. Many patients with septic shock demonstrate depressed vasopressor sensitivity to catecholamines[19] and do not appropriately respond to corticotropin stimulation.[20] Mortality was shown to be higher in septic-shock patients with baseline cortisol levels less than 34 μg/dL (938 mmol/L) which did not increase after corticotropin stimulation greater than 9 μg/dL (248 nmol/L).[20]

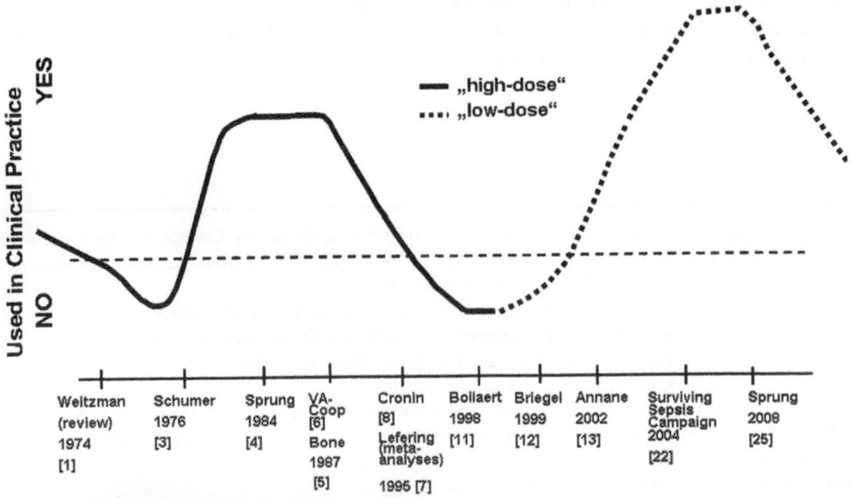

Fig. 1. The use of corticosteroids for patients in septic shock over the years. *From* Sprung CL, Goodman S, Weiss YG. Corticosteroid treatment of patients in septic shock. In: Vincent JL, editor. Yearbook of intensive care and emergency medicine. Springer; 2009. p. 753–60.

Various studies noted improved hemodynamic parameters after steroid therapy.[10,11,13–15] Bollaert and colleagues[10] studied patients in late septic shock with hydrocortisone given intravenously 100 mg every 8 hours for at least 5 days to assess steroid ability to improve hemodynamics. Patients receiving corticosteroids had greater shock reversal at days 7 and 28.[10] Briegel and colleagues[11] evaluated hyperdynamic septic shock patients treated with hydrocortisone (100 mg followed by 0.18 mg/kg/hr intravenously for 6 days) and subsequent tapering. Patients treated with corticosteroids required less vasopressor therapy and had a trend for a quicker reversal of organ dysfunction.[11] Overall shock reversal and mortality, however, did not change.[11] Keh and colleagues[13] performed a crossover study in which patients receiving vasopressors were treated with hydrocortisone (100 mg followed by 10 mg/hr intravenously for 3 days) or a placebo. Patients given corticosteroid therapy had a decrease in the dose and duration of norepinephrine therapy with a concomitant increase in blood pressure.[13] Oppert and colleagues[14] evaluated patients with early hyperdynamic septic shock; patients received intravenous hydrocortisone 50 mg followed by 0.18 mg/kg/hr until shock reversal and subsequent tapering or placebo. Patients treated with corticosteroids had a shorter duration of vasopressor therapy.[14] Cicarelli and colleagues[15] evaluated patients in septic shock who received either dexamethasone (0.2 mg/kg intravenously every 36 hours for 5 days) or placebo. Patients receiving dexamethasone therapy had less time on vasopressors, a significant decrease in mortality at day 7, and a trend for a lower 28-day mortality.[15]

In patients with early, severe septic shock, Annane and colleagues[12] evaluated low-dose hydrocortisone therapy in a multicenter, randomized, placebo-controlled, double-blind study. Patients were randomized within 8 hours of shock and received either intravenous hydrocortisone 50 mg every 6 hours and enteral fludrocortisone (50 μg/d) for 7 days, or placebo. Patients were classified as "nonresponders" or "responders" to a 250 μg corticotropin stimulation test with nonresponders being defined by an increase in cortisol ≤9 μg/dL (248 nmol/L).[12] There were 299 patients analyzed in the study. The primary source of infection was the lungs. Patients treated with steroids had more reversal of shock (57%) than patients receiving placebo (40%); the reversal was also more rapid.[12] The 28-day mortality was decreased by corticosteroid therapy in the overall patient population (61% vs 55%) and the nonresponder group of patients (63% vs 53%).[12] There was a similar incidence of adverse events in both study groups (22% vs 21%). These studies provided evidence that septic shock patients had impaired adrenal reserve and that corticosteroid replacement could reverse shock and improve survival. The Surviving Sepsis Campaign[21] and two meta-analyses[22,23] recommended the use of low-dose hydrocortisone for patients with septic shock based primarily on the Annane study.[12] The use of corticosteroids for septic shock patients again became extremely common (see **Fig. 1**).

THE CORTICUS STUDY

As the previous Annane study[12] evaluated patients with severe septic shock and inclusion criteria of a systolic blood pressure of less than 90 mmHg for more than 1 hour despite aggressive fluid and vasopressor therapy, which is found in a very small percentage of septic shock patients, the Corticus study[24] evaluated more typical septic shock patients who did not have to have a systolic blood pressure of less than 90 mmHg for more than 1 hour. The Corticus study evaluated the use of hydrocortisone and corticotropin testing in septic shock patients in a multicenter, randomized, placebo-controlled, double-blind study. In the Corticus study patients could be septic and in shock for up to 72 hours. Analysis was performed in 499 patients. The primary source of infection was the gastrointestinal tract. At baseline, 99% of patients were receiving vasopressors and the study drug was started within 12 hours in 77% of patients. The Corticus study demonstrated no differences in 28-day mortality in patients receiving hydrocortisone versus placebo respectively in nonresponders (39% vs 36%), responders (29% vs 29%), or all patients (34% vs 32%). There was no difference in the overall shock-reversal in patients receiving hydrocortisone versus placebo in the three groups of patients: nonresponders (76% vs 70%), responders (85% vs 77%), or all patients (80% vs 74%). In those patients who did reverse their shock, reversal occurred quicker in patients treated with hydrocortisone compared with placebo in all the three groups. In all patients, shock reversal occurred within 3.3 days in the patients treated with hydrocortisone and 5.8 days in placebo patients. Unfortunately, patients receiving hydrocortisone had a greater incidence of superinfections including new sepsis or septic shock. There was, however, no increased incidence of neuromuscular weakness.[24]

ADVERSE EFFECTS OF STEROIDS

As noted above, corticosteroid use in the critically ill can lead to adverse effects. Acute complications include superinfection, hyperglycemia, muscular weakness, hypernatremia, upper-gastrointestinal bleeding, arrhythmias, psychosis, and poor wound healing.[1] Some commentators have noted that previous steroid studies showed superinfections when high-dose steroids were used; whereas more recent studies with low-doses of steroids did not. Although some of the recent studies did not show an increased incidence of superinfections,[10,12] the Corticus study using steroids in low-doses did show an increased rate of superinfection, including new sepsis or septic shock.[24] Intensely ill patients are susceptible to viral infections and not only to bacterial infections. Heininger and colleagues[25] demonstrated that critically ill septic patients are more prone to develop cytomegalovirus infections. Jaber and colleagues[26] showed that cytomegalovirus infection was associated with steroid use in ICU nonimmunosuppressed patients with fever for more than 72 hours. Patients with cytomegalovirus infections had a greater mortality, longer duration of mechanical ventilation, and longer ICU length-of-stay.

Studies have also noted a higher incidence of the development of critical illness polyneuromyopathy in critically ill patients receiving corticosteroid therapy.[16,17] The weakness may be related to the administration of higher doses of corticosteroids as the Corticus study (stress-dose steroids)[24] did not show evidence of muscular weakness in patients receiving low-doses of steroids.

Some doctors believe that corticosteroids given to patients in septic shock may help to prevent the development of the acute respiratory distress syndrome (ARDS). A recent meta-analysis[27] demonstrated just the opposite, patients receiving corticosteroid therapy had a subsequent higher rate of ARDS development (ARDS developed in 37% patients treated with corticosteroids and 17% of patients receiving placebo; odds ratio 1.55 [95%CrI 0.58–4.05]). The meta-analysis suggested a weakly increased risk of death associated with corticosteroid therapy in those patients who developed ARDS (mortality in 52% patients treated with corticosteroids and 39% of patients receiving placebo; odds ratio 1.52 [95%CrI 0.30–5.94]).[27]

MECHANISM OF CORTICOSTEROID ACTION IN REVERSING SHOCK

The Corticus study demonstrated no differences in mortality, overall shock reversal, or effect of steroids in patients who were nonresponders or responders to a corticotropin stimulation test.[24] Many critically ill patients may not respond to a corticotropin stimulation test but this does not indicate that they have relative adrenal insufficiency or require corticosteroid therapy. Critically ill patients may have critical-illness–related corticosteroid insufficiency, which can be secondary to a decrease in adrenal steroid production or tissue resistance to steroids.[28] The Corticus study results suggest that the septic shock reversal that is hastened by corticosteroid treatment may be unrelated to adrenal insufficiency; the mechanism may be related to vascular hyporeactivity.[29,30] The glucocorticoid effects on vascular tone have been long recognized.[31] That corticosteroid therapy of septic shock patients reverses the depressed vasopressor sensitivity to catecholamines supports the role of steroids in affecting vasomotor tone.[19]

RECONCILING THE ANNANE AND SPRUNG STUDIES

The two recent, largest studies of steroid use in septic shock patients came to opposite conclusions after studying different patient populations. Differences between the two studies can be seen in **Table 1** and include for Annane and colleagues[12] and Sprung and colleagues[24] respectively: entry window, inclusion criteria systolic blood pressure less than 90 mmHg, additional treatment with fludrocortisone, duration of treatment, weaning, SAPS II severity scores, nonresponders to corticotropin, effects of corticosteroids according to the response to corticotropin, increased risk of superinfection, and study occurring after practice guidelines recommending steroids were published.

Despite the recent findings, some doctors continue to believe strongly in the use of steroids for septic shock patients. This may be related to the fact that many shock patients respond shortly after receiving a dose of corticosteroids with reversal of their shock. However, they may develop superinfections much later when it is not so evident that the infection is caused by the steroids. Physicians must remember that, although 80% of overall patients treated with corticosteroids in the Corticus study had shock reversal, 74% of patients receiving placebo also reversed their shock.[24] Recent meta-analyses have shown that corticosteroids reverse shock at day 7 but do not increase 28-day survival (**Figs. 2** and **3**).[28] It is interesting that a substudy of the recent Vasopressin and Septic Shock Trial[32] evaluated vasopressin infusion, corticosteroid treatment, and septic shock mortality.[33] In the 76% of patients receiving

Table 1
Differences in Annane[12] and Corticus[24] studies

	Annane	Corticus
Entry window	8 hours	72 hours
SBP < 90 mmHg	>1 hour	<1 hour
Treatment	Fludrocortisone	None
Treatment duration	7 days	11 days
Weaning	No	Yes
SAPS II score	59 ± 21	49 ± 17
Nonresponders	229 (77%)	233 (47%)
Steroid effect by		
Corticotropin response	Yes	No
Superinfection	No	Yes
Practice or guidelines	None	Steroids used

SAPS II severity scores mean ±SD.

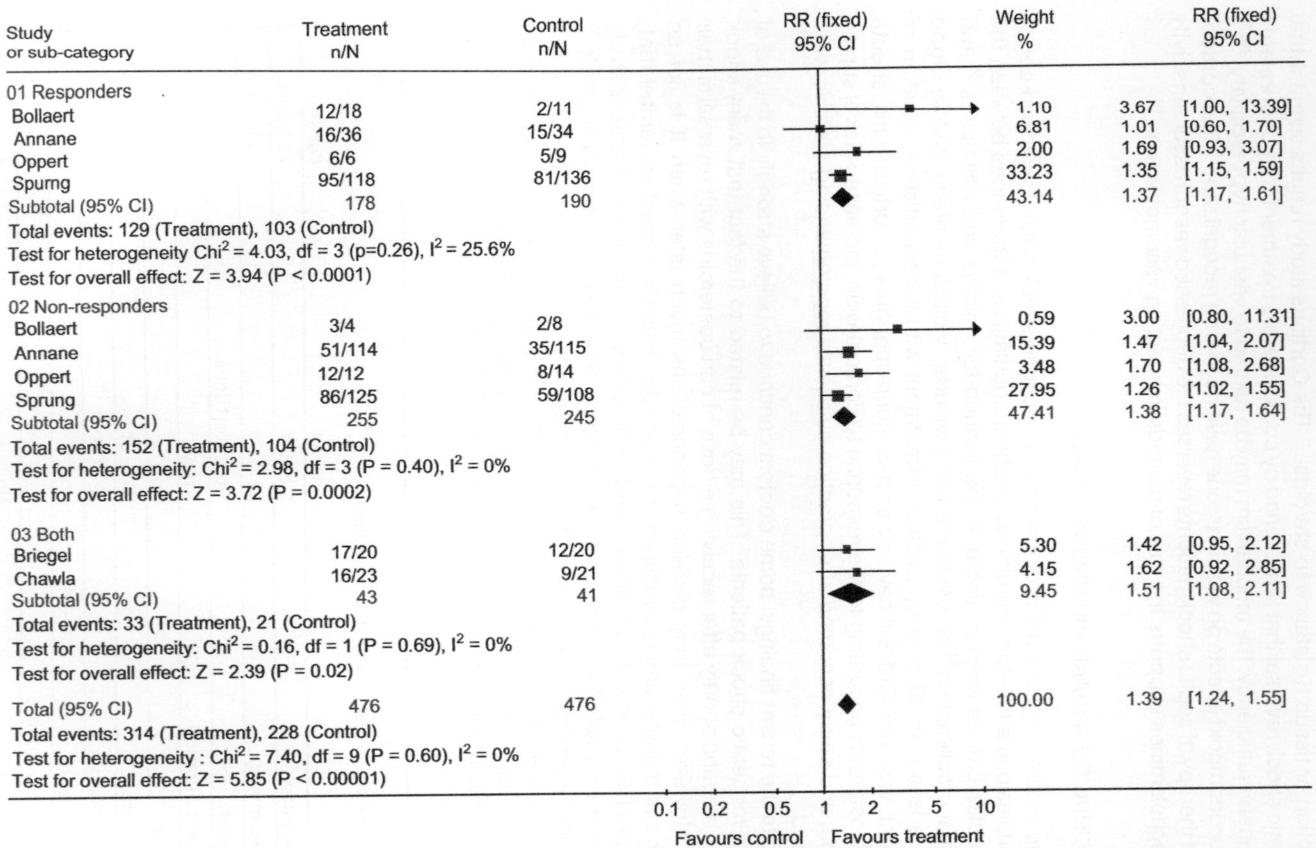

Fig. 2. Meta-analysis of treatment with hydrocortisone on shock reversal at day 7 in patients with septic shock grouped by response to adrenocorticotropic hormone. RR, relative risk; 95% CI, 95% confidence interval. (*From* Marik PE, Pastores SM, Annane D, et al. Recommendations for the diagnosis and management of corticosteroid insufficiency in critically ill adult patients: consensus statements from an international task force by the American College of Critical Care Medicine. Crit Care Med 2008;36:1942; with permission.)

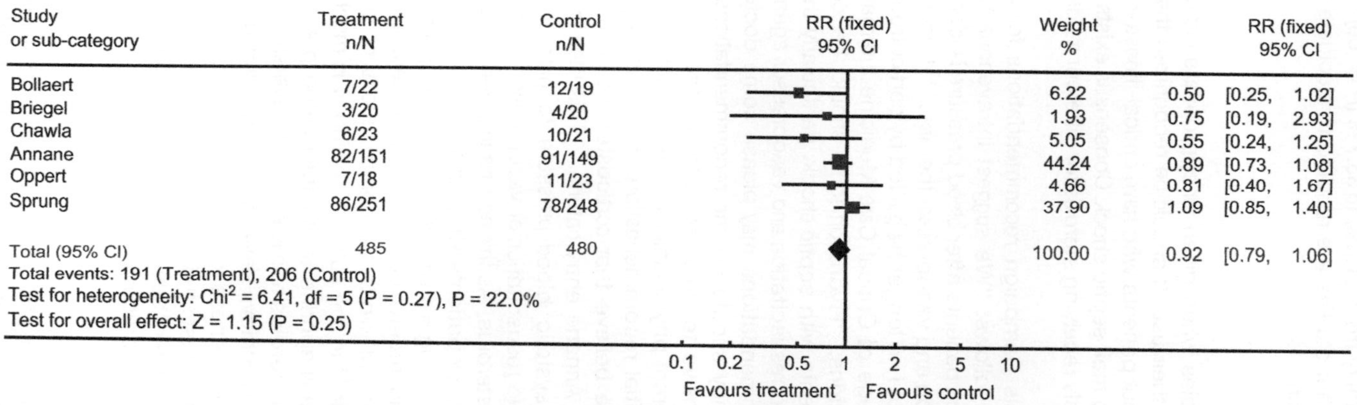
Study or sub-category
Treatment n/N
Control n/N
RR (fixed) 95% CI
Weight %
RR (fixed) 95% CI
Bollaert 7/22 12/19 6.22 0.50 [0.25, 1.02]
Briegel 3/20 4/20 1.93 0.75 [0.19, 2.93]
Chawla 6/23 10/21 5.05 0.55 [0.24, 1.25]
Annane 82/151 91/149 44.24 0.89 [0.73, 1.08]
Oppert 7/18 11/23 4.66 0.81 [0.40, 1.67]
Sprung 86/251 78/248 37.90 1.09 [0.85, 1.40]
Total (95% CI) 485 480 100.00 0.92 [0.79, 1.06]
Total events: 191 (Treatment), 206 (Control)
Test for heterogeneity: Chi² = 6.41, df = 5 (P = 0.27), P = 22.0%
Test for overall effect: Z = 1.15 (P = 0.25)
0.1 0.2 0.5 1 2 5 10
Favours treatment
Favours control

Fig. 3. Meta-analysis of treatment with hydrocortisone on 28-day survival in patients with septic shock. RR, relative risk; 95% CI, 95% confidence interval. (*From* Marik PE, Pastores SM, Annane D, et al. Recommendations for the diagnosis and management of corticosteroid insufficiency in critically ill adult patients: consensus statements from an international task force by the American College of Critical Care Medicine. Crit Care Med 2008;36:1942; with permission.)

steroids, vasopressin compared with norepinephrine decreased 28-day mortality from 35.9% to 44.7% (P = .03); whereas, in patients who did not receive steroids, vasopressin increased 28-day mortality from 21.3% to 33.7% (P = .06).[35] As these results were a post hoc analysis, further studies are required to elucidate the interaction of corticosteroids and vasopressin.

RECOMMENDATIONS

Steroids are life-saving therapies when given for appropriate indications. However, serious injury can occur after their use. It should be recognized that the controversy over the use of steroids is about patients who have critical-illness–related corticosteroid insufficiency secondary to their septic shock. Consensus exists for corticosteroid treatment for patients previously receiving steroids for different medical disorders who develop septic shock.

The recent Surviving Sepsis Campaign recommendations for corticosteroids in septic shock patients are as follows: "We suggest intravenous hydrocortisone be given only to adult septic shock patients after blood pressure is identified to be poorly responsive to fluid resuscitation and vasopressor therapy."[34] Recommendations also state that steroid therapy should no longer be guided by corticotropin stimulation test results.[21] The American College of Critical Care Medicine International Task Force issued similar recommendations: "Hydrocortisone should be considered in the management strategy of patients with septic shock, particularly those patients who have responded poorly to fluid resuscitation and vasopressor agents."[28]

Although these new recommendations may please some doctors because they have guidance as to what they should do, the recommendations are too general. What exactly "poorly responsive to fluid resuscitation and vasopressor therapy" means is not very clear. Different physicians may treat or not treat the same patient with septic shock. As the initial recommendations to use low-dose steroids came from the Annane study,[12] we believe that corticosteroids should only be used in patients who meet the initial Annane entry criteria.[12] This means that only patients who do not increase their systolic blood pressure to greater than or equal to 90 mmHg with aggressive fluid resuscitation or vasopressor therapy after more than 1 hour should receive corticosteroids. As this occurs in a very small number of septic shock patients, most septic shock patients whose systolic blood pressure is increased to greater than or equal to 90 mmHg with aggressive fluid resuscitation or vasopressor therapy within 1 hour should not receive corticosteroids. Potential benefits of a shorter duration of septic shock are not worth the complications of superinfection, new sepsis, and new septic shock.[24] In the authors' opinion, it is much better to receive an additional 2 days of norepinephrine to maintain blood pressure and perfusion than to be treated with corticosteroids to hasten shock reversal and suffer complications.[24] Alternatively, one could achieve similar results by using low-dose vasopressin to increase the vascular responsiveness to norepinephrine.[32] Therefore, based on the Corticus study,[24] which is the largest study of corticosteroids in septic shock patients and represents the preponderance of septic shock patients, the majority of patients in septic shock should not receive corticosteroids.

SUMMARY

Steroid therapy in patients with septic shock has been controversial for decades. Although treatment with high-doses of corticosteroids for patients with septic shock has been shown not to be beneficial, it was believed that therapy with low-doses would be helpful. Recent studies document that steroids are beneficial only in adult septic shock patients whose blood pressure is poorly responsive to fluid resuscitation and vasopressor therapy. For the majority of septic shock patients, corticosteroids should not be used, as the benefit of reversing shock is not worth the complications of superinfection, new sepsis, and septic shock. Finally, steroid therapy should not be guided by corticotropin test results.

REFERENCES

1. Schein RMH, Sprung CL. The use of corticosteroids in the sepsis syndrome. Critical Care - State of the Art 1986; The Society of Critical Care Medicine, Fullerton (CA); 1986;7:131–49.
2. Schumer W. Steroids in the treatment of clinical septic shock. Ann Surg 1976;184:333–41.
3. Sprung CL, Caralis PV, Marcial EH, et al. The effects of high-dose corticosteroids in patients with septic shock. A prospective, controlled study. N Engl J Med 1984;311:1137–43.
4. Bone RC, Fisher CJ Jr, Clemmer TP, et al. A controlled clinical trial of high-dose methylprednisolone in the treatment of severe sepsis and septic shock. N Engl J Med 1987;317:653–8.
5. The Veterans Administration Systemic Sepsis Cooperative Study Group. Effect of high-dose glucocorticoid therapy on mortality in patients with clinical signs of systemic sepsis. N Engl J Med 1987;317:659–65.
6. Lefering R, Neugebauer EAM. Steroid controversy in sepsis and septic shock: a meta-analysis. Crit Care Med 1995;23:1294–303.
7. Cronin L, Cook DJ, Carlet J, et al. Corticosteroid treatment for sepsis: a critical appraisal and meta-analysis of the literature. Crit Care Med 1995;24:1430–9.
8. Slotman GJ, Fisher CJ Jr, Bone RC, et al. Detrimental effects of high-dose methylprednisolone sodium succinate on serum concentrations of hepatic and renal function indicators in severe sepsis and septic shock. The Methylprednisolone Severe Sepsis Study Group. Crit Care Med 1993;21:191–5.
9. Lamberts SWJ, Bruining HA, de Jong FH. Corticosteroid therapy in severe illness. N Engl J Med 1997;337:1285–92.
10. Bollaert PE, Charpentier C, Levy S, et al. Reversal of late septic shock with supraphysiologic doses of hydrocortisone. Crit Care Med 1998;26:645–50.
11. Briegel J, Frost H, Haller M, et al. Stress doses of hydrocortisone reverse hyperdynamic septic shock: a prospective, randomized, double-blind, single center study. Crit Care Med 1999;27:723–32.
12. Annane D, Sebille V, Charpentier C, et al. Effect of treatment with low doses of hydrocortisone and fludrocortisone on mortality in patients with septic shock. JAMA 2002;288:862–70.
13. Keh D, Boehnke T, Weber-Cartens S, et al. Immunologic and hemodynamic effects of "low-dose" hydrocortisone in septic shock: a double-blind, randomized, placebo-controlled, crossover study. Am J Respir Crit Care Med 2003;167(4):512–20.
14. Oppert M, Schindler R, Husung C, et al. Low-dose hydrocortisone improves shock reversal and reduces cytokine levels in early hyperdynamic septic shock. Crit Care Med 2005;33:2457–64.
15. Cicarelli DD, Viera JE, Martin Besenor FE. Early dexamethasone treatment for septic shock patients: a prospective randomized clinical trial. Sao Paulo Med J 2007;125:237–41.

16. De Jonghe B, Sharshar T, Lefaucheur JP, et al. Paresis acquired in the intensive care unit: a prospective multicenter study. JAMA 2002;288:2859–67.
17. Herridge MS, Cheung AM, Tansey CM, et al. One-year outcomes in survivors of the acute respiratory distress syndrome. N Engl J Med 2003;348:683–93.
18. Bone RC. The pathogenesis of sepsis. Ann Intern Med 1991;115:457–69.
19. Annane D, Bellissant E, Sebille V, et al. Impaired pressor sensitivity to noradrenaline in septic shock patients with and without impaired adrenal reserve. Br J Clin Pharmacol 1998;46:589–97.
20. Annane D, Sebille V, Trocke G, et al. A 3-level prognostic classification of septic shock based on cortisol level and cortisol response to corticotropin. JAMA 2000; 283:1038–45.
21. Dellinger P, Carlet JM, Masur H, et al. Surviving Sepsis Campaign guidelines for the management of severe sepsis and septic shock. Crit Care Med 2004;32: 858–73.
22. Annane D, Bellissant E, Bollaert PE, et al. Corticosteroids for severe sepsis and septic shock: a systematic review and meta-analysis. BMJ 2004;329:480–8.
23. Minneci PC, Deans KJ, Banks SM, et al. Meta-analysis: the effects of steroids on survival and shock during sepsis depends on the dose. Ann Intern Med 2004; 141:47–56.
24. Sprung CL, Annane D, Keh D, et al, for the Corticus Study Group. The CORTICUS randomized, double-blind, placebo-controlled study of hydrocortisone therapy in patients with septic shock. N Engl J Med 2008;358:111–24.
25. Heininger A, Jahn J, Engel C, et al. Human cytomegalovirus infections in nonimmunosuppressed critically ill patients. Crit Care Med 2001;29:541–7.
26. Jaber S, Chanques G, Borry J, et al. Cytomegalovirus infection in critically ill patients. Chest 2005;127:233–41.
27. Peter JV, John P, Graham PL, et al. Corticosteroids in the prevention and treatment of acute respiratory distress syndrome (ARDS) in adults: meta-analysis. Br Med J 2008;336:1006–9.
28. Marik PE, Pastores SM, Annane D, et al. Clinical practice guidelines for the diagnosis and management of corticosteroid insufficiency in critical illness: recommendations of an international task force. Crit Care Med 2008;36:1937–49.
29. Silverman HJ, Penaranda R, Orens JB, et al. Impaired beta-adrenergic receptor stimulation of cyclic adenosine monophosphate in human septic shock: Association with myocardial hyporesponsiveness to catecholamines. Crit Care Med 1993;21:31–9.
30. Saito T, Takanashi M, Gallagher E, et al. Corticosteroid effect on early beta-adrenergic down-regulation during circulatory shock: hemodynamic study and beta-adrenergic receptor assay. Intensive Care Med 1995;21:204–10.
31. Perla D, Marmorston J. Suprarenal cortical hormone and salt in the treatment of pneumonia and other severe infections. Endocrinology 1940;27:367–74.
32. Russell JA, Walley KR, Singer J, et al. Vasopressin versus norepinephrine infusion in patients with septic shock. N Engl J Med 2008;358:877–87.
33. Russell JA, Walley KR, Gordon AC, et al. Interaction of vasopressin infusion, corticosteroid treatment and mortality of septic shock. Crit Care Med 2009;37:811–8.
34. Dellinger RP, Levy MM, Carlet JM, et al. Surviving Sepsis Campaign Guidelines Committee. Surviving Sepsis Campaign: International guidelines for management of severe sepsis and septic shock: 2008. Crit Care Med 2008;36: 296–327.

Genetic Polymorphisms in Sepsis

Allen Namath, MD[a], Andrew J. Patterson, MD, PhD[b,*]

KEYWORDS

• Sepsis • Polymorphism • Predisposition
• Genetic variation • Gene

Host predisposition influences risk of[1] and outcome during sepsis.[1,2] Genetic polymorphisms represent interindividual genetic variability and may help to explain host predisposition. This article is meant to serve as a summary of scientific advances from the past 5 years with regard to genetic polymorphisms in sepsis. It is also meant to highlight some of the discoveries that may improve our ability to identify vulnerable patients at earlier time points in sepsis, when interventions are more likely to have a positive effect. The intention of this article is not to minimize the importance of nongenetic factors and elements extrinsic to the host in determining the susceptibility to and consequences of sepsis. Indeed, sepsis is a multifactorial process.

The past decade has witnessed important advances in our understanding of the human genome and in our ability to evaluate patterns of synchronized gene expression changes. The convergence of engineering, computer science, and genetics has facilitated these advances. Whether these advances will allow us to discern the mechanisms of sepsis remains to be seen. In the immediate future, they are more likely to facilitate the division of sepsis into disease subsets with common molecular footprints that benefit from similar therapeutic interventions. Technological advances have significantly improved our ability to characterize the physiologic effect of genetic polymorphisms. Computer technology has facilitated associational studies linking polymorphisms to specific patient outcomes. During the next 10 years, the greatest advances in sepsis research may come from the development of prediction techniques, techniques that allow us to identify patients at highest risk for developing sepsis, techniques with the potential to facilitate cost-effective preventive medicine strategies. Included in this article is a synopsis of the technologies likely to facilitate these techniques.

[a] Division of Pulmonary and Critical Care Medicine, Santa Clara Valley Medical Center, 751 South Bascom Avenue, San Jose, CA 95128, USA
[b] Department of Anesthesia, Stanford University Medical Center, 300 Pasteur Drive, Stanford, CA 94305, USA
* Corresponding author.
E-mail address: ajpanes@stanford.edu (A.J. Patterson).

Crit Care Clin 25 (2009) 835–856
doi:10.1016/j.ccc.2009.06.004
criticalcare.theclinics.com
0749-0704/09/$ – see front matter

IS SEPSIS AN APPROPRIATE DISEASE FOR GENETIC POLYMORPHISM STUDIES?

More than 20 years ago, Sørensen and colleagues[3] reported that adult adoptees had a 5.81-fold increased risk of dying from infection if one of their biologic parents died of infection before the age of 50. This risk exceeded the relative risk (RR) of dying of cancer or cardiovascular disease, suggesting a significant but unspecified genetic susceptibility to mortal infections, and by extension, to sepsis. Ten genes have now been associated with the development of more than 30 infectious diseases.[4] Given the worldwide attention to recent H5N1 and H1N1 influenza outbreaks, it is noteworthy that for patients dying of influenza, the relative risk of dying of influenza is elevated in second (RR 1.22, $P<.0001$) and even third-generation relatives (RR 1.16, $P<.0001$) for whom the environmental commonality is reduced.[5]

THE EVOLUTION OF POLYMORPHISM STUDIES

Sequencing of the human genome has underscored how similar we are as members of a species. Investigations of genetic polymorphisms have illustrated how unique we are as individuals. During the past 15 years, approximately 10 million polymorphisms have been identified in the human genome. In some instances, rare genetic diseases have been shown to result from uncommon polymorphisms in otherwise highly conserved gene sequences. Conversely, many frequently occurring disorders may be attributable to common polymorphisms. Enough people develop sepsis to reasonably hypothesize that response to sepsis is related to common polymorphisms; that is, it would be reasonable to hypothesize that heterogeneity in sepsis manifestations and outcomes might be explained by single nucleotide polymorphisms (SNPs).

CANDIDATE GENE VERSUS GENOME-WIDE ASSOCIATION STUDY DESIGNS

Two study designs have been commonly used for sepsis investigations. In the first design, specific candidate genes were the focus of attention. In the second design, broad surveys of the entire genome were performed. Sepsis-related polymorphism studies have most commonly focused on one or more polymorphisms for specific genes whose protein products are elements of biologic pathways implicated in sepsis. These have included pro- and antiinflammatory cytokines, innate immunity, and coagulation/fibrinolysis pathways. Using this approach, groups of patients with specific polymorphisms have been compared with groups without them. For instance, burn patients with and without tumor necrosis factor (TNF)-α -308A polymorphisms have been compared for development of severe sepsis.[6]

Genome-wide association (GWA) studies have been used to compare patient populations. At the time of this article, no GWA study that focused on patients with sepsis has been published. In contrast to candidate gene studies, GWA investigations analyze large representative sets of genetic markers derived from the human haplotype map (HapMap) in search of those markers associated with a chosen phenotype, usually a disease. Current chip technology allows 500,000 such markers to be analyzed in parallel. GWA studies of traits such as eye color[7] and skeletal height[8] as well as studies of common diseases[9] have pointed to genetic loci whose associations with disease have been of modest strength. On track to potentially yield the first GWA study targeting sepsis in humans, the Wellcome Trust has established a case-control consortium for GWA studies, including 120,000 samples and 13 diseases, of which one is bacteremia.[10]

BENEFITS AND LIMITATIONS OF TARGETED VERSUS GENOME-WIDE STUDIES

Targeted studies of candidate genetic loci are hypothesis-driven, require fewer study subjects, and are typically less expensive and more rapid than genome-wide studies. The hypothesis in such studies is based on biologic plausibility. Therefore, identified associations are generally biologically plausible. Ideally, intermediate phenotypes occur in these investigations (eg, predefined messenger RNA [mRNA] or protein levels). In such cases, positive results can quickly point toward options for pharmaceutical interventions. On the other hand, there are already more than 20 genes whose polymorphisms have been implicated in sepsis. Consequently, the impact of an additional SNP study can only be to add another member to the list for future studies that might demonstrate cause and effect.

In contrast, GWA studies cast a much wider net, are not bound by a specific hypothesis, and have the potential to discover genetic loci associated with sepsis that would be difficult to predict using known pathways. These studies rely on associations between a phenotype, such as sepsis, and polymorphic loci but not necessarily genes. Many SNPs do not reside within protein-encoding regions of the genome, which raises questions of gene expression variability through transcription, RNA stability, RNA splicing, and other translation effects.

SEPSIS-RELATED GENETIC POLYMORPHISMS

In the last 6 years, more than 30 genes have had their respective polymorphisms studied for relationships to sepsis and critical infection or inflammation. Fifty-eight such studies are summarized in **Table 1** as a nonexhaustive representation of this body of work. Of the 58 studies, 28 included an intermediate phenotype such as mRNA or protein levels of either the targeted gene itself or others in the putative pathway. Biologic plausibility is enhanced when a given polymorphism is associated with a clinical phenotype and an intermediate phenotype concordantly. For example, the IRAK1 1595C SNP has been associated with higher levels of NFκB in peripheral blood cells treated with lipopolysaccharide (LPS) and has associated odds ratios for septic shock, ventilator dependence, and 60-day mortality all greater than 2.5 with P values all less than or equal to .05.[11] Six studies presented in **Table 1** assessed intermediate phenotypes only, commonly measuring select protein levels in response to endotoxin or pathogen exposure. One of the benefits of these studies was that they started with well-defined moments of exposure, which is obviously difficult to accomplish in studies of clinical sepsis. Consequently, these investigations facilitated tracking of temporally associated changes. Many of the genes investigated so far belong to familiar sepsis-related groups including pro- and antiinflammatory cytokines, coagulation, and innate immunity. TNF-α polymorphisms were widely examined in multiple contexts encompassing burn injuries, esophagectomy, neonatal sepsis, smoke inhalation, meningococcal disease, and LPS infusion. Protein C polymorphism studies highlighted the importance of haplotype analyses, in which SNP combinations have phenotypic associations beyond those seen with a single allele.[12] Genes with other roles were studied, including leukocyte rolling via selectins, apoptosis by caspase 12, and complement activating C-reactive protein (CRP). Polymorphisms in mitochondrial DNA may also play a role in sepsis through putative variation in handling oxidative stress. A small subset of the studies presented in **Table 1** is discussed later in greater detail.

Table 1
Associations between gene polymorphisms and intermediate and clinical phenotypes related to sepsis

Gene or Locus	Sequence Polymorphism(s)	Study Species	Study Size	Intermediate Phenotype	Clinical Phenotype	Odds Ratio or Other Risk (*P* Value)	References
APOE	APOE3TR, APOE4TR	Mouse	94	Cytokine levels after cecal ligation and puncture (CLP)	Mortality after CLP	Increased mortality in APOE4TR (.039)	17
Caspase 12	125C	Human	1167	7 cytokine levels after ex vivo LPS	Severe sepsis	7.8-fold ↑ in homozygotes (.005)	20
CD14	-159C	Human	288	None	Severe sepsis after burn injury	1.668 (.047)	6
CD14	-260T	Human	293	None	Multiple blood stream infections	13% ↑ in homozygotes (.022)	21
CD14	-260T	Human	44	CD14 expression in sepsis and after LPS	Sepsis	-260T SNP associated with higher membrane-bound CD14 in early sepsis	22
CD14	-260T	Human	85	None	Critical illness (sepsis and other causes), mortality	TT genotype favored survival (.042)	23
CRP	-717G	Human	147	CRP concentration	Bacteremia, mortality	Strong association with mortality from *S pneumoniae*, no effect on CRP level	19
CRP	1444C	Human	91	CRP, cytokine, D-dimer, prothrombin fragments after LPS	Temperature after LPS infusion	Higher temperature, cytokine, coagulation markers (<.05)	24

CXCL2	-665(AC)n, -437G	Human	535	None	Severe sepsis	Only -665(AC)n associated, OR, 3.65 (.0006)	25
CXCL2	-665(AC)n	Human	183	None	Mortality, ARDS, multiorgan failure in severe sepsis	32%↓ mortality in homozygotes vs noncarriers (.018)	26
DDAHII	-449C	Human	57	ADMA, IL-6 levels	Sepsis mortality, day 1 and day 7 SOFA scores	-449G: ↑ADMA levels at days 1 & 7 (.03, .04); no clinical association	27
DEFB1	-44G	Human	368	None	Severe sepsis and mortality	Sepsis OR, 1.9 (.0049); death OR, 2.4 (.002)	28
E-selectin	128R	Human	157	E-selectin, TNF, IL-6, thrombin generation after LPS infusion	None	30%↑ thrombin generation in 128R (<.01)	14
Factor V	Factor V leiden (FVL)	Human (pediatric patients)	53	None	Sepsis, severe sepsis	No association seen	29
Factor V	FVL	Human (H) and mouse (M)	1690 patients	Biomarkers of coagulation, inflammation	Human sepsis mortality, mortality benefit of APC, mouse mortality s/p endotoxin	FVL mortality benefit 13.9% vs 27.9% (.013)H 19% vs 57% (.008)M biomarkers/APC effect unchanged	30
Fibrinogen	-148T	Human	73	TNF-α, IL-6, D-dimer, prothrombin F(1+2) levels after LPS	None	56%↓TNF-α Other markers unchanged	31

(continued on next page)

Table 1
(continued)

Gene or Locus	Sequence Polymorphism(s)	Study Species	Study Size	Intermediate Phenotype	Clinical Phenotype	Odds Ratio or Other Risk (*P* Value)	References
Protein C	-1641A/-1654C haplotype	Human (Chinese Han)	563	None	Sepsis, mortality, organ dysfunction	-1641A/-1654C associated with sepsis mortality: 35 vs 23% (.008)	12
Protein C	-1654C/-1641G (CG)	Human (pediatric)	288	None	Systemic meningococcemia, sepsis	CG allele sepsis OR, 3.43 pressors OR, 6.61	53
Protein Z	79A	Human	123	None	Sepsis and sepsis-related mortality	(AA genotype) Sepsis OR, 4.5 (CI, .45–46); no mortality association	54
TIRAP/Mal	S180L	Human(H) Mouse(M)	1160	TLR2 signal transduction (M)	Bacteremia (B), pneumococcal bacteremia (PB)	OR for heterozygote advantage: B - 0.34 (.003) PB - 0.30 (.024)	55
Toll-like receptor 1 (TLR1)	-7202G	Human	999	Cytokine production	Sepsis, organ dysfunction & death (ODD), sepsis related acute lung injury (ALI)	Increased cytokine production ODD OR, 1.82 ALI OR, 3.4	56
TLR2	-16,933AA	Human	252	Bacteremia, gram-positive vs gram-negative infection	Sepsis, septic shock, 28-d survival	↑bacteremia, not with shock or mortality	1

TLR4	896G	Human	598	None	Posttrauma SIRS or complicated sepsis	Reduced risk of complicated sepsis OR, 0.3 (.008)	57
TLR4	299gly	Human	209	Peripheral blood monocyte IL-10 levels	*Candida albicans* blood stream infection	Candidemia OR, 3 Higher IL-10 levels	58
TLR4	299gly 399Ile	Human (pediatric)	494	None	Pneumococcal sepsis	Both polymorphisms less common in septic patients OR, 0.3	59
TLR4	896G	Human	288	None	Severe sepsis after burn injury	2.943 (.027)	6
TNF-α	-308A	Human	288	None	Severe sepsis after burn injury	2.602 (.013)	6
TNF-α	-308A	Human	2601	TNF secretion, macrophage TNF mRNA	Meningococcal disease and death	No effect on death + disease OR, 1.93; higher TNF/mRNA	60
TNF-α	-308A	Human	411	None	Sepsis and mortality	-308A significantly higher in sepsis, worse outcomes	61
TNF-α	-308A	Human	69	None	Shock/death after burn injury	Death OR, 10.7 (.034) (CI, 1.2–95.5)	62
TNF-α	-308A	Human	200	TNF, IL-6, IL-10, IL-18 levels after LPS infusion	None	No association between SNP and cytokine levels	63

(*continued on next page*)

Table 1
(continued)

Gene or Locus	Sequence Polymorphism(s)	Study Species	Study Size	Intermediate Phenotype	Clinical Phenotype	Odds Ratio or Other Risk (*P* Value)	References
TNF-α	-308G	Human	197	None	Infection after esophagectomy	Higher infection rates (.021)	64
TNF-α	-308A	Human	87	IL-6, TNF, D-dimer, temperature after LPS infusion	None	No association between SNP and cytokines or D-dimer	65
TNF-α	-308A	Human	169	None	Early onset sepsis in neonates	No association	66
TNF-α	-308A	Human	213	TNF and TNF-receptor levels	Sepsis outcomes	No association	67
TNF-α	-308A	Human	159	None	Severe sepsis and mortality after burn or smoke inhalation injury	OR, 4.5 for severe sepsis, no association for mortality	68
TREM-1	rs7768162, rs9471535, rs2234237	Human	314	None	Severe sepsis	No association	69

Abbreviations: ↑, increase; ↓, decrease; ADMA, asymmetric dimethylarginine; APC, activated protein C; ARDS, acute respiratory distress syndrome; CI, confidence interval; DIC, disseminated intravascular coagulation; MIF, migration inhibitory factor; NA, not available; OR, odds ratio; SIRS, systemic inflammatory response syndrome; SOFA, sequential organ failure assessment; s/p, status post.

E-SELECTIN

Selectins are surface proteins expressed by vascular endothelial cells, and they mediate leukocyte rolling. The Ser128Srg SNP of E-selectin is associated with stent restenosis.[13] Jilma and colleagues[14] investigated the effect of the Ser128Arg SNP of E-selectin on inflammation and coagulation in human volunteers receiving LPS infusions. Of 157 individuals, 40 (25.5%) were Ser128Arg heterozygotes (3 homozygotes). Within 8 hours of LPS infusion, markers of coagulation were increased in Ser128Arg individuals compared with genotype controls. Prothrombin fragment levels were increased 50% to 80% and D-dimer levels were doubled. Levels of interleukin (IL)-6 and TNF-α were unchanged over the same period. Although the effects of this SNP in frankly septic patients have not been determined, it appears to confer procoagulant effects in the presence of LPS independent of other inflammatory pathways.

APOLIPOPROTEIN E

Apolipoprotein E (ApoE) is involved in cholesterol metabolism and immune modulation. In humans it exists in 3 isoforms (ApoE2, ApoE3, and ApoE4) differing from each other by amino acids at positions 112 and 158: Cys112-Cys158 (ApoE2), Cys112-Arg158 (ApoE3), and Arg112-Arg158 (ApoE4). Fourteen percent of the population is estimated to have the ApoE4 genotype, with which there is an associated increased inflammatory response to cardiopulmonary bypass.[15] After 2 groups of mice expressing human ApoE3 or ApoE4 were exposed to LPS, the ApoE4 group showed higher levels of IL-6 and TNF-α.[16] Wang and colleagues[17] in 2009 have demonstrated increased mortality in ApoE4 mice compared with ApoE3 mice after cecal ligation and puncture. Their data suggest that the mortality effect could be attenuated by simultaneous administration of an ApoE-mimetic peptide.[17]

CRP

CRP is an acute phase reactant typically elevated in conditions of infection or inflammation. It activates complement-mediated opsonization and can modulate inflammatory cytokine production. Healthy adult volunteers who were either hetero- or homozygous for CRP 1444C/T polymorphism showed higher basal levels of serum CRP, relative to those who were heterozygous for 286 C/T/A.[18] In 2006, Marsik and colleagues[24] exposed 91 healthy volunteers to LPS infusions. These investigators confirmed basal CRP differences reflecting the 1444C/T polymorphism and showed that wild-type 1444CC homozygotes had higher fevers, higher TNF-α, IL-6, D-dimer, and prothrombin fragment concentrations following LPS administration.[18]

Of 147 bacteremic patients, those with the 717GG genotype had a mortality odds ratio of 9.6 compared with 717AA and 717AG individuals. In the study by Marsik and colleagues, there was no association between 30-day mortality and SNPs at 1444 or 1059. The increased mortality associated with 717GG was seen predominantly in those cases of bacteremia due to *Streptococcus pneumoniae* as opposed to *Escherichia coli, Staphylococcus aureus*, or β-hemolytic *streptococcus.*[19] The 717 genotype did not appear to influence CRP levels (see **Table 1**).

CONSORTIA-BASED PROJECTS CATALYZE SEPSIS RESEARCH

It has been more than 20 years since the US Congress first approved funding for the Human Genome Project, which involved sequencing of all 3 billion bases in the human genome. Numerous countries on several continents contributed to the project's success by providing data and technology. Primary questions addressed by this project were (1) How do our genes function? (2) How is one individual's genome different from another's? (3) Do genes behave differently in different organs? (4) Is there a genetic contribution to common diseases? (5) What is the genomic identity of the microbial environment within each of us? The Human Genome Project was the first successful consortium-based genome project. As such, it served as a proof of principle.

Numerous consortium-based genome projects have followed the Human Genome Project. For instance, the International HapMap Project[70] characterized approximately 10 million SNPs across the human genome using samples from 270 individuals from Asia, Europe, and Africa. Most SNP chips used today are products of this project. With regard to sepsis and polymorphisms, the International HapMap Project has the potential to be of tremendous value. For instance, in the future when single SNPs are associated with sepsis, the HapMap may show other SNPs that are in linkage disequilibrium, providing a more comprehensive explanation as to why individuals differ in their responses to infection and inflammation. It is likely that large-scale multi-SNP analyses of sepsis will not be feasible without HapMap data.

The Wellcome Trust Case Control Consortium (WTCCC) supports GWA studies examining 13 disease conditions. Its goal is to analyze 120,000 samples. Diseases in this study that are relevant to sepsis include those involving breakdown of the barrier between host and microbial environment and those involving pathologic inflammatory states, such as ulcerative colitis, Barrett esophagus, and esophageal carcinoma. Studies involving invasive infection include investigations of visceral leishmaniasis.[10] Studies associated with the WTCCC may provide insight with regard to how pathogens penetrate host defenses more readily in certain individuals and how inflammation can be protective or deleterious in different individuals.

The Encyclopedia of DNA Elements (ENCODE) project aims to systematically identify all genes, promoters, and other regulators of transcription as well as elements regulating chromosomal structure and function. One percent of the genome (30 megabases) has been completed so far, whereas a full analysis of the genome has begun.[71] Protein coding genes number in the tens of thousands out of a genome of 3 billion bases. However, most of the bases analyzed so far in this project are transcribed. This finding raises many questions about the roles of most transcripts. ENCODE will be a significant resource for sepsis transcriptomics and may reveal additional factors that determine how individuals respond to infection and inflammation.

To better understand the link between clinical phenotype (ie, the clinical manifestation of sepsis) and genotype, intermediate phenotypes such as gene expression levels may be useful. The Genotype-Tissue Expression (GTEx) project collects tissue samples from various organs in subjects who are densely genotyped.[72] Expression levels of genes in a given tissue that correlate strongly with genotype variations are considered expression quantitative trait loci (eQTLs).[73] The initial GTEx project focused on 160 individuals, but it may increase to 1000. It should be emphasized that sepsis is a dynamic disease that evolves over a period of hours and even days. Expression data may compliment genotyping data in diseases like sepsis by capturing "snapshots" of the disease process at specific points in time. Renal failure,[74] acute respiratory distress syndrome (ARDS),[74] myocardial depression,[75] and cholestatic hepatic insufficiency[76] are variably associated with sepsis. Analyzing gene expression changes in these disease states may provide insight with regard to why and how multi-organ dysfunction occurs in sepsis.

Genome sequencing offers the finest level of detail in terms of genotypic differences between individuals. The 1000 Genomes Project based in England, China, and the United States aims to sequence the genomes of approximately 1200 people, with the information housed in a public-access database.[77] This project should permit analysis of polymorphisms in sequence or copy number that occur at lower frequencies than those in the HapMap. It may lead to disease associations (including associations with sepsis) otherwise unrecognized by other approaches. It is likely that in some circumstances, the sepsis phenotype correlates with structural variations in the genome that are not in linkage disequilibrium with common SNPs. Should GWA studies be completed for septic patients, the 1000 Genomes Project might provide a reference framework for resequencing loci of interest.

Unlike many other common diseases examined for genetic underpinnings, sepsis has an obligatory partnership with nonhost pathogens, particularly bacteria. Even in the nondisease state, there are tenfold more microbial cells in the human body than host cells. The Human Microbiome Project (HMP) aims to better characterize this complex interaction by building a reference collection of more than 1000 microbial genomes from human microenvironments including skin, nasopharynx, oropharynx, and gastrointestinal and urogenital tracts.[78] The degree to which we share common or disparate microbiomes may influence our view of sepsis variability. How the body regulates and reacts to the microbiome could provide a baseline for comparison to the presumed dysregulation in sepsis.

WILL TECHNOLOGICAL ADVANCEMENTS RESHAPE EXPERIMENTAL QUESTIONS?

Commercially available chip-based platforms (Illumina[79] [San Diego, CA] and Affymetrix[80] [Santa Clara, CA]) contain from 1 to 1.8 million genetic markers, including SNPs and probes for copy number variation. These platforms allow massive parallel polymorphism analyses for any given sample. Using these platforms, an extraordinarily wide net can be cast in terms of the number of genes potentially analyzed in a sepsis study. Studies involving large numbers of sepsis patients can, therefore, yield significant associations between distinct SNPs and sepsis. Unfortunately, at this time, applying complex technology such as commercially available chip-based arrays to large sepsis study populations is prohibitively expensive. In addition, although 1 million SNPs per assay is an extremely large number, it is still a small percentage of the total number of SNPs in the human genome. Consequently, sepsis research in the near term may have to remain focused while it awaits the development of more cost-effective technology.

Because the number of SNPs implicated in sepsis-related or otherwise biologically plausible pathways remains fewer than 100, a more cost-effective approach to studying sepsis might be to scale down from 1,000,000 element chips to one-SNP-one-well reactions. A single sample/SNP could be analyzed in 1 reaction (or several hundred) in a multiwell plate (Applied Biosystems [Carlsbad, CA] and Fluidigm [San Francisco, CA]).[81,82] Fluorescence labeling of probes could allow for color association with given SNP alleles. Cost reduction would be extended by reducing reagent consumption through microfluidics plates.

The opposite approach would be to work with companies and investigators developing the next generation technology to pursue a "sequencing everything" strategy, bypassing representative polymorphisms and characterizing the complete genotype for each sample. This approach would be sensitive and might overcome concerns related to missing rare SNPs that are not represented on existing chips but have strong phenotypic effects.

Complete Genomics (Mountain View, CA) can now provide a complete human genome sequence as a service, bypassing investment in new sequencing capital equipment and reagents. Helicos (Cambridge, MA) and Pacific Biosciences (Menlo Park, CA)[83] have developed technology to sequence single molecules of DNA with enormous throughput capabilities. Using a zero-mode waveguide nanostructure array, a single sequencing reaction occurring in a zeptoliter (10^{-21} L) can produce 400 kilobases of sequence data per day. Fourteen thousand reactions arrayed in parallel could generate onefold sequence coverage of a diploid human genome in 24 hours.[84] Clarke and colleagues[85] have distinguished unlabeled individual nucleotides by passing them through a modified α-hemolysin protein nanopore containing cyclodextrin. These investigators identified bases by their unique interference with an electrical current passing through the pore. They used an exonuclease to cleave single bases from the DNA strand to be sequenced on 1 side of the pore. Using this approach, base identification took only milliseconds, implying label-free, single-molecule detection and fast sequencing amenable to parallel construction.[84]

ETHICAL AND SOCIAL ISSUES GERMANE TO HUMAN GENOMIC STUDIES

Although polymorphism studies have the potential to provide tremendous insight into types and mechanisms of sepsis, such investigations may have unintended consequences. The information obtained from individuals might also reveal their risk for serious nonsepsis diseases, such as malignancy[86] and autoimmune diseases.[87] Some polymorphism-associated traits, such as mental illness[88] and drug abuse,[89] could confer unwanted social stigma. For example, although the TNF-α -308 polymorphism has been associated with sepsis,[60,61] it has also been associated with earlier onset of Alzheimer disease,[90] multiple sclerosis,[91] schizophrenia,[88] asthma,[92] systemic lupus erythematosus,[87] prostate cancer,[86] and preterm premature rupture of membranes.[93] IL-10 polymorphisms are associated with sepsis mortality[38] and sudden infant death syndrome.[94] Targeted studies of select polymorphisms might reduce the number of unintended discoveries. Standardized reporting of the strength of associations might minimize unwarranted concern over very weak cause-effect relationships. However, these issues will need to be considered to ensure public support for this type of research.

Unlike patients with other chronic or less acute diseases, septic patients often require surrogate decision makers (SDMs) to provide consent for study enrollment. Freeman and colleagues[95] have shown that 90% to 95% of SDMs are receptive to genetic testing to explain familial or ethnic traits, but 77% to 80% are reluctant to permit such testing if results could be accessed by employers or insurance providers.

SUMMARY

The number of genetic polymorphisms shown to play a role in sepsis continues to increase. At the same time, platforms for genetic sequencing and expression analysis are being refined, allowing unprecedented data generation. International databases may soon facilitate synchrony of genotypic and phenotypic data using enormous numbers of septic patients. If this occurs, 2 strategies for investigating polymorphisms in sepsis are likely to gain favor. In the first strategy, sepsis will continue to be viewed as a single entity. High-throughput genetic techniques will be used to evaluate numerous polymorphisms, each with fractional disease responsibility. Nongenetic variables, such as pathogen characteristics, underlying host medical conditions, and type and timing of resuscitation, will be considered cofactors. Using this approach, principal components that predict susceptibility to and outcomes during sepsis are likely to be identified.

In the second strategy, sepsis will be divided into subtypes based on the concentration of specific variables. Categories will be based on features like the presence or absence of specific polymorphisms, gram-positive or gram-negative staining of causative organisms, age and comorbid conditions of the host, recent administration of chemotherapeutic agents, and hospital setting (ie, community vs teaching institution). Each category will be used to create homogenous sepsis subgroups for detailed evaluation. This approach will increase the odds of finding single dominant factors responsible for predilection and/or outcome within well-defined groups among those with sepsis.

Several elements will be essential for the success of both these strategies. Firstly, databases that are extremely detailed will have to be generated. Secondly, better clinical information technology systems will be needed to facilitate large-scale phenotyping. Thirdly, standardization of protocols will need to take place to ensure uniformity of data sets.

If the rapid advances in technology and informatics continue, they may catalyze paradigm shifts with regard to how clinicians address sepsis. Clinicians may change their focus from aggressive uniform treatment strategies to rapid stratification and subcategorization, with subsequent aggressive targeted therapeutic interventions. Advances in technology have the potential to change our primary goal in sepsis from rapid treatment to prevention for those most at risk. The cost savings to the US health care systems from such changes could be substantial.

REFERENCES

1. Sutherland AM, Walley KR, Russell JA. Polymorphisms in CD14, mannose-binding lectin, and Toll-like receptor-2 are associated with increased prevalence of infection in critically ill adults. Crit Care Med 2005;33(3):638–44.
2. Henckaerts L, Nielsen KR, Steffensen R, et al. Polymorphisms in innate immunity genes predispose to bacteremia and death in the medical intensive care unit. Crit Care Med 2009;37(1):192–201, e191–3.
3. Sørensen T, Nielsen G, Andersen P, et al. Genetic and environmental influences on premature death in adult adoptees. N Engl J Med 1988;318(12):727–32.
4. Burgner D, Jamieson SE, Blackwell JM. Genetic susceptibility to infectious diseases: big is beautiful, but will bigger be even better? Lancet Infect Dis 2006;6(10):653–63.
5. Albright FS, Orlando P, Pavia AT, et al. Evidence for a heritable predisposition to death due to influenza. J Infect Dis 2008;197(1):18–24.
6. Barber RC, Chang LY, Arnoldo BD, et al. Innate immunity SNPs are associated with risk for severe sepsis after burn injury. Clin Med Res 2006;4(4):250–5.
7. Kayser M, Liu F, Janssens AC, et al. Three genome-wide association studies and a linkage analysis identify HERC2 as a human iris color gene. Am J Hum Genet 2008;82(2):411–23.
8. Soranzo N, Rivadeneira F, Chinappen-Horsley U, et al. Meta-analysis of genome-wide scans for human adult stature identifies novel Loci and associations with measures of skeletal frame size. PLoS Genet 2009;5(4):e1000445.
9. Torkamani A, Topol EJ, Schork NJ. Pathway analysis of seven common diseases assessed by genome-wide association. Genomics 2008;92(5):265–72.
10. Available at: http://wtccc.org.uk. Accessed May 15, 2009.
11. Arcaroli J, Silva E, Maloney JP, et al. Variant IRAK-1 haplotype is associated with increased nuclear factor-kappaB activation and worse outcomes in sepsis. Am J Respir Crit Care Med 2006;173(12):1335–41.
12. Chen QX, Wu SJ, Wang HH, et al. Protein C -1641A/-1654C haplotype is associated with organ dysfunction and the fatal outcome of severe sepsis in Chinese Han population. Hum Genet 2008;123(3):281–7.

13. Mlekusch W, Exner M, Schillinger M, et al. E-Selectin and restenosis after femoropopliteal angioplasty: prognostic impact of the Ser128Arg genotype and plasma levels. Thromb Haemost 2004;91(1):171–9.
14. Jilma B, Marsik C, Kovar F, et al. The single nucleotide polymorphism Ser128Arg in the E-selectin gene is associated with enhanced coagulation during human endotoxemia. Blood 2005;105(6):2380–3.
15. Grocott HP, Newman MF, El-Moalem H, et al. Apolipoprotein E genotype differentially influences the proinflammatory and anti-inflammatory response to cardiopulmonary bypass. J Thorac Cardiovasc Surg 2001;122(3):622–3.
16. Lynch JR, Tang W, Wang H, et al. APOE genotype and an ApoE-mimetic peptide modify the systemic and central nervous system inflammatory response. J Biol Chem 2003;278(49):48529–33.
17. Wang H, Christensen DJ, Vitek MP, et al. APOE genotype affects outcome in a murine model of sepsis: implications for a new treatment strategy. Anaesth Intensive Care 2009;37(1):38–45.
18. Jones J, Chen LS, Baudhuin L, et al. Relationships between C-reactive protein concentration and genotype in healthy volunteers. Clin Chem Lab Med 2009; 47(1):20–5.
19. Eklund C, Huttunen R, Syrjanen J, et al. Polymorphism of the C-reactive protein gene is associated with mortality in bacteraemia. Scand J Infect Dis 2006; 38(11–12):1069–73.
20. Saleh M, Vaillancourt JP, Graham RK, et al. Differential modulation of endotoxin responsiveness by human caspase-12 polymorphisms. Nature 2004;429(6987): 75–9.
21. Baier RJ, Loggins J, Yanamandra K. IL-10, IL-6 and CD14 polymorphisms and sepsis outcome in ventilated very low birth weight infants. BMC Med 2006;4:10.
22. de Aguiar BB, Girardi I, Paskulin DD, et al. CD14 expression in the first 24h of sepsis: effect of -260C>T CD14 SNP. Immunol Invest 2008;37(8):752–69.
23. D'Avila LC, Albarus MH, Franco CR, et al. Effect of CD14 -260C>T polymorphism on the mortality of critically ill patients. Immunol Cell Biol 2006;84(4):342–8.
24. Marsik C, Sunder-Plassmann R, Jilma B, et al. The C-reactive protein (+)1444C/T alteration modulates the inflammation and coagulation response in human endotoxemia. Clin Chem 2006;52(10):1952–7.
25. Flores C, Maca-Meyer N, Perez-Mendez L, et al. A CXCL2 tandem repeat promoter polymorphism is associated with susceptibility to severe sepsis in the Spanish population. Genes Immun 2006;7(2):141–9.
26. Villar J, Perez-Mendez L, Flores C, et al. A CXCL2 polymorphism is associated with better outcomes in patients with severe sepsis. Crit Care Med 2007; 35(10):2292–7.
27. O'Dwyer MJ, Dempsey F, Crowley V, et al. Septic shock is correlated with asymmetrical dimethyl arginine levels, which may be influenced by a polymorphism in the dimethylarginine dimethylaminohydrolase II gene: a prospective observational study. Crit Care 2006;10(5):R139.
28. Chen QX, Lv C, Huang LX, et al. Genomic variations within DEFB1 are associated with the susceptibility to and the fatal outcome of severe sepsis in Chinese Han population. Genes Immun 2007;8(5):439–43.
29. Sipahi T, Pocan H, Akar N. Effect of various genetic polymorphisms on the incidence and outcome of severe sepsis. Clin Appl Thromb Hemost 2006;12(1):47–54.
30. Kerlin BA, Yan SB, Isermann BH, et al. Survival advantage associated with heterozygous factor V Leiden mutation in patients with severe sepsis and in mouse endotoxemia. Blood 2003;102(9):3085–92.

31. Kovar FM, Marsik C, Jilma B, et al. The fibrinogen -148 C/T polymorphism influences inflammatory response in experimental endotoxemia in vivo. Thromb Res 2007;120(5):727–31.
32. Manocha S, Russell JA, Sutherland AM, et al. Fibrinogen-beta gene haplotype is associated with mortality in sepsis. J Infect 2007;54(6):572–7.
33. Kee C, Cheong KY, Pham K, et al. Genetic variation in heat shock protein 70 is associated with septic shock: narrowing the association to a specific haplotype. Int J Immunogenet 2008;35(6):465–73.
34. Chapman SJ, Khor CC, Vannberg FO, et al. IkappaB genetic polymorphisms and invasive pneumococcal disease. Am J Respir Crit Care Med 2007;176(2):181–7.
35. Sabelnikovs O, Nikitina-Zake L, Vanags I. Association of IL-6 promoter polymorphism -174C/G with outcome in severe sepsis. Crit Care 2008;12:462.
36. Sutherland AM, Walley KR, Manocha S, et al. The association of interleukin 6 haplotype clades with mortality in critically ill adults. Arch Intern Med 2005; 165(1):75–82.
37. Gu W, Du DY, Huang J, et al. Identification of interleukin-6 promoter polymorphisms in the Chinese Han population and their functional significance. Crit Care Med 2008;36(5):1437–43.
38. Wattanathum A, Manocha S, Groshaus H, et al. Interleukin-10 haplotype associated with increased mortality in critically ill patients with sepsis from pneumonia but not in patients with extrapulmonary sepsis. Chest 2005;128(3):1690–8.
39. Stanilova SA, Miteva LD, Karakolev ZT, et al. Interleukin-10-1082 promoter polymorphism in association with cytokine production and sepsis susceptibility. Intensive Care Med 2006;32(2):260–6.
40. Gordon AC, Waheed U, Hansen TK, et al. Mannose-binding lectin polymorphisms in severe sepsis: relationship to levels, incidence, and outcome. Shock 2006; 25(1):88–93.
41. Smithson A, Munoz A, Suarez B, et al. Association between mannose-binding lectin deficiency and septic shock following acute pyelonephritis due to Escherichia coli. Clin Vaccine Immunol 2007;14(3):256–61.
42. Yende S, Angus DC, Kong L, et al. The influence of macrophage migration inhibitory factor gene polymorphisms on outcome from community-acquired pneumonia. FASEB J 2009;23: [epub ahead of print].
43. Temple SE, Cheong KY, Price P, et al. The microsatellite, macrophage migration inhibitory factor -794, may influence gene expression in human mononuclear cells stimulated with E. coli or S. pneumoniae. Int J Immunogenet 2008;35(4–5): 309–16.
44. Gomez R, O'Keeffe T, Chang LY, et al. Association of mitochondrial allele 4216C with increased risk for complicated sepsis and death after traumatic injury. J Trauma 2009;66(3):850–7 [discussion: 857–858].
45. Baudouin SV, Saunders D, Tiangyou W, et al. Mitochondrial DNA and survival after sepsis: a prospective study. Lancet 2005;366(9503):2118–21.
46. Yang Y, Shou Z, Zhang P, et al. Mitochondrial DNA haplogroup R predicts survival advantage in severe sepsis in the Han population. Genet Med 2008;10(3): 187–92.
47. Gao L, Grant A, Halder I, et al. Novel polymorphisms in the myosin light chain kinase gene confer risk for acute lung injury. Am J Respir Cell Mol Biol 2006; 34(4):487–95.
48. Brenmoehl J, Herfarth H, Gluck T, et al. Genetic variants in the NOD2/CARD15 gene are associated with early mortality in sepsis patients. Intensive Care Med 2007;33(9):1541–8.

49. Garcia-Segarra G, Espinosa G, Tassies D, et al. Increased mortality in septic shock with the 4G/4G genotype of plasminogen activator inhibitor 1 in patients of white descent. Intensive Care Med 2007;33(8):1354–62.
50. Binder A, Endler G, Muller M, et al. 4G4G genotype of the plasminogen activator inhibitor-1 promoter polymorphism associates with disseminated intravascular coagulation in children with systemic meningococcemia. J Thromb Haemost 2007;5(10):2049–54.
51. Russell JA, Wellman H, Walley KR. Protein C rs2069912 C allele is associated with increased mortality from severe sepsis in North Americans of East Asian ancestry. Hum Genet 2008;123(6):661–3.
52. Walley KR, Russell JA. Protein C -1641 AA is associated with decreased survival and more organ dysfunction in severe sepsis. Crit Care Med 2007; 35(1):12–7.
53. Binder A, Endler G, Rieger S, et al. Protein C promoter polymorphisms associate with sepsis in children with systemic meningococcemia. Hum Genet 2007;122(2): 183–90.
54. Sipahi T, Kuybulu A, Ozturk A, et al. Protein Z G79A polymorphism in patients with severe sepsis. Clin Appl Thromb Hemost 2009; [epub ahead of print].
55. Khor CC, Chapman SJ, Vannberg FO, et al. A Mal functional variant is associated with protection against invasive pneumococcal disease, bacteremia, malaria and tuberculosis. Nat Genet 2007;39(4):523–8.
56. Wurfel MM, Gordon AC, Holden TD, et al. Toll-like receptor 1 polymorphisms affect innate immune responses and outcomes in sepsis. Am J Respir Crit Care Med 2008;178(7):710–20.
57. Shalhub S, Junker CE, Imahara SD, et al. Variation in the TLR4 gene influences the risk of organ failure and shock posttrauma: a cohort study. J Trauma 2009; 66(1):115–22 [discussion: 122–113].
58. Van der Graaf CA, Netea MG, Morre SA, et al. Toll-like receptor 4 Asp299Gly/ Thr399Ile polymorphisms are a risk factor for Candida bloodstream infection. Eur Cytokine Netw 2006;17(1):29–34.
59. Yuan FF, Marks K, Wong M, et al. Clinical relevance of TLR2, TLR4, CD14 and FcgammaRIIA gene polymorphisms in Streptococcus pneumoniae infection. Immunol Cell Biol 2008;86(3):268–70.
60. Read RC, Teare DM, Pridmore AC, et al. The tumor necrosis factor polymorphism TNF (-308) is associated with susceptibility to meningococcal sepsis, but not with lethality. Crit Care Med 2009;37(4):1237–43.
61. Nakada TA, Hirasawa H, Oda S, et al. Influence of toll-like receptor 4, CD14, tumor necrosis factor, and interleukin-10 gene polymorphisms on clinical outcome in Japanese critically ill patients. J Surg Res 2005;129(2):322–8.
62. Shalhub S, Pham TN, Gibran NS, et al. Tumor necrosis factor gene variation and the risk of mortality after burn injury: a cohort study. J Burn Care Res 2009;30(1): 105–11.
63. Taudorf S, Krabbe KS, Berg RM, et al. Common studied polymorphisms do not affect plasma cytokine levels upon endotoxin exposure in humans. Clin Exp Immunol 2008;152(1):147–52.
64. Azim K, McManus R, Brophy K, et al. Genetic polymorphisms and the risk of infection following esophagectomy. Positive association with TNF-alpha gene -308 genotype. Ann Surg 2007;246(1):122–8.
65. Kovar FM, Marsik C, Cvitko T, et al. The tumor necrosis factor alpha -308 G/A polymorphism does not influence inflammation and coagulation response in human endotoxemia. Shock 2007;27(3):238–41.

66. Schueller AC, Heep A, Kattner E, et al. Prevalence of two tumor necrosis factor gene polymorphisms in premature infants with early onset sepsis. Biol Neonate 2006;90(4):229–32.
67. Gordon AC, Lagan AL, Aganna E, et al. TNF and TNFR polymorphisms in severe sepsis and septic shock: a prospective multicentre study. Genes Immun 2004; 5(8):631–40.
68. Barber RC, Aragaki CC, Rivera-Chavez FA, et al. TLR4 and TNF-alpha polymorphisms are associated with an increased risk for severe sepsis following burn injury. J Med Genet 2004;41(11):808–13.
69. Chen Q, Zhou H, Wu S, et al. Lack of association between TREM-1 gene polymorphisms and severe sepsis in a Chinese Han population. Hum Immunol 2008; 69(3):220–6.
70. Available at: http://www.hapmap.org. Accessed May 12, 2009.
71. Birney E, Stamatoyannopoulos JA, Dutta A, et al. Identification and analysis of functional elements in 1% of the human genome by the ENCODE pilot project. Nature 2007;447(7146):799–816.
72. Available at: http://nihroadmap.nih.gov/GTEx/index.asp. September 9, 2008. Accessed May 6, 2009.
73. Gibson G, Weir B. The quantitative genetics of transcription. Trends Genet 2005; 21(11):616–23.
74. Schrier RW, Wang W. Acute renal failure and sepsis. N Engl J Med 2004;351(2): 159–69.
75. Parker MM, Shelhamer JH, Bacharach SL, et al. Profound but reversible myocardial depression in patients with septic shock. Ann Intern Med 1984;100(4):483–90.
76. Geier A, Fickert P, Trauner M. Mechanisms of disease: mechanisms and clinical implications of cholestasis in sepsis. Nat Clin Pract Gastroenterol Hepatol 2006; 3(10):574–85.
77. Available at: http://www.1000genomes.org. Accessed May 12, 2009.
78. Available at: http://nihroadmap.nih.gov/hmp. Accessed May 17, 2009.
79. Available at: http://www.illumina.com. Accessed May 21, 2009.
80. Available at: http://www.affymetrix.com. Accessed May 20, 2009.
81. Available at: http://www.fluidigm.com. Accessed May 25, 2009.
82. Available at: http://www.AppliedBiosystems.com. Accessed June 22, 2009.
83. Korlach J, Marks PJ, Cicero RL, et al. Selective aluminum passivation for targeted immobilization of single DNA polymerase molecules in zero-mode waveguide nanostructures. Proc Natl Acad Sci U S A 2008;105(4):1176–81.
84. Eid J, Fehr A, Gray J, et al. Real-time DNA sequencing from single polymerase molecules. Science 2009;323(5910):133–8.
85. Clarke J, Wu H, Jayasinghe L, et al. Continuous base identification for single-molecule nanopore DNA sequencing. Nat Nanotechnol 2009;4(4):265–70.
86. Oh BR, Sasaki M, Perinchery G, et al. Frequent genotype changes at -308, and 488 regions of the tumor necrosis factor-alpha (TNF-alpha) gene in patients with prostate cancer. J Urol 2000;163(5):1584–7.
87. Rood MJ, van Krugten MV, Zanelli E, et al. TNF-308A and HLA-DR3 alleles contribute independently to susceptibility to systemic lupus erythematosus. Arthritis Rheum 2000;43(1):129–34.
88. Boin F, Zanardini R, Pioli R, et al. Association between -G308A tumor necrosis factor alpha gene polymorphism and schizophrenia. Mol Psychiatry 2001;6(1):79–82.
89. Berrettini WH, Persico AM. Dopamine D2 receptor gene polymorphisms and vulnerability to substance abuse in African Americans. Biol Psychiatry 1996; 40(2):144–7.

90. Alvarez V, Mata IF, Gonzalez P, et al. Association between the TNF-alpha -308 A/G polymorphism and the onset age of Alzheimer disease. Am J Med Genet 2002;114:574–7.
91. Braun N, Michel U, Ernst BP, et al. Gene polymorphism at position -308 of the tumor-necrosis-factor-alpha (TNF-alpha) in multiple sclerosis and its influence on the regulation of TNF-alpha production. Neurosci Lett 1996;215(2):75–8.
92. Li Kam Wa TC, Mansur AH, Britton J, et al. Association between -308 tumour necrosis factor promoter polymorphism and bronchial hyperreactivity in asthma. Clin Exp Allergy 1999;29(9):1204–8.
93. Kalish RB, Vardhana S, Gupta M, et al. Polymorphisms in the tumor necrosis factor-alpha gene at position -308 and the inducible 70 kd heat shock protein gene at position +1267 in multifetal pregnancies and preterm premature rupture of fetal membranes. Am J Obstet Gynecol 2004;191(4):1368–74.
94. Opdal SH. IL-10 gene polymorphisms in infectious disease and SIDS. FEMS Immunol Med Microbiol 2004;42(1):48–52.
95. Freeman BD, Kennedy CR, Coopersmith CM, et al. Genetic research and testing in critical care: surrogates' perspective. Crit Care Med 2006;34(4):986–94.

Performance Improvement in the Management of Sepsis

Christa Schorr, RN, MSN

KEYWORDS

• Guidelines • Sepsis • Bundles • Severe sepsis
• Performance improvement • Surviving Sepsis Campaign

There is abundant evidence of variation in the practice of medicine.[1] Despite our professed interest in providing best patient care, studies suggest that less than 60% of patients receive appropriate evidence based care.[2] Large variability in clinical practice plus the increasing awareness that certain processes of care are associated with improved medical outcomes has led to the development of clinical practice guidelines in a variety of areas related to infection and sepsis.[3] Initially, guidelines were controversial, but now data exist that support guideline use with some studies showing a statistically significant reduction in costs, length of hospital stay, and mortality.[4–9]

At a time when we are engaged in research to find new effective therapies for perceived areas of need, it is interesting that we are not grabbing the low hanging fruit, which is the effective timely delivery of existing accepted therapies.[10] Unfortunately, it may take 15 to 20 years for a newly proven therapy to become standard of care.[11] This process can be facilitated by transforming guidelines to key performance indicators, building protocols around these indicators and providing performance feedback by way of indicator measurement. This model is readily adaptable to severe sepsis because evidence-based guidelines exist in this area. Furthermore, there is general agreement among health care professionals, hospital management, and biostatisticians that severe sepsis is an area worthy of targeting performance improvement (PI).

GUIDELINE ADVANCEMENT TO CLINICAL PRACTICE

The quality of the data used to develop clinical guidelines has improved over time.[3] More than half of the guidelines published before 2000 were not based on randomized controlled trials.[12] Evidence from positive clinical trials fails to rapidly change clinical practice patterns and the persistent gap between intended and actual clinical behavior is marked.[13,14]

Division of Critical Care Medicine, Department of Medicine, Cooper University Hospital, One Cooper Plaza, 3 Dorrance, Camden, NJ 08103, USA
E-mail address: schorr-christa@cooperhealth.edu

Crit Care Clin 25 (2009) 857–867
doi:10.1016/j.ccc.2009.06.005
criticalcare.theclinics.com
0749-0704/09/$ – see front matter

Implementation of clinical practice guidelines in sepsis is challenging for many institutions for a variety of reasons including lack of administrative support, staff resistance, unfamiliar equipment, and inability to apply sepsis education in the clinical setting. Severe sepsis guideline implementation may be facilitated by delivering small blocks of information, building on initial successes, and using the bundle approach.

The Institute for Health Care Improvement (IHI) has pioneered the creation of valid and feasible process measures of quality of care for critically ill patients, developed standard data collection tools, and allowed institutions to enter data and monitor performance. For organizations new to quality improvement science, the IHI Web site introduces the model for improvement with an extensive Web site based education program.[15] Educational programs are designed to increase awareness and agreement with the recommendations. The use of decision support tools assists in standardizing assessment and interventions in a specific patient population.[3] Change bundles facilitate achievement of indicator performance measures and provide a feedback mechanism to clinicians with the improvement process. They have been demonstrated to be applicable to severe sepsis.[16]

Bundles are selected sets of interventions or processes of care distilled from evidence-based practice guidelines and targeted to be achieved over a fixed period of time. Bundles should act as a cohesive unit to ensure all steps of care are consistently delivered. The Surviving Sepsis Campaign (SSC) and the IHI used key recommendations from the 2004 SSC Guidelines for the Management of Severe Sepsis and Septic Shock to develop sepsis bundles containing a core set of quality indicators.[17,18] The SSC/IHI sepsis bundles are an innovative step in improving outcomes in severe sepsis. It is likely that the greatest opportunity to improve patient outcomes comes not from discovering new treatments but from more effective delivery of existing, best practice therapies.[10]

As new evidence is published, as experience is gained with the bundles, and as experts ponder how up-to-date sepsis guidelines should be best translated into the bundles, sepsis bundles will be optimized.

Bringing Sepsis Bundles into a PI Program

The SSC/IHI PI program includes not only bundles but also software for data collection, storage and analysis, and educational tools. This program facilitates integration of the SSC guidelines into clinical practice with performance measurement and feedback.[19] Bundles, when instituted over the same time frame for a specific diagnosis or process, are likely to improve outcome.[15] The sepsis bundles consist of a set of quality indicators to precisely evaluate a hospital's performance with respect to disease care. This allows hospitals to objectively assess the quality of care being rendered to the patient with severe sepsis at their institution.

The SSC sepsis resuscitation bundle is scored over 6 hours and includes blood cultures, antibiotics, and early goal-directed resuscitation indicators (**Fig. 1**). Three indicators in this bundle apply to all patients with severe sepsis: measure lactate, obtain blood cultures before antibiotics, and timely administration of antibiotics. One combined indicator (fluid challenge and maintaining adequate mean arterial blood pressure) applies only to patients with hypotension or a lactate greater than 4.0 mmol/L. The final two indicators apply only to patients with hypotension persisting after fluid challenge or a lactate greater than >4.0 mmol/L (CVP $\geq$ 8 mmHg and $ScvO_2 \geq 70\%$).

Severe Sepsis Bundles:

Sepsis Resuscitation Bundle
(To be accomplished as soon as possible and scored over first 6 hours):

1. Serum lactate measured.
2. Blood cultures obtained prior to antibiotic administration.
3. From the time of presentation, broad-spectrum antibiotics administered within 3 hours for ED admissions and 1 hour for non-ED ICU admissions.
4. In the event of hypotension and/or lactate > 4 mmol/L (36 mg/dl):
   a) Deliver an initial minimum of 20 ml/kg of crystalloid (or colloid equivalent*).
   b) Apply vasopressors for hypotension not responding to initial fluid resuscitation to maintain mean arterial pressure (MAP) ≥ 65 mm Hg.
5. In the event of persistent hypotension despite fluid resuscitation (septic shock) and/or lactate > 4 mmol/L (36 mg/dl):
   a) Achieve central venous pressure (CVP) of ≥ 8 mm Hg.
   b) Achieve central venous oxygen saturation ($ScvO_2$) of ≥ 70%.**

Sepsis Management Bundle
(To be accomplished as soon as possible and scored over first 24 hours):

1. Low-dose steroids* administered for septic shock in accordance with a standardized hospital policy.
2. Drotrecogin alfa (activated) administered in accordance with a standardized hospital policy.
3. Glucose control maintained ≥ lower limit of normal, but < 150 mg/dl (8.3 mmol/L).
4. Inspiratory plateau pressures maintained < 30 cm H_2O for mechanically ventilated patients.

See the individual chart measurement tool for an equivalency chart.

****Achieving a mixed venous oxygen saturation (SvO_2) of 65% is an acceptable alternative.***

Fig. 1. The SSC 6 hour Severe Sepsis Resuscitation Bundle and the 24 hour Severe Sepsis Management Bundle. (*From* Surviving Sepsis Campaign. Townsend SR, Dellinger RP, Levy MM, et al, editors. Surviving Sepsis Campaign: Implementing the Surviving Sepsis Campaign. Des Plaines, IL: Society of Critical Care Medicine, International Sepsis Forum, and European Society of Intensive Care Medicine; 2005.)

The SSC sepsis management bundle consists of indicators for consideration of low dose steroids in septic shock and drotrecogin alfa in severe sepsis (see **Fig. 1**). Both of these indicators are somewhat unique in that they are not scored based on whether they are accomplished, but instead based on documentation that they were considered in line with hospital policy. The third indicator is glucose control with a threshold less than 150 mg/dL (8.3 mmol/L). Glucose control is somewhat controversial and since 2004 the SSC has been concerned about tight glycemic control outside of well-resourced institutions. Recent literature supports avoidance of tight glycemic control, with a threshold of keeping blood glucose less than 110 mg/dL. The final indicator in the sepsis management bundle is maintaining inspiratory plateau pressure less than or equal to 30 cm H_2O for patients who are mechanically ventilated.

Establishing a Sepsis Protocol

Implementation of a sepsis performance program is customized based on institutional support and available resources (**Fig. 2**).[19]

Critical steps prior to protocol implementation

- Obtain administrative support
- Evaluate interdepartmental interactions
- Develop and relay a firm understanding of the goals
- Establish a formal interactive relationship with the emergency department and the critical care unit
- Collaborate with the general/internal medicine team
- Identify champions/unit protocol leaders
- Provide a unit-, hospital-, and system-wide education campaign

From Schorr C. Value of protocolization and sepsis performance improvement programs in early identification of sepsis handbook: Early Diagnosis of Sepsis. France. Biomerieux Education; 2007. p. 130–9.

Goal achievement requires continuous data collection and feedback. Strategies to improve performance should be aimed at constant process evaluation for ways to

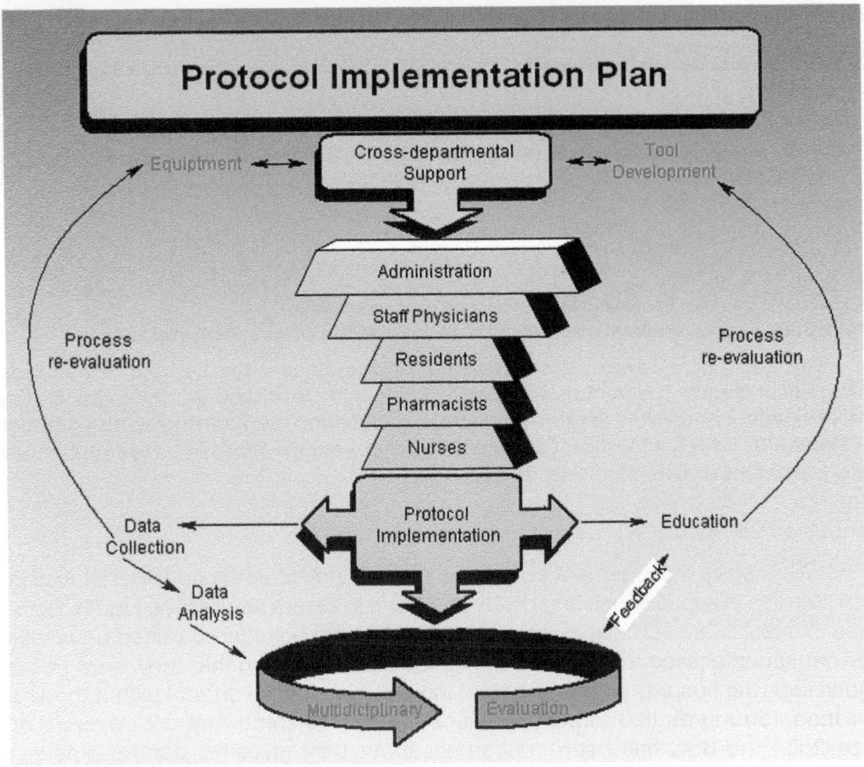

Fig. 2. An approach to protocol implementation. (*From* Biomerieux. Townsend SR, Dellinger RP, Levy MM, et al, editors. Surviving Sepsis Campaign: Implementing the Surviving Sepsis Campaign. Des Plaines, IL: Society of Critical Care Medicine, International Sepsis Forum, and European Society of Intensive Care Medicine; 2005.)

engender needed change. Protocols can be successful when education, commitment, behavior modification and maintenance are observed by proficient healthcare practitioners. Recognizing achievements may be observed over a period of months to years. Success of a program is reliant upon the people implementing the sepsis bundle protocol and the process put in place to achieve the goals.[20] Recent publications show the potential for successful local implementation of a protocol that when judged, based on historical controls, demonstrates improved outcome in sepsis.[21,22]

PI can be observed when there is

- Interdepartmental collaboration
- Multidisciplinary involvement
- Recognized behavior change
- Decreased variation in clinical management
- Efficient and effective treatment delivered
- Achievement of performance goals
- Decreased mortality
- Reduction in resources
- Decreased costs

From Schorr C. Value of protocolization and sepsis PI programs in early identification of sepsis handbook: Early Diagnosis of Sepsis. France. Biomerieux Education; 2007. p. 130–9.

Early Diagnosis and Identification for Protocol Application

Reducing the time to diagnose severe sepsis is thought to be a critical component of reducing mortality from sepsis-related multiple organ dysfunction.[23] Screening for severe sepsis should be employed throughout the hospital and should not be delayed pending ICU admission. Although the ICU team is often the initiator of the program and plays an important ongoing leadership role, the battleground for improving outcome in severe sepsis is likely to be the emergency department (ED) and the hospital floors, where the critical early care of the patient with severe sepsis is usually delivered.

PI PROCESS

Improvement in the process of care through increasing compliance with sepsis quality indicators is the goal of a severe sepsis PI program. Evaluating the steps in the process including personnel, environmental issues, and availability of supplies can help identify barriers to achieve success.[24] Severe sepsis patient management requires multidisciplinary (physicians, nurses, pharmacy, respiratory and administration) and multispecialty (medicine, surgery, and emergency medicine) collaboration to maximize the chance for success.[24]

The Role of Collaboration

The benefits of collaboration include a foundation of support through team building and knowledge transfer among clinicians. On a local level, individual hospitals or system collaboration is essential. It is estimated that one half of sepsis hospitalizations originate in the ED.[25,26] For this reason, a partnership between the ED and ICU may be the first key component in the sepsis PI program. Establishing support from key department leaders (ICU and ED) is crucial. Interdepartmental collaboration and communication can facilitate seamless steps in the continuum of care and lead to the ultimate success of the program.

Developing an Educational Program

A hospital-wide education initiative can be implemented over a designated period of time, employing lectured instruction, simulated instruction, and circulation of written resources. Educational sessions should be conducted by a member of the sepsis PI team. Multidisciplinary sessions should include, at a minimum, medical and nursing staff. Education may be provided through unit-based in-services, departmental conferences, and staff meetings. Sepsis bundle education posters may be displayed in key patient care areas, resource pocket cards can be distributed to medical and nursing staff, and use of a simulation mannequin replicating sepsis cases can be included in the educational efforts.

Data Collection

Prior to initiating a PI program, a method to collect and measure performance should be in place. Collecting data within the first 24 hours of presentation can help facilitate rapid identification of performance measures and the ability to discuss compliance with the clinical staff that were involved with the care of the patient being scored. Retrospective chart review may provide significant information, but does not allow the clinicians to easily recall the barriers that may have led to inability to meet specific indicators. Data collection may occur at the bedside or in medical records with a hard-copy data collection sheet or in real time with a laptop computer and wireless coupling with the hospital server, which has the PI software database program embedded. The latter is preferred as a one-step process and can be accomplished in line with the recommended daily screening process for patients that qualify for data entry as previously described. It is important to work with information technology at each hospital to ensure optimization of the program and data-backup capability.

Evaluating Process Improvement

Evaluation of process change requires consistent data collection, measurement of the indicators, and feedback to facilitate the continuous path to PI. Ongoing educational sessions provide feedback of indicator compliance and can help identify areas for additional PI efforts.

OVERCOMING CHALLENGES IN THE CHANGE PROCESS

Limitations for Changing Behavior

Changing clinicians' behavior in response to published data has long been a recognized failure in medical practice. There are several factors that might be predicted to motivate clinicians to change, including quality of the evidence, magnitude of the treatment effect, precision of the treatment effect, risk/benefit ratio, and the cost analysis.[3,27] These variables have recently been integrated into evidence-based medicine grading systems and determines strength of recommendation.[28] Physiologic rationale for a new intervention and how easy it is to apply a new intervention are the factors that drive the rate at which clinicians adapt guidelines into new standards of care. In general, for a clinician to voluntarily follow a guideline recommendation, he or she must be aware of them, agree with the recommendation, and have the ability to use it.[15] If any of these are lacking, voluntary, self-motivated change will not be possible. Hospital decree and governmental regulation, such as pay for performance, can also enact change in behavior but is less desirable than self-motivated change. Medical executives who want to accelerate the rate of diffusion of innovations, such as instituting the team model in the ICU, need to accomplish the following: find and support innovators, invest in early adopters of the innovation, make early adopter activity observable, trust and enable reinvention, create room for change, and lead by example.

Creating Successful Change

There are several levels of participation in creating successful change in behavior. The working team should be multiprofessional and knowledgeable about specific aims, the current local work processes, the associated literature, and any environmental issues that will be affected by changes. Active working teams are responsible for daily planning, documentation, communication, education, and evaluation of activities. A leadership group or person within the team (champion or champions) helps remove barriers, provides resources, monitors global progress, and gives suggestions from an institutional perspective. The working team needs someone with authority in the organization to overcome barriers and leadership needs to understand how the proposed changes will affect various parts of the system. Providers and stakeholders in the sepsis PI program must be kept informed through feedback, and be assured that their responses are respected.

SOLUTIONS: APPLYING THE PLAN-DO-STUDY-ACT CYCLE

Efforts to improve care can be tedious and discouraging at times. However, observed improvement in sepsis quality performance and outcomes can be extremely satisfying. Individual hospitals may have challenges unique to their center or a specific unit. Implementation of a rapid cycle change program may help identify barriers and aid in improving one quality indicator at a time with an overall improvement in bundle compliance. The Plan-Do-Study-Act (PDSA) cycle of implementing change is an effective method of testing change by developing a plan to test the change, enacting the change, and observing the effects, followed by determining what further improvements need to be made.[16] Problems that may be identified and entered into a severe sepsis PDSA cycle include ED overcrowding, difficulty obtaining central venous access and delays in ordering, delivery, and administration of antibiotics.

At the time of executing the SSC PI program at our institution, limited resources and overcrowding in the ED created opposition from the ED staff for early implementation of the sepsis bundles. Baseline data discovered a low percentage of qualifying patients receiving early goal-directed therapy and delays in administration of antibiotics. The medical directors of the ED and ICU established a policy launching a collaborative approach to patients qualifying for the sepsis bundles. According to the policy, the ED staff is responsible for early patient identification and the ICU staff will assist or assume care of the patient requiring early goal-directed therapy if ED resources limit ED capability to accomplish this goal. Additionally, promoting early critical care consults and expediting rapid transfer to the ICU has assisted in improved indicator compliance.

We initiated a PDSA cycle geared toward decreasing time to antibiotics. This is a good starter and institutional improvement is likely (ie, low hanging fruit). We identified all cases of severe sepsis entered into the SSC database receiving antibiotics more than 3 hours after ED triage to determine the reason for delay. The causes for delay included delay in patient identification, ordering and administering antibiotics, and miscommunication among the healthcare practitioners. Ongoing evaluation of individual cases continues. However, after identifying barriers to early antibiotic delivery and educating health care deliveries on best ways to overcome these barriers, a rapid improvement was observed and continued over the subsequent six month period.

DATA COLLECTION CHALLENGES AND SOLUTIONS

Screening for Protocol Entry Versus Screening for Database Entry

Each day, screening for protocol entry should be a hospital-wide process. This needs to be differentiated from routine screening for identification of patients who meet the definition of severe sepsis for the purpose of scoring performance. The first type of

Chart record – use patient label. Do not remove from chart

Evaluation for Severe Sepsis Screening Tool

<u>Instructions:</u> Use this optional tool to screen patients for severe sepsis in the emergency department, on the wards, or in the ICU.

1. Is the patient's history suggestive of a new infection?

- ☐ Pneumonia, empyema
- ☐ Urinary tract infection
- ☐ Acute abdominal infection
- ☐ Meningitis
- ☐ Skin/soft tissue infection
- ☐ Bone/joint infection
- ☐ Wound infection
- ☐ Bloodstream catheter infection
- ☐ Endocarditis
- ☐ Implantable device infection
- ☐ Other ____________

___ **Yes** ___**No**

2. Are any two of following signs & symptoms of infection both present and new to the patient? <u>Note</u>: laboratory values may have been obtained for inpatients but may not be available for outpatients.

- ☐ Hyperthermia > 38.3 °C (101.0 °F)
- ☐ Hypothermia < 36 °C (96.8°F)
- ☐ Tachycardia > 90 bpm
- ☐ Tachypnea > 20 bpm
- ☐ Acutely altered mental status
- ☐ Leukocytosis (WBC count >12,000 µL–1)
- ☐ Leukopenia (WBC count < 4000 µL–1)
- ☐ Hyperglycemia (plasma glucose >120 mg/dL) in the absence of diabetes

___ **Yes** ___**No**

If the answer is yes to both either question 1 and 2, *suspicion of infection* is present:

- ✓ Obtain: **lactic acid, blood cultures,** CBC with differential, basic chemistry labs, bilirubin.
- ✓ At the physician's discretion obtain: UA, chest x-ray, amylase, lipase, ABG, CRP, CT scan.

3. Are any of the following organ dysfunction criteria present at a site remote from the site of the infection that are not considered to be chronic conditions? <u>Note</u>: the remote site stipulation is waived in the case of bilateral pulmonary infiltrates.

- ☐ SBP < 90 mmHg or MAP < 65 mmHg
- ☐ SBP decrease > 40 mm Hg from baseline
- ☐ Bilateral pulmonary infiltrates with a new (or increased) oxygen requirement to maintain SpO2 > 90%
- ☐ Bilateral pulmonary infiltrates with PaO2/FiO2 ratio < 300
- ☐ Creatinine > 2.0 mg/dl (176.8 mmol/L) or Urine Output < 0.5 ml/kg/hour for > 2 hours
- ☐ Bilirubin > 2 mg/dl (34.2 mmol/L)
- ☐ Platelet count < 100,000
- ☐ Coagulopathy (INR >1.5 or aPTT >60 secs)
- ☐ Lactate > 2 mmol/L (18.0 mg/dl)

___ **Yes** ___**No**

If *suspicion of infection* is present AND *organ dysfunction* is present, the patient meets the criteria for SEVERE SEPSIS and should be entered into the severe sepsis protocol.

Date: ____/____/____ (circle: dd/mm/yy or mm/dd/yy) Time: ____: ____ (24 hr. clock)

Version 7.12.2005

Fig. 3. The SSC Screening Tool for database Entry. (*From* Surviving Sepsis Campaign. Schorr C. Value of protocolization and sepsis PI programs in early identification of sepsis handbook: Early Diagnosis of Sepsis. France. Biomerieux Education 130–39, 2007.)

screening needs to be done by all hospital practitioners who are involved with the treatment of sepsis. Improvement in this area means earlier identification and more timely and appropriate treatment. The second type of screening is performed by an individual or individuals who work with the data entry part of the PI program to identify patients that qualify for entering into the PI database. In many hospitals, this is done daily, Monday through Friday, with a review of patients admitted over the weekend generally completed on Monday. The SSC screening tool for database entry is shown in **Fig. 3**. Many hospitals elect to do screening only on ICU service patients with the assumption that the great majority of patients who develop severe sepsis in a hospital will be admitted to the ICU service. Obviously, an occasional patient will be treated in the ED or hospital wards and improves and does not require ICU admission. These patients may be missed as part of the database, but their prevalence is constant over time.

Identifying Time Zero

Time zero (T0) is the time that starts the clock ticking for scoring performance in the treatment of severe sepsis. An effective PI program has time-sensitive indicators, such as time to antibiotics and time to achieve hemodynamic targets. This requires a reproducible T0 across patients entered into the database. For patients who are diagnosed with severe sepsis in the ED, the assumption is made that the patient presented with the capability for achieving this diagnosis and T0 is the time of presentation to the ED (triage time). There will be occasional patients that develop severe sepsis after arrival and, therefore, penalize health care practitioners in their ability to achieve time-based indicators, but the alternative of ascertaining a time of onset during an ED stay, when data collection is not in real time, is a less attractive alternative. Fortunately, this occurrence will be constant over time and because performance is graded over time with improvement evaluation based on historical controls, the penalty is the same for comparator groups. For patients originating from a unit other than the ED, T0 is ideally ascertained from review of hospital records annotating the date and time of resuscitation and management of severe sepsis. If the resuscitation and management of severe sepsis was not annotated, the default T0 for patients developing severe sepsis on the ward is the ICU admission date and time. For patients admitted to the ICU with a diagnosis other than sepsis, who subsequently develop severe sepsis, T0 is ascertained from ICU records using the date and time annotated as the beginning of the management and resuscitation effort.[19,29]

Clinical Endpoints

PI evaluation is based on process change (ie, increased compliance with achieving indicators either using achievement, yes or no, or using time to achievement), ICU stay, hospital stay, and hospital mortality. It is more appropriate to use all-cause mortality as opposed to sepsis mortality because it is often difficult to ascertain mortality as being unrelated to severe sepsis, and the all-cause mortality is totally objective with no chance of bias (ie, easy to say that patient is either alive or dead).

SUMMARY

Sepsis guidelines, although creating a base to allow change in health care practitioner behavior, do not, in and of themselves, effect change. Change only comes with institution of a PI program, converting a core of key goals of guideline recommendations to quality indicators, and giving feedback on performance. These quality indicators are tracked before or during (recommended approach) initiation of hospital-wide education to evaluate baseline performance. When combining multispecialty and multidisciplinary champions in the ED, hospital wards, ICU, and hospital administrative leadership with timely performance feedback, case failure analysis, and re-education, an opportunity to succeed in decreasing mortality in severe sepsis can be achieved. Sepsis bundle indicators require updating as new evidence emerges and new guidelines are published.[30,31]

REFERENCES

1. Andersen TF, Mooney G. Medical practice variations: where are we? In: Anderson TF, Mooney G, editors. The challenges of medical practice variations. Basingstoke, Hampshire, United Kingdom: Macmillan Press; 1990. p. 1–15.
2. McGlynn EA, Asch SM, Adams J, et al. The quality of health care delivered to adults in the United States. N Engl J Med 2003;348:2635–45.
3. Cinel I, Dellinger RP. Guidelines for severe infections: are they useful? Curr Opin Crit Care 2006;12(5):483–8.
4. Gleason PP, Meehan TP, Fine JM, et al. Associations between initial antimicrobial therapy and medical outcomes for hospitalized elderly patients with pneumonia. Arch Intern Med 1999;159:1562–72.
5. Stahl JE, Barza M, DesJardin J, et al. Effect of macrolides as part of initial empiric therapy on length of stay in patients hospitalized with community-acquired pneumonia. Arch Intern Med 1999;159:2576–80.
6. Kortgen A, Niederprum P, Bauer M, et al. Implementation of an evidence based "standard operating procedure" and outcome in septic shock. Crit Care Med 2006;34:943–9.
7. Nguyen HB, Corbett SW, Steele R, et al. Implementation of a bundle of quality indicators for the early management of severe sepsis and septic shock is associated with decreased mortality. Crit Care Med 2007;35:1105–12.
8. Shorr AF, Micek ST, Jackson WL, et al. Economic implications of an evidence-based sepsis protocol: can we improve outcomes and lower costs? Crit Care Med 2007;35:1257–62.
9. Zambon M, Ceola M, Almeida-de-Castro R, et al. Implementation of the Surviving Sepsis Campaign guidelines for severe sepsis and septic shock: we could go faster. J Crit Care 2008;23(4):455–60.
10. Pronovost PJ, Nolan T, Zeger S, et al. How can clinicians measure safety and quality in acute care? Lancet 2004;363:1061–7.
11. The Institute of Medicine. Committee on Quality of Health Care in America. Crossing the quality chasm: a new health system for the 21st century. Washington, D.C.: National Academy Press; 2001.
12. Cabana MD, Rand CS, Powe NR, et al. Why don't physicians follow clinical practice guidelines? A framework for improvement. JAMA 1999;282:1458–65.
13. Nathwani D, Rubinstein E, Barlow G, et al. Do guidelines for community-acquired pneumonia improve the cost-effectiveness of hospital care? Clin Infect Dis 2001; 32:728–41.
14. Giannakakis IA, Haidich AB, Contopoulos-Ioannidis DG, et al. Citation of randomized evidence in support of guidelines of therapeutic and preventive interventions. J Clin Epidemiol 2002;55:545–55.
15. A resource from the Institute of Healthcare Improvement. Available at: http://www.ihi.org. Last accessed October 16, 2008.
16. Gao F. Will sepsis care bundles improve patient outcome? Adv Sepsis 2006;5(3):94–6.
17. Dellinger RP, Carlet JM, Masur H, et al. Surviving Sepsis Campaign guidelines for management of severe sepsis and septic shock. Crit Care Med 2004;32:858–73.

18. Dellinger RP, Carlet JM, Masur H, et al. Surviving Sepsis Campaign Management Guidelines Committee: Surviving Sepsis Campaign guidelines for management of severe sepsis and septic shock. Intensive Care Med 2004;30:536–55.
19. Townsend SR, Dellinger RP, Levy MM, et al, editors. Surviving Sepsis Campaign: implementing the surviving sepsis campaign. Des Plaines (IL): Society of Critical Care Medicine, International Sepsis Forum, and European Society of Intensive Care Medicine; 2005;8:24–5.
20. Schorr C. Value of protocolization and sepsis performance improvement programs in early identification of sepsis handbook: early diagnosis of sepsis. France: Biomerieux Education; 2007. p. 130–9.
21. Trzeciak S, Dellinger RP, Abate NL, et al. Translating research to clinical practice: a 1-year experience with implementing early goal-directed therapy for septic shock in the emergency department. Chest 2006;129:225–32.
22. Jones AE, Focht A, Horton JM, et al. Prospective external validation of the clinical effectiveness of an emergency department-based early goal-directed therapy protocol for severe sepsis and septic shock. Chest 2007;132(2):425–32.
23. Cinel I, Dellinger RP. Current treatment of severe sepsis. Curr Infect Dis Rep 2006;8:358–65.
24. Schorr C, Trzeciak S, Dellinger RP, et al. Surviving Sepsis campaign (SSC) performance improvement program: demonstration of process change [abstract]. Crit Care Med 2006;34(Suppl:12)A107.
25. Strehlow MC, Emond SD, Shapiro NI, et al. National study of emergency department visits for sepsis, 1992 to 2001. Ann Emerg Med 2006;48(3):326–31.
26. Wang HE, Shapiro NI, Angus DC, et al. National estimates of severe sepsis in United States emergency departments. Crit Care Med 2007;35(8):1928–36.
27. Levy MM, Provonost PJ, Dellinger RP, et al. Sepsis change bundles: converting guidelines into meaningful change in behavior and clinical outcome. Crit Care Med 2004;32(Suppl):S595–7.
28. Jaeschke R, Guyatt GH, Dellinger RP, et al. Use of GRADE grid to reach decisions on clinical practice guidelines when consensus is elusive. BMJ 2008;337: a744.
29. Surviving Sepsis Campaign. Available at: http://www.survivingsepsis.org. Last accessed October 16, 2008.
30. Dellinger RP, Levy MM, Carlet JM, et al. Surviving Sepsis Campaign: international guidelines for management of severe sepsis and septic shock: 2008. Crit Care Med 2008;36(1):296–327.
31. Dellinger RP, Levy MM, Carlet JM, et al. Surviving Sepsis Campaign: international guidelines for management of severe sepsis and septic shock: 2008. Intensive Care Med 2008;34(1):17–60.

Multicenter Clinical Trials in Sepsis: Understanding the Big Picture and Building a Successful Operation at Your Hospital

R. Phillip Dellinger, MD, MSc[a,b,*], Christa Schorr, RN, MSN[c],
Stephen Trzeciak, MD[a,b]

KEYWORDS

- Clinical trial design • Clinical coordinating center
- Contract research organization • Informed consent
- Research collaboration • Conflicts of interest

For a multicenter sepsis clinical trial to be successfully carried out, there must be functionality at the investigative center level and integration among the investigative center, the sponsor, and other groups put in place to facilitate the overall trial process (such as a contract research organization [CRO] or a clinical coordinating center [CCC]). For the investigative site to be successful an understanding of the big picture of the trial is useful. Since sepsis is a disease that crosses multiple areas of the hospital, collabroation among those areas is essential for success.

UNDERSTANDING THE BIG PICTURE

The Environment for Clinical Trials in Sepsis

The general consensus is that clinical trials in severe sepsis are very difficult for a multitude of reasons.[1–4] Perhaps the main reason is that even a beneficial therapeutic intervention in this condition may not be evident because of a small "signal-to-noise" ratio

Funding Support: None.

[a] Robert Wood Johnson Medical School, University of Medicine and Dentistry of New Jersey, NJ, USA

[b] Division of Critical Care Medicine, Cooper University Hospital, One Cooper Plaza, 393 Dorrance, Camden, NJ 08103, USA

[c] Department of Medicine, Cooper University Hospital, Camden, NJ, USA

* Corresponding author. Robert Wood Johnson Medical School, University of Medicine and Dentistry of New Jersey, New Jersey.

E-mail address: dellinger-phil@cooperhealth.edu (R.P. Dellinger).

Crit Care Clin 25 (2009) 869–879
doi:10.1016/j.ccc.2009.08.003 criticalcare.theclinics.com
0749-0704/09/$ – see front matter

in this severely ill population who is at risk for morbidity and mortality by many other noninvestigational factors. It is possible that previous trials with experimental agents that failed to show significant outcome benefit may have actually been beneficial yet the signal of benefit was overwhelmed by the signal-to-noise ratio.[5] To maximize success, the best approach is to do conservative sample size estimates. As sepsis research continues to evolve, it is increasingly being recognized that tailoring an investigational therapy to subjects with the greatest capacity to respond (ie, akin to a "personalized medicine" strategy) may increase the likelihood of a positive trial. Along these lines, using biomarkers to personalize subject enrollment such that the phenotype of the subject enrolled matches the known activity of the intervention seems logical.[6] Enrolling subjects who have reduced biologic plausibility of responding to a specific intervention is more likely to result in no observed treatment effect. In the future, the ability to identify specific genotypes of septic patients by using rapid genetic testing and enrolling patients who would be expected to have the biology targeted by the intervention may be useful.[7–9]

Preclinical/Phase I/II Trials in Severe Sepsis Research

Why have so many Phase III clinical trials in sepsis failed?[10] Where is the problem? Is it our preclinical data or are animal models not appropriate?[11] Is the sepsis intervention field a hopeless mire of redundancy of molecular mechanisms that makes attacking one point in the cascade futile? What should new strategies for success be?[12]

Existing animal models likely do provide useful information but are specifically designed to limit the heterogeneity of the many variables that are present in human sepsis that affect outcome other then the intervention at hand.[13] There is large variability of physiology, genetics, immunology, and host response to infection from one original species to another, and all animal models, with the possible exception of the chimpanzee, have substantial differences from human sepsis.[2] The focus of animal studies is on young healthy animals without underlying diseases. They enter the septic insult healthy. The method by which severe sepsis is induced in the animal may affect the success or failure of the therapeutic agent being tested. Timing and magnitude of injury and the causative pathogen are carefully controlled in the animal experiment. The situation in the intensive care unit with human sepsis is markedly different where extremely variable genetic makeup exists, and the patient is often malnourished, elderly, or immunocompromised. No two patients with severe sepsis are identical. Even with relatively precise inclusion criteria there may be great biologic heterogeneity among patients enrolled. The limitations of the randomized controlled trial in this environment are significant.[14] It is likely that previous biologically active therapies that failed in clinical trials were beneficial in some patients and harmful in others. The causative microorganism is highly variable and the onset in pace of illness is uncontrolled and often poorly defined. Extrapolation on dosing and efficacy of agents based on preclinical studies is therefore imprecise and often inaccurate.

Selecting Patient Population for Enrollment

As mentioned earlier, patients with severe sepsis are very heterogeneous and their outcome is often determined by conditions other then the septic insult. The best definition for sepsis and severe sepsis remains a matter of debate, and, as a result, defining the patient who meets the intent of the research study (ie, the "spirit" of the study) is often challenging. Challenges defining the optimal target population could result in significant numbers of subjects who do not actually meet the intent of the study and yet must be included in the intent-to-treat analysis. When a highly motivated and well-organized clinical evaluation committee of sepsis experts is used to evaluate all subjects enrolled in a study, blinded to treatment allocation, data have supported drug benefit despite failure of the intent-to-treat population analysis to show benefit. A clinical evaluation committee can also answer important questions about the robustness of a positive trial and support for effect or lack of effect in subgroups.[15] The standard end point for sepsis clinical trials is mortality. Targeting the more severely ill septic patient increases the chance to show mortality benefit; however, patients who are highly likely to die regardless of the addition of a new beneficial therapy must be excluded.

Contract Research Organization

Initially, pharmaceutical and device companies used CROs for a limited aspect of the conduct of a clinical trial in severe sepsis, perhaps monitoring for regulatory compliance.[16] Today sepsis trials are more likely to have a full-service CRO totally engaged with the clinical trial to include sitting at the table during study planning, working with the sponsor for Food and Drug Administration (FDA) submissions to sanction the trial, assisting in site selection and site monitoring for regulatory compliance (site visits for review for proper reporting of adverse events and completion of case report forms), facilitating subject recruitment, safety surveillance and reporting, and data management and biostatistics. With this expanded role, CROs are taking on more and more of the regulatory and ethical risks and responsibilities related to the conduct of the sepsis clinical trial. CROs are unique from the sponsor in that they are not interested in the outcome of the study but nevertheless, similar to the sponsors as to strict regulation by state and federal research regulatory bodies. CROs are steeped in operational procedures. They are graded by their industry employer based not only on services provided for trial oversight but the professional working relationships established with investigative groups at both academic and community-based clinical sepsis research programs. In the end, whether the previously mentioned functions are performed directly by the sponsor or indirectly through a CRO, in the end it is all about data integrity.

The Clinical Coordinating Center

The late 1980s saw the blossoming of large industry clinical trials in the area of severe sepsis. It is interesting to look at how conduct of these clinical trials has evolved. Clearly the trials are bigger and the expectations for success are targeted more toward absolute mortality reductions of 6% to 8% as opposed to the lofty goals set earlier. Another change has been more sponsor oversight of patients entered into the clinical trial. In the late 1980s and into the mid-1990s most industry-sponsored large clinical trials relied totally on the expertise and commitment of the primary investigator for selecting subjects who met both the letter and the intent of the targeted patient population. The emergence of CCCs beginning in the mid-1990s likely represents a major advancement in ensuring quality subject selection. The CCC consists of a group of sepsis experts, intimately familiar with the clinical trial design and letter/intent of inclusion/exclusion criteria, ideally participating in that trial (especially if there are unique characteristics of the trial) who are available 24 hours a day, 7 days a week to approve study enrollment. In addition, the CCC can serve in other roles by answering questions that come up after enrollment that are more relevant for trial medical expertise as opposed to administrative (for which the CRO would suffice). A CCC can also serve as a resource to the clinical research organization for questions concerning severe sepsis and trial conduct. The complexity and capabilities of the CCC will likely continue to grow in the future as a centralized process becomes increasingly more

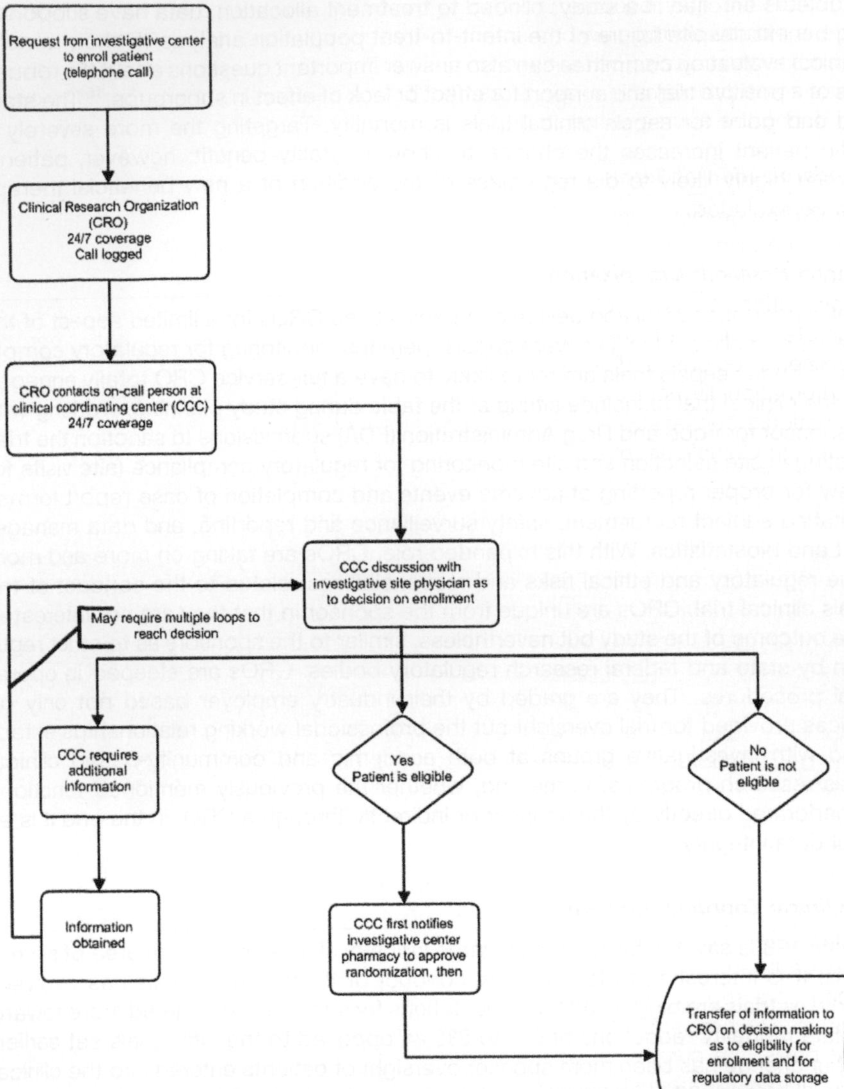

Fig. 1. Interaction among the investigative center, CRO, and CCC during potential patient enrollment is shown.

desirable. **Fig. 1** demonstrates interactions among the investigative site, the CRO, and the CCC.

Needs and Priorities of Industry Sponsor

The industry sponsor has two important goals that may in fact compete with each other. First is to enroll quality patients to enhance the chance of observing a treatment effect and the second is avoiding being so precise in trying to achieve this goal that enrollment is difficult and the study is prolonged.[17] When a study is prolonged because of difficulty in enrolling, the fixed costs of sponsoring the study also is extended and may become untenable. When this occurs during the clinical trial, options include adding new centers and enrolling more patients from quality centers. Amendments may also be required to make enrollment criteria more lenient, but may create some problems in analysis, as the study will have a change in patient population during the course of the study.

Standardization of Sepsis Trial Entry Criteria and Protocol Management

Despite the general consensus that specific biomarker criteria would be optimal for patient enrollment in clinical trials, clinical criteria continue to be the primary route of patient selection for severe sepsis trials. Some similarity in enrollment criteria exists across different study protocols; however, heterogeneity is marked. A problem likely of greater relevance is the wide variation in treatment of severe sepsis across centers, geographic regions, and continents. Of potential utility to address this problem would be internationally accepted criteria for diagnosis of severe sepsis and generalized international consensus on basic core protocol management. The Surviving Sepsis Campaign Guidelines for the management of severe sepsis and septic shock represents an attempt to provide a template for some standardization of management.[18]

SUCCEEDING AT YOUR HOSPITAL

Why Participate as an Investigator in Multicenter Clinical Trials in Sepsis?

The most appropriate answer to this question is an altruistic one, to advance knowledge of sepsis and improve care of the septic patient. Unless one believes that the research study is potentially beneficial as to improving our understanding of sepsis or demonstrating benefit of a new therapy, then participation as a member of the primary research team (primary investigator, co-investigator, research nurse, or research coordinator) is not justified. When key members of the research team are hesitant about the value of a study, a formula for failure has been put in place.

Another reason to participate is to gain experience in an area that will enhance job qualifications. Having experience in sepsis multicenter clinical trials is a desirable capability for many job opportunities in medicine for physicians and nurses. This is even more so the case if that experience is associated with proven success. A less altruistic, but still important, reason for participation in industry-sponsored clinical research in sepsis is to generate research revenue. Because most of the costs of setting up a sepsis clinical research program are fixed (research coordinator and/or assistant salaries) and most multicentered trials are funded on a per-patient enrollment basis, the number of patients enrolled over time determines financial loss or financial gain for the institution.

A final reason for participation is to become a co-author for the publication of the trial results. Being co-author on a multicenter trial publication usually comes about when one or more members of that research team participate in the design and planning of a multicenter clinical trial in sepsis. This occurs when a center gains experience and participates in multiple trials over time, building a reputation of success. Participating in sepsis clinical trial design, especially if that site also participates in the trial as an enrollment site, offers a good chance that someone from that site will be represented on abstract or manuscript publication.

Essentials for Success

The essentials for success in a multicenter sepsis trial are the following: (1) a dedicated and experienced investigative team; (2) an appropriate volume of patients at that hospital that meet entry criteria for the sepsis study; (3) having total or partial

Box 1
Essentials for success

- Dedicated/experienced investigative team
- Adequate number of patients meeting entry criteria
- Access to enroll eligible patients
- Effective screening process
- Personnel available and capable of consent and initiation of enrollment

administrative control over the clinical care of the patients targeted for enrollment (or a positive relationship with the primary caregiver for these patients); (4) a screening process in place that will identify most eligible patients during the enrollment period; and (5) personnel who are dedicated and available to complete the consent and initial enrollment process, which is typically the most resource-intensive phase of the clinical trial (**Box 1**).

Dedication and experience

A dedicated research team is essential. This is very similar to an exercise program where it is often difficult to initiate the exercise but once the exercise is completed there is great gratification of the accomplishment. In clinical sepsis research it is impossible to pre-plan days to the needs of screening/enrollment of a research subject and even more difficult to work into the evening after an afternoon decision is made to enroll a research subject. However the development of severe sepsis is an unscheduled, emergent, and time-sensitive event, and flexibility on the part of the study team is necessary.

Sponsors are always seeking proven experienced investigators and investigative sites. Experience in multicenter sepsis clinical trials is however somewhat of a "catch 22." To get clinical research experience, occasionally sponsors need to take a chance on an investigative center. A potential solution to this problem is, especially for a physician, to gain experience as a subinvestigator during a clinical training program. Sponsors may consider taking a chance on a physician who may come from a highly experienced institution and was a successful subinvestigator in a prior clinical trial. Having either a research coordinator or physician with experience, even if the other component of the duo is not experienced, is usually enough to convince a sponsor of likely success. When neither component is experienced, the best option is to start small with observational study or minimal risk noninterventional protocols. Once a proven track record in these studies is achieved, obtaining a position as a site in an interventional trial is more likely. Importantly, one mandatory element for any site participating in a clinical trial is the demonstration of experience with human subjects protection including training in the principles of Good Clinical Practice (GCP) and requirements for conducting FDA-regulated trials.

Available patients who are suitable candidates for study

There is nothing more frustrating for the sponsor or for a hospital sepsis research team than to be involved with a study and discover there is an inadequate pool of patients who qualify for enrollment. This may come as a result of poor planning by the sponsor as to the prevalence of these patients (in which case amendments usually follow to make patient enrollment easier) or poor initial assessment by the clinical investigative team of their hospital patient population. Common practice is for the sponsor or organization administrating the trial to have a site feasibility survey completed by the potential primary investigator or research coordinator that forces the prospective site to assess availability of the planned target population and prevalence of these patients at their hospital.

Ability to approach and attempt to enroll suitable subjects

The presence of adequate numbers of sepsis patients in the planned target population does not necessarily mean that these patients can be approached. To approach a patient or patient's family (the usual case) for a severe sepsis research trial, permission from the primary care provider or primary service is needed. This may come in the form of a blanket approval from an individual group or department. If approaching potential subjects is not preapproved, then the primary caregiver is approached for permission on a case-by-case basis. Regardless of prior permission, the primary attending should still be made aware the patient is being approached for enrollment. Enrollment of sepsis patients in a closed unit when the sepsis research is being done by the ICU team is obviously very different (easier) when compared with enrollment in an open unit. To provide an accurate estimate of the number of patients who could potentially be enrolled, considerable advance thought and discussion among physicians and physician groups who admit patients to the ICU is needed. When an ICU patient database is available, the projection of how many patients will qualify is made easier.

At Cooper we have had the Project Impact (Cerner) database in place since 2001 and have almost 12,000 ICU admissions in our database. All patients admitted to the ICU have extensive data capture that allows us to query and match entry criteria for a sepsis trial to our ICU patient population over the past 8 years. Recently we have assisted industries interested in pursuing multicenter clinical trials in critical care by projecting how many patients would qualify for a study over 1 year from a representative tertiary care referral center medical/surgical ICU like Cooper.

Effective timely screening

Research personnel generally work 40-hour weeks, whereas critical care trial enrollment is not necessarily a 40-hour a week process that conforms to fixed schedules. Solutions to overcome this coverage problem include overlapping schedules as well as on-call off-hours coverage by trained subinvestigators (eg, nurses, resident physicians, or medical students). At Cooper University Hospital we have an instant messaging system that broadcasts study-related information (eg, presence and location of a potential study subject, next scheduled research activity on an enrolled subject) to handheld devices for all study personnel via E-mail or text messages. An example of a typical message exchange is shown in **Fig. 2**. This allows immediate notification of key research team members when a potential sepsis research subject is identified or research activities need to be performed. The notifications can be sent by other members of the research team, or by any member of the clinical staff who identifies a potential sepsis subject during his or her clinical duties. The requested criteria for triggering the research team's notification is intentionally made very broad so that clinicians who may have encountered a patient with severe sepsis do not have to have the typically long list of inclusion/exclusion criteria committed to memory. Following this initial notification, a member of the research team goes to the bedside to apply inclusion/exclusion criteria and perform the in-depth detailed screening required for enrollment in the trial. In this type of system, clinicians who are not members of the research team can still be an important source of subject identification without specific regard (and consumption of time) as to inclusion and exclusion criteria for a trial.

----- Original Message -----

From: Doe, John
To: SEPSIS
Sent: Monday August 10, 2009 15:08
Subject: ED 5

Elderly female with hypotension after 20 ml/kg IVF.

WBC 15.2
Lactate 2.6
Plt 233

Treatment includes abx.

-----Original Message-----
From: Jones, Bob
Sent: Monday, August 10, 2009 3:09 PM
To: SEPSIS
Subject: Re: ED 5

Nice job John! Rachel will screen for studies shortly.
Rachel will need to see INR for ZOPAT study as that is our current priority for enrollment.

-----Original Message-----
From: Rooney, Rachel
Sent: Monday, August 10, 2009 3:27 PM
To: SEPSIS
Subject: FW: ED 5

Excluded for ZOPAT study with DIC score not qualifying.
I believe she is eligible for ARGOT.
Can one of the co-investigators come and verify qualification for ARGOT.
Family is currently available as far as consent if the patient qualifies.

-----Original Message-----
From: Cotton, Chris
Sent: Thursday, August 10, 2009 3:29 PM
To: SEPSIS
Subject: RE: ED 5

On the way

-----Original Message-----

From: Cotton, Chris
Sent: Thursday, August 10, 2009 4:10 PM
To: SEPSIS
Subject: RE: ED 5
Not a candidate for ARGOT due to liver disease.
Qualifies for Rob's microcirculation study. Will attempt to get consent.
Harry or Richard, are either of you available for the microcirculation studies through the night?

-----Original Message-----
From: Heart, Harry
Sent: Thursday, August 10, 2009 4:17 PM
To: SEPSIS
Subject: RE: ED 5

I am available and Richard did the last late night work.
Let me know if you get consent.

-----Original Message-----
From: Cotton, Chris
Sent: Thursday, August 10, 2009 5:15 PM
To: SEPSIS
Subject: RE: ED 5
Got consent. We are a go!

Fig. 2. A simulated but representative E-mail exchange during screening and eventual patient enrollment is shown. The acronyms of the sepsis studies and the names of the indi viduals are fictitious.

Collaboration Between the Emergency Department and the Intensive Care Unit

Essentially all sepsis clinical research studies have a limited time from qualification for study entry to initiating study therapy, which severely impacts the ability for the research team to obtain informed consent before the time window expires. This time may range from 12 to 36 hours after qualification. With these short timelines it is important to have a sepsis research program in which screening begins in the emergency department (ED). Collaboration between the ICU and ED and participation of both ED and ICU physicians as co-investigators is ideal. Likewise, knowledge and support of the program by physicians and nurses in both ED and ICU bolsters a program's success. Inservices and other education programs in both areas are often useful.

Obtaining Written Informed Consent in Sepsis Trials

The great majority of consent for severe sepsis trials will come from a surrogate (either next of kin or other legally authorized representative). With a limited amount of time for eligibility for most sepsis clinical trials, locating the surrogate can become a limiting step. Obtaining written informed consent for critical care research has become more challenging over recent years, perhaps because of increased scrutiny by the lay public of research intentions. In most institutions, the informed consent document itself has grown incredibly complex and long.[19] Certain basic principles of consent exist. The patient or surrogate must be presented with and understand a fair representation of risk/benefit ratio. Working on the side of the investigator is that a regulatory agency (such as the FDA or The European Regulatory Authority) would not allow clinical sepsis trials to go forward when preclinical data favor risk over benefit. Nevertheless, it is important for the research subject to understand that the possibility of worse outcome through participation cannot be ruled out. The appearance of the consenter to the patient and family can make a difference in "yes" or "no," and ability to gain consent may hinge on appearance of experience, quiet confident demeanor, and perhaps some gray hair. Despite a well-rationalized clinical research study, the right characteristics of the attempted consenter, and correct approach, consent is still often not obtained.

Conflicts of Interest

Over the past 10 years there has been a heightened awareness of potential financial conflicts of interest in industry-sponsored trials.[20,21] Participation in industry-sponsored clinical research as an investigator is problematic when the investigator has ownership or stock in the sponsor, as this clearly represents a conflict of interest with the trial results. In that scenario, the investigator is discouraged from study involvement. Although the receipt of paid consultancies, honoraria, or other payments to an investigator from the sponsor must be clearly identified to the local institutional review board (IRB) and at their discretion to the potential subject, these relationships are not necessarily exclusionary for participation in a trial. Whether or not the presence of the relationship should preclude an investigator's participation in a trial is typically decided by the local IRB or by local institutional policies on conflict of interest with industry.

Institutional Review Board

To get an industry clinical trial going at an institution requires working with the IRB and the local grants and contracts office. The IRB should be viewed as an ally and not as an impediment to clinical research. A properly functioning IRB can be tremendously

5. Dellinger RP, Parrillo JE. Mediator modulation therapy of severe sepsis and septic shock: does it work? Crit Care Med 2004;32(4):282–6.
6. Marshall JC, Reinhart K. Biomarkers of sepsis. Crit Care Med 2009;37(7):2290–8.
7. Cariou A, Chiche JD, Charpentier J, et al. The era of genomics: impact on sepsis and clinical trial design. Crit Care Med 2002;30(5):S341–8.
8. Majetschak M, Obertacke U, Schade U, et al. Tumor necrosis factor gene polymorphisms, leukocyte function, and sepsis susceptibility in blunt trauma patients. Clin Diagn Lab Immunol 2002;9(6):1205–11.
9. Stassen NA, Breit CM, Norfleet LA, et al. IL-18 promoter polymorphisms correlate with the development of post-injury sepsis. Surgery 2003;134(2):351–6.
10. Kaplan BI, Tipirneni P. Lessons for the future: a review of sepsis past and present. IDrugs 2007;10(4):264–9.
11. Opal SM, Cross AS. The use of immunocompromised animals as models for human septic shock. Shock 2005;24(1):64–71.
12. Cohen J, Guyatt G, Bernard GR, et al. New strategies for clinical trials in patients with sepsis and septic shock. Crit Care Med 2001;29(4):880–6.
13. Dyson A, Singer M. Animal models of sepsis: why does preclinical efficacy fail to translate to the clinical setting? Crit Care Med 2009;37(Suppl 1):S30–7.
14. Glasser SP, Howard G. Clinical trial design issues: at least 10 things you should look for in clinical trials. J Clin Pharmacol 2006;46(10):1106–15.
15. Dhainaut JF, Laterre PF, Larosa SP, et al. The clinical evaluation committee in a large multicenter phase 3 trial of drotrecogin alfa (activated) in patients with severe sepsis (PROWESS): role, methodology, and results. Crit Care Med 2003;31(9):2291–301.
16. Beach JE. Clinical trials integrity: a CRO perspective. Account Res 2001;8(3):245–60.
17. Peelen L, Peek N, de Jonge E, et al. The use of a registry database in clinical trial design: assessing the influence of entry criteria on statistical power and number of eligible patients. Int J Med Inf 2007;76(2–3):176–83.
18. Dellinger RP, Levy MM, Carlet JM, et al. Surviving sepsis campaign: international guidelines for management of severe sepsis and septic shock: 2008. Crit Care Med 2008;36(1):296–327 and Intensive Care Med 2008;34(1):17–60.
19. Fost N, Levine R. The dysregulation of human subjects research. JAMA 2007;298(18):2196–8.
20. Bekelman JE, Li Y, Gross CP. Scope and impact of financial conflicts of interest in biomedical research: a systematic review. JAMA 2003;289(4):454–65.
21. Silverman HJ, Lemaire F. Ethics and research in critical care. Intensive Care Med 2006;32(11):1697–705.

Index

Note: Page numbers of article titles are in **boldface** type.

Crit Care Clin 25 (2009) 881–889
doi:10.1016/S0749-0704(09)00100-6
critical care.theclinics.com
0749-0704/09/$ – see front matter

United States Postal Service

Statement of Ownership, Management, and Circulation
(All Periodicals Publications Except Requestor Publications)

1. Publication Title Critical Care Clinics	2. Publication Number 0 0 0 - 7 0 8	3. Filing Date 9/15/09
4. Issue Frequency Jan, Apr, Jul, Oct	5. Number of Issues Published Annually 4	6. Annual Subscription Price $222.00
7. Complete Mailing Address of Known Office of Publication (*Not printer*) (*Street, city, county, state, and ZIP+4®*) Elsevier Inc. 360 Park Avenue South New York, NY 10010-1710		Contact Person Stephen Bushing Telephone (Include area code) 215-239-3688

8. Complete Mailing Address of Headquarters or General Business Office of Publisher (*Not printer*)

Elsevier Inc., 360 Park Avenue South, New York, NY 10010-1710

9. Full Names and Complete Mailing Addresses of Publisher, Editor, and Managing Editor (*Do not leave blank*)

Publisher (*Name and complete mailing address*)

John Schrefer, Elsevier, Inc., 1600 John F. Kennedy Blvd. Suite 1800, Philadelphia, PA 19103-2899

Editor (*Name and complete mailing address*)

Patrick Manley, Elsevier, Inc., 1600 John F. Kennedy Blvd. Suite 1800, Philadelphia, PA 19103-2899

Managing Editor (*Name and complete mailing address*)

Catherine Bewick, Elsevier, Inc., 1600 John F. Kennedy Blvd. Suite 1800, Philadelphia, PA 19103-2899

10. Owner (*Do not leave blank. If the publication is owned by a corporation, give the name and address of the corporation immediately followed by the names and addresses of all stockholders owning or holding 1 percent or more of the total amount of stock. If not owned by a corporation, give the names and addresses of the individual owners. If owned by a partnership or other unincorporated firm, give its name and address as well as those of each individual owner. If the publication is published by a nonprofit organization, give its name and address.*)

Full Name	Complete Mailing Address
Wholly owned subsidiary of	4520 East-West Highway
Reed/Elsevier, US holdings	Bethesda, MD 20814

11. Known Bondholders, Mortgagees, and Other Security Holders Owning or Holding 1 Percent or More of Total Amount of Bonds, Mortgages, or Other Securities. If none, check box → ☐ None

Full Name	Complete Mailing Address
N/A	

12. Tax Status (*For completion by nonprofit organizations authorized to mail at nonprofit rates*) (*Check one*)
The purpose, function, and nonprofit status of this organization and the exempt status for federal income tax purposes:
☐ Has Not Changed During Preceding 12 Months
☐ Has Changed During Preceding 12 Months (*Publisher must submit explanation of change with this statement*)

PS Form 3526, September 2007 (Page 1 of 3 (Instructions Page 3)) PSN 7530-01-000-9931 **PRIVACY NOTICE:** See our Privacy policy in www.usps.com

13. Publication Title: Critical Care Clinics

14. Issue Date for Circulation Data Below: July 2009

15. Extent and Nature of Circulation		Average No. Copies Each Issue During Preceding 12 Months	No. Copies of Single Issue Published Nearest to Filing Date
a. Total Number of Copies (*Net press run*)		2105	2100
b. Paid Circulation (By Mail and Outside the Mail)	(1) Mailed Outside-County Paid Subscriptions Stated on PS Form 3541. (*Include paid distribution above nominal rate, advertiser's proof copies, and exchange copies*)	1014	958
	(2) Mailed In-County Paid Subscriptions Stated on PS Form 3541 (*Include paid distribution above nominal rate, advertiser's proof copies, and exchange copies*)		
	(3) Paid Distribution Outside the Mails Including Sales Through Dealers and Carriers, Street Vendors, Counter Sales, and Other Paid Distribution Outside USPS®	411	391
	(4) Paid Distribution by Other Classes Mailed Through the USPS (e.g. First-Class Mail®)		
c. Total Paid Distribution (*Sum of 15b (1), (2), (3), and (4)*)		1425	1349
d. Free or Nominal Rate Distribution (By Mail and Outside the Mail)	(1) Free or Nominal Rate Outside-County Copies Included on PS Form 3541	87	86
	(2) Free or Nominal Rate In-County Copies Included on PS Form 3541		
	(3) Free or Nominal Rate Copies Mailed at Other Classes Through the USPS (e.g. First-Class Mail)		
	(4) Free or Nominal Rate Distribution Outside the Mail (Carriers or other means)		
e. Total Free or Nominal Rate Distribution (Sum of 15d (1), (2), (3) and (4)		87	86
f. Total Distribution (Sum of 15c and 15e)		1512	1435
g. Copies not Distributed (See instructions to publishers #4 (page #3))		593	665
h. Total (Sum of 15f and g)		2105	2100
i. Percent Paid (15c divided by 15f times 100)		94.25%	94.01%

16. Publication of Statement of Ownership

☐ If the publication is a general publication, publication of this statement is required. Will be printed in the October 2009 issue of this publication. ☐ Publication not required

17. Signature and Title of Editor, Publisher, Business Manager, or Owner

Stephen R. Bushing

Stephen R. Bushing – Subscription Services Coordinator

Date: September 15, 2009

I certify that all information furnished on this form is true and complete. I understand that anyone who furnishes false or misleading information on this form or who omits material or information requested on the form may be subject to criminal sanctions (including fines and imprisonment) and/or civil sanctions (including civil penalties).

PS Form 3526, September 2007 (Page 2 of 3)

Printed and bound by CPI Group (UK) Ltd, Croydon, CR0 4YY
14/10/2024
01773700-0001